PEDIATRIC ANDROLOGY

CLINICS IN ANDROLOGY

E.S.E. HAFEZ, *series editor*

VOLUME 7

series ISBN 90-247-2333-7

PEDIATRIC ANDROLOGY

edited by

S.J. KOGAN
Bronx, New York, U.S.A.

and

E.S.E. HAFEZ
Detroit, Michigan, U.S.A.

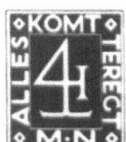

1981

MARTINUS NIJHOFF
THE HAGUE/BOSTON/LONDON

Distributors:

for the United States and Canada

Kluwer Boston, Inc.
190 Old Derby Street
Hingham, MA 02043
USA

for all other countries

Kluwer Academic Publishers Group
Distribution Center
P.O. Box 322
3300 AH Dordrecht
The Netherlands

This volume is listed in the Library of Congress Cataloging in Publication Data

ISBN-13: 978-94-010-3721-1   e-ISBN-13:978-94-010-3719-8
DOI: 10.1007/978-94-010-3719-8

Very special thanks and appreciation are expressed to Mrs. E. Marash for her skill and patience in typing and collating this volume, and to Mrs. M. Scheffer, M. D'Alo, K. Maguire and L. Rust for their assistance.

TABLE OF CONTENTS

VIII

CONTRIBUTORS

BERCU, B.B.: Neonatal and Pediatric Medicine Branch, National Institute of Health, 9000 Rockville Pike, Bethesda, MD 20205, USA

BIERICH, J.R.: University-Kinderklinik, Rumelinstrasse 19–23, D-7400 Tubingen, West Germany

BUDZIK, G.P.: Departments of Surgery and Biological Chemistry, Harvard Medical School, Boston, MA 02114, USA

CUNHA, G.R.: Department of Anatomy, University of Colorado, Health Sciences Center, 4200 East Ninth Avenue, Denver, CO 80262, USA

DEVINE, C.J. JR.: Department of Urology, Eastern Virginia Medical School, 700 Botetourt Street, Post Office Box 1980, Norfolk, VA 23501, USA

DONAHOE, P.K.: Pediatric Surgical Research Laboratories, Harvard Medical School, Boston, MA 02114, USA

FAIMAN, C.: Department of Medicine, The University of Manitoba, Health Sciences Centre, General Centre Room G4, 700 William Avenue, Winnipeg, Manitoba R3E 0Z3, Canada

FUJII, H.: Department of Anatomy, University of Colorado, 4200 East Ninth Avenue, Denver, CO 80260, USA

GAUTIER, T.: Universidad Nacional, Pedro Henriquez Urena, Department of Pediatrics, Santa Domingo, Dominican Republic

GONZALEZ-SERVA, L.: Department of Urology, Eastern Virginia Medical School, 700 Botetourt Street, Norfolk, VA 23501, USA

GORSKI, R.A.: Departments of Anatomy and Brain, Research Institute, University of California at Los Angeles, School of Medicine, Room AK 01, Los Angeles, USA

HADŽISELIMOVIĆ F.: Department of Pediatrics, Kinderspital Basel, Romergasse 8, 4005 Basel, Switzerland

HAFEZ, E.S.E.: Department of Gynecology/Obstetrics, C.S. Mott Center for Human Growth and Development, Wayne State University School of Medicine, Detroit, MI 48201, USA

HIGHAM E.: Department of Psychology, John Hopkins Hospital and University, Baltimore, MD 21205, USA

HORTON, C.E.: Department of Plastic Surgery, Eastern Virginia Medical School, 700 Botetourt Street, Norfolk, VA 23501, USA

IMPERATO-MCGINLEY J.: Department of Medicine/Division of Endocrinology, The New York Hospital, Cornell University Medical Center, 525 East 68th Street, New York, NY 10021, USA

JACOBSON, C.D.: Department of Anatomy, University of California at Los Angeles, School of Medicine, The Center for Health Sciences 73–235, Los Angeles, CA 90024, USA

KOGAN, S.J.: Department of Surgery, Division of Pediatric Urology, Albert Einstein College of Medicine, Bronx, NY 10461, USA

KROOVAND, R.L.: Department of Pediatric Urology, Wayne State University School of Medicine, Children's Hospital of Michigan, 3901 Beaubien Boulevard, Detroit MI 48201, USA

LEVINE, L.S.: Department of Pediatrics, Division of Pediatric Endocrinology, The New York Hospital, Cornell University Medical Center, 525 East 68th Street, Room N-236, New York, NY 10021, USA

MORIKAWA, Y.: Department of Pediatric Surgery, Massachusetts General Hospital, 32 Fruit Street, Boston, MA 02114, USA

NAMKUNG, P.C.: Department of Obstetrics-Gynecology, BB 638 University Hospital RH 20, University of Washington School of Medicine, Seattle, WA 98195, USA

NEUBAUER, B.L.: Department of Anatomy, University of Colorado, Health Sciences Center, 4200 East Ninth Avenue, Denver, CO 80262, USA

NEW, M.I.: Department of Pediatrics, Division of Pediatric Endocrinology, The New York Hospital, Cornell University Medical Center, 525 East 68th Street, New York, NY 10021, USA

PERLMUTTER, A.D.: Department of Pediatric Urology, Wayne State University School of Medicine, Children's Hospital of Michigan, 3901 Beaubien Boulevard, Detroit, MI 48201, USA

PETERSON, R.E.: Department of Medicine/Division of Endocrinology, The New York Hospital, Cornell University Medical Center, 525 East 68th Street, New York, NY 10021, USA

PETRA, P.H.: Department of Obstetrics-Gynecology and Biochemistry and Laboratory Medicine, BB 632 University Hospital RH 20, University of Washington School of Medicine, Seattle, WA 98195, USA

RAJFER, J.: Division of Urology, University of California at Los Angeles School of Medicine, Los Angeles, CA 90024, USA

REESE, B.A.: Department of Anatomy, University of Colorado, 4200 East Ninth Avenue, Denver, CO 80262, USA

REYES, F.I.: Department of Obstetrics/Gynecology, The University of Manitoba, Woman's Centre S021, 735 Notre Dame Avenue, Winnipeg, Manitoba R3E OL8, Canada

ROBBOY, S.J.: Department of Pathology, Harvard Medical School, Boston, MA 02114, USA

SAENGER, P.: Montefiore Hospital and Medical Center and Albert Einstein College of Medicine, Bronx, NY 10467, USA

SHANNON, J.M.: Department of Anatomy, University of Colorado, Health Sciences Center, 4200 East Ninth Avenue, Denver, CO 80262, USA

SMAIL, P.J.: Department of Pediatrics, The University of Manitoba Health Sciences Centre, Children's Hospital, 685 Bannatyne Avenue, Winnipeg, Manitoba R3E OW1, Canada

STECKER, J.F. JR.: Department of Urology, Eastern Virginia Medical School, 700 Botetourt Street, Norfolk, VA 23501, USA

STURLA, E.: Department of Medicine/Division of Endocrinology, The New York Hospital, Cornell University Medical Center, 525 East 68th Street, New York, NY 10021, USA

SWANN, D.A.: Department of Surgery, Massachusetts General Hospital, Shriners Burns Institute, Boston, MA 02114, USA

WACKSMAN, J.: Department of Surgery, Division of Urology, Children's Hospital Medical Center, Elland and Bethesda Avenue, Cincinnati, OH 45229, USA

WACHTEL, S.S.: Cornell University Graduate School of Medical Sciences, Cornell University, 1300 York Avenue at 69th Street, New York, NY 10021, USA

WELCH, W.R.: Department of Pathology, Boston Hospital for Women and Harvard Medical School, Boston, MA 02114, USA

WINTER, J.S.D.: Department of Pediatrics, Health Sciences Centre, Children's Hospital Room CN 103, 685 Bannatyne Avenue, Winnipeg, Manitoba R3E OW1, Canada

FOREWORD

The subject matter in this volume was derived from papers presented at the Pediatric Andrology session of the 1st Pan American Congress of Andrology held in Caracas, Venezuela in February 1979, as well as from selected additional manuscripts of interest in this field. Prior to this session, identification of a distinct discipline and specialty devoted to *pediatric* andrology had not occurred, nor had it been conceptualized.

Pediatric andrology encompasses many different areas: disorders of sexual development, structural disease of the genital organs, normal and abnormal puberty, undescended testes, genital tumors, gonadal function and its relationship to growth, virilization, fertility and gender identity all represent areas of specific interest, to name but a few.

Andrology itself is a unique field, bringing together clinicians and basic scientists with diverse backgrounds. It should be noted that between one-half and three-quarters of the clinicians contributing to this issue conduct basic research as well. It has been this unique blend of basic research and clinical medicine which has done much to unravel many of these problems characteristic of this field.

Why a separate discipline of *pediatric* andrology? Firstly, because many of the diseases first manifest in adulthood have their beginnings in childhood, or for that matter, at conception. Secondly, because children are not just miniature adults; their anatomy, physiology and mentality are different, as well as their medical problems, both andrologic and otherwise. The discipline of pediatric andrology represents an input from individuals who have a knowledge of the problems *unique* to children, and who are skilled in dealing with these problems.

It is hoped that this volume will serve as a vehicle for communication between individuals who work in different specialty fields of interest, who all have a common interest in the problems unique to pediatric andrology, and that future volumes may be able to serve a similar function as well.

S.J. KOGAN, M.D.
Bronx, New York
December 1980

1. SEX DIFFERENTIATION OF MALE GENITALIA

E.S.E. HAFEZ

The sex of the fetus is an inherited characteristic carried by the genetic material of the X- and Y-chromosomes. The combination of the sex chromosomes is fixed at the time of fertilization and is normally transmitted unchanged to all subsequent somatic cells of a given individual. Although a specific sex is thus built into the cells, the transfer of the sex determining genes seems to have been discharged by the formation of the ovary or testis.

1. FETAL SEXUAL DIFFERENTIATION

1.1. Indifferent (ambisexual) stage

The indifferent stage refers to the initial period of development prior to differentiation of gonads or genitalia. During the indifferent stage, about 20 mesonephric tubules are present. The cranial group, numbering from 5 to 12, persists and establishes direct contact with the developing rete testes during the third month; whereas the caudal tubules, which do not connect with the rete testes, eventually fragment, separate from the Wolffian duct and degenerate to form the vestigial paradidymis (Cunha and Lung, 1979). The indifferent stage may first be recognized in an embryo of 5 mm crown–rump length (approximately 28 days after ovulation). The indifferent stage continues until testicular differentiation is recognizable, which occurs at about 15 mm (between 6 and 7 weeks).

The mesonephros is derived from the intermediate mesoderm and is located on the posterior abdominal wall within a longitudinal mass of mesenchyme, which projects downward into the coelomic cavity. This mass, the urogenital ridge, contains the mesonephros, the developing gonad, the suprarenal gland and the Wolffian or mesonephric duct (Fig. 1).

On the lateral aspect of the urogenital ridge is the developing Müllerian duct represented as an invagination of the coelomic epithelium (Cunha and Lung, 1979) (Fig. 2).

During sex differentiation in the male fetus, the gonads develop into fetal testis; the mesonephric tubules differentiate into ductuli efferentes, and the Wolffian ducts form the fetal epididymis, vas deferens, seminal vesicle and ejaculatory duct (Fig. 3, Table 1).

Male fetuses castrated before sexual differentiation will develop as females. Testosterone restores male development. Androgens act locally, as shown by the effects of localized implants of androgens or by unilateral castration, to regulate the development of the Wolffian duct which differentiates into epididymis, ductus deferens and seminal vesicles. On the other hand, the development of external genitalia is regulated by blood-borne androgens.

1.2. The duct system

Müllerian ducts develop as invaginations of the coelomic epithelium on the lateral surface of the

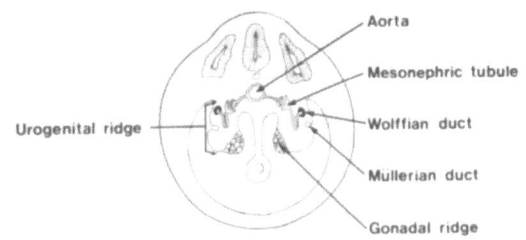

Figure 1. Diagrammatic illustration of the structures of the ambisexual stage can be recognized. Projecting from the dorsal wall of the coelomic cavity is the urogenital ridge which contains the mesonephros, the Wolffian duct and the developing gonad. On the lateral aspect of the urogenital ridge is the developing Müllerian duct which is represented as an invagination of the coelomic epithelium (Cunha and Lung, 1979).

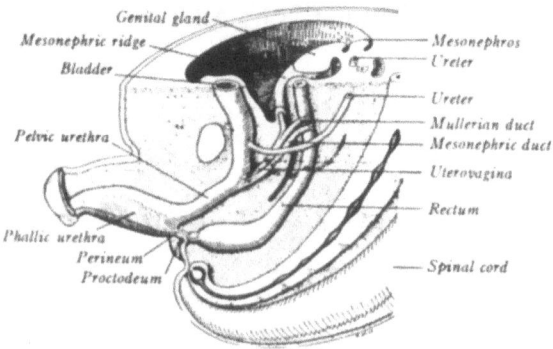

Figure 2. Model illustrating the caudal portion of a nine-week-old human embryo. (Reproduced from Arey, 1965.)

urogenital ridges. The Müllerian ducts grows caudally down the urogenital ridge parallel to the Wolffian duct and crosses anterior to the Wolffian duct, fuses with the Müllerian duct of the opposite side and joins the urogenital sinus, which is derived from the ventral aspect of the cloaca (O'Rahilly, 1973). The Wolffian duct acts as a guide for the caudal growth of the Müllerian duct (Gruenwald, 1941; Didier, 1968). The temporal relationships of fetal differentiation of the duct system, fetal gonads and the external genitalia are summarized in Tables 2 and 3. The development of the derivatives of the mesonephric apparatus are shown for 3- and 4-month male fetuses (Fig. 4).

1.3. Fetal gonad

The indifferent gonad differentiates into an ovary or a testis by 6–7 weeks (15 mm crown–rump length).

Table 1. Male sex differentiation under genetic and hormonal influences.

Fetal origin	Differentiated genitalia
Mesonephric tubules	Ductuli efferenti
Wolffian ducts	Epididymis Ductuli deferenti Seminal vesicle Ejaculatory ducts
Urogenital sinus	Prostate Bulbourethral glands Most urethra
Müllerian ducts	Degenerate, except for vestigial remnants cranially (the appendix of the testes) and caudally (the prostatic utricle)

In the testis, the original epithelial cords, which can now properly be designated as seminiferous cords, continue to expand and convolute. They are then separated from the epithelium by a thin layer of mesenchyme cells that constitute a true tunica albuginea. Primary epithelial cords become seminiferous cords shortly after their separation from the germinal epithelium, as the cords enlarge and the tunica albuginea condenses. Gonadal development is initiated as a thickening of the coelomic epithelium (the gonadal ridge) on the medial side of the mesonephros. This thickened coelomic epithelium as well as the underlying mesenchyme forms the somatic or extragerminal portion of the gonad.

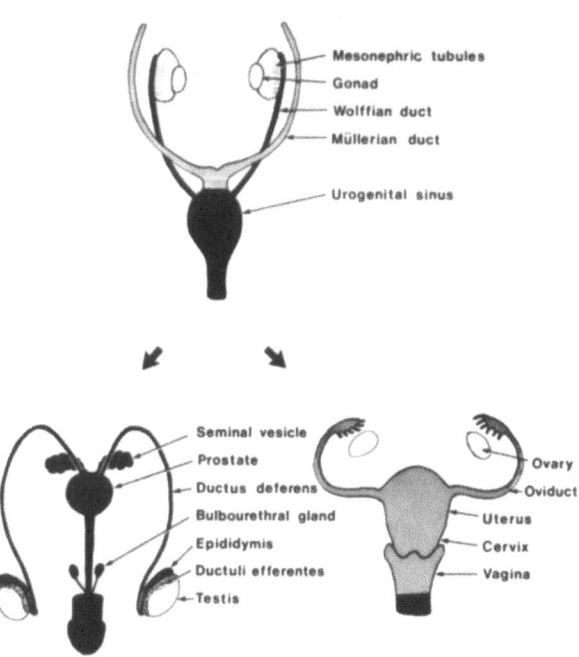

Figure 3. In the ambisexual stage, the gonads are undifferentiated, and the Wolffian and Müllerian ducts extend from the gonads caudally to the urogenital sinus. Mesonephric tubules are associated with the gonads and the cranial portion of the Wolffian duct. During masculine sex differentiation, the gonads develop into testes, and the mesonephric tubules form the ductuli efferentes. The Wolffian ducts differentiate into ductus epididymis, ductus deferens, seminal vesicles, and ejaculatory ducts. The urogenital sinus forms the prostate, bulbourethral glands, and most of the urethra. Müllerian ducts degenerate in males except for the caudal portions which contribute to the formation of the prostatic utricle and cranial portions which form the vestigial appendix of the testes. In females, the gonads differentiate into ovaries, and Müllerian ducts form the oviducts, uterus, cervix and upper portion of the vagina. The remainder of the vagina and all of the urethra are derived from the urogenital sinus. In females, the Wolffian ducts and mesonephric tubules degenerate but are represented as vestigial structures: the epoophoron, paroophoron, and Gartner's duct (Cunha and Lung, 1979).

Table 2. Summary of fetal differentiation of male reproductive organs. (Data from: Gillman 1948; Van Wagenen and Simpson, 1965; Barnes, 1968; Gier and Marion, 1970; Narbaitz, 1974; Winter et al., 1977; Cunha and Lung, 1979)

Organ	Fetal differentiation
Gonadal ridge	Special types of large, periodic acid–Schiff and alkaline phosphatase positive cells, the primordial germ cells, are apparently responsible for initiating the processes which lead to the formation of the gonadal ridge and subsequently its differentiation into testis or ovary. Such cells arise in the yolk sac, migrating through the mesenchyme of the midgut wall and dorsal mesentery into the area lateral to the dorsal aorta and ventral to the mesonephric tubules.
Urogenital sinus	The cloacal membrane, which originally obturates the caudal end of the cloaca, disappears by the seventh week, when the partition has been completed. At this time or shortly after, two portions can be distinguished in the urogenital sinus: the tubular cephalic portion connected with the bladder (pelvic urethra) and the open groove at the base of the genital tubercle (phallic urethra). The pelvic portion receives the Wolffian and Müllerian ducts in its dorsal wall, the growing sinus produces the resorption of part of the Wolffian ducts in such a way that a small zone of the sinus and the bladder is temporarily lined with Wolffian epithelium.
Testis	The differentiation of the testis first becomes recognizable on morphologic grounds in an embryo 14–16 mm crown–rump length (6–7 weeks postovulation). The medullary cords of the indifferent gonad acquire a prominence and might now be referred to as seminiferous tubules. During the same period the cortex degenerates, the germ cells disappear from the cortical area and in a male fetus of about 8 weeks postovulatory, the sex gland becomes a recognizable testis. At about 10 weeks the interstitial cells acquire characteristics which allow their identification. By the time the fetus reaches 50 mm (about 11 weeks), these begin to increase enormously, and separate the seminiferous tubules. This relative increase of the interstitial material continues until the fetus reaches about 160–190 mm (5–6 months) when the interstitial cells suddenly shrink and degenerate. The functional significance of this phenomenon in relation to the development of the sex ducts must be kept in mind.
Mesonephros	A pronephric rudiment develops along the dorsal body wall, from the nephrotoma along somite 5 or 6 to somites 8–11, mesonephros developing caudal to the pronephros. The mesonephric duct is continuous with the pronephric duct which proceeds to grow caudally beyond the pronephros as a tubular structure posterior to somite 9 or 10. The mesonephromeres, approximately 50, differentiate progressively several hours after the tip of the mesonephric duct passes over the particular region. The metanephros begins differentiation from the nephrotome lateral to somite 28 shortly after the last mesonephromere is formed.
Epididymis	Wolffian duct cranial to the ductuli efferentes degenerates, portion of Wolffian duct that connects with ductuli efferentes grows rapidly and becomes the highly convoluted ductus epididymis, the epididymis, which in the newborn may reach an overall length of 20 mm.
Vas deferens	Portion of the Wolffian duct, after testicular descent, traverses the inguinal canal, enters the pelvis, and converges on the base of the bladder, where it expands to form the ampulla.
Ejaculatory duct	The Wolffian duct beyond the point where the duct of the seminal vesicle joins the ampulla is the ejaculatory duct. It traverses the tissues of the prostate and terminates in the prostate urethra; termini of ejaculatory ducts open on sides of the verumontanum to act as flap valves preventing refluxing of urine from the urethra.
Prostate	Formed from the upper part of the urogenital sinus near where it is joined by the Müllerian and Wolffian ducts. Development of the primitive prostatic cords appears to be dependent on the production of androgens by the fetal testes; prostatic cord formation is initiated shortly after testes begin secretion of these hormones; prostatic cords arise as five groups from the prostatic urethra; first (middle) lobe, originates from the posterior wall of the urethra between the bladder neck and the openings of the ejaculatory ducts and prostatic utricle. Second end third [(lateral) lobes] arise on either side of the verumontanum; Fourth, or posterior lobe, arises from the area caudal to the verumontanum; fifth, (anterior lobe) is derived from the cords budding from the anterior urethral wall; as epithelial cords grow, they branch extensively, forming tubules that extend toward the prostatic capsule.
External genitalia	Like the other portions of the genital tract, the external genitalia pass through a bisexual period before specialized differentiation begins at about 50 mm (2 months). At early stages the external genitalia are constituted by (1) a genital tubercle or phallus, (2) the urethral groove which is limited laterally by the two urethral folds, and (3) the genital swellings (scrotolabial swellings) which appear on either side of the phallus. The urogenital sinus opens into the urethral groove. The under surface of the phallus is composed of a urethral plate which is a proliferation of sinus epithelium.

Table 3. Fetal development of male genitalia. (Data from Glenister, 1962; Arey, 1965; Hamilton and Mossman, 1972; Moore, 1977)

Fetal stage (weeks)	Fetal development
4	Development of mesonephros begins.
5	Maximal development of mesonephros, 40 mesonephric kidney tubules, kidney.
6	Urorectal septum appears and division of the cloaca is completed during the seventh week of gestation.
7	Mesonephros begins to degenerate in a cranio-caudal direction; testis and ovary become distinct.
8	Mesonephros almost completely degenerates and disappears. Its duct and a few tubules persist, which either contribute to the development of genital ducts in males or form vestigial remnants in females.
11	Glands of Littre (urethral glands) appear.
12	Mesenchyme condensation assumes primitive shape of prostate gland; short cords of epithelial cells appear and grow outwards from urogenital sinus, which now may be called the prostatic urethra.
13	Very small lumen is formed, incompletely canalizing the primitive utricular cord. Seminal vesicles appear; their primordia arise as outpocketings of the lower portion of the Wolffian ducts in the vicinity of the urogenital sinus.
14	The epithelial cords of the rete testes begin to canalize and establish connections with the mesonephric tubules; prostatic utricle is a pouch situated between the openings of the ejaculatory ducts at the apex of the verumontanum. Its upper or cranial portion is derived from the caudal remnants of the Müllerian ducts, while its lower or caudal part is derived from the mixed epithelium. Differentiation of the utricle begins from a median cord of cells derived from the fusion of two solid epithelial rudiments; a solid cord of cells from the fused Müllerian ducts and a sinu-utricular cord derived from the Müllerian tubercle (a proliferation of epithelium from the dorsal wall of the urogenital sinus).
14	Active differentiation of seminal vesicle, branches emerging from the central lumen. The glands themselves begin to bend in a knee-like fashion, posteriorly toward the prostate; the seminal vesicles begin to fold and coil upon themselves. The initial folds are generally in a dorsal-ventral plane, but later the terminal ends may coil laterally; terminal portions of the branches of glands of Littre. Muscular development of vas deferens and expansion and convolution of ampulla.
15	Solid buds of bulbourethral glands appear, on both sides of the urogenital sinus among longitudinal folds of the mucosa. The primordial ducts arise in proximity to each other from the posterior wall of the penile urethra in the region of the bulb of the penis.
16	The tip of the solid bud expands to form a knob-like structure, which becomes the future glandular portion. The narrower proximal portion, the primitive bulbourethral duct, develops a lumen first at its junction with the urogenital sinus.
17	Bulbourethral glands grow upwards (cranially) toward the bladder, paralleling the differentiating urethra. Although the ducts of the bulbourethral glands arise from the bulbar portion of the penile urethra, the glandular portions become extrabulbar and lie close to the membranous urethra.
20	Mesonephric tubules become highly convoluted and are then called the ductuli efferentes. Distinct muscle layers are developed, particularly in outer areas of prostate, where the tubules from lateral group can be readily distinguished by virtue of their larger diameters; enlargement of lumen of prostatic utricle to extend as an elongated pouch between the ejaculatory ducts upwards to the limit of the prostatic capsule.
22	Glandular branches of bulbourethral glands become more numerous and acquire lumens, forming definite alveoli that open directly into the ducts; the epithelium is composed of irregularly distributed patches of clear mucous cells interspersed among cuboidal cells.
25	Seminal vesicles essentially assume their adult morphology, both in terms of general architecture and branching of the glandular epithelium.

Primordial germ cells, will ultimately give rise to the gametes and arise in an extragonadal site from the endoderm of the allantois, yolk sac, and possibly the hindgut, and later migrate into the developing gonad (Witschi, 1948).

The gonadal primordia formed during the early part of the fifth week remain undifferentiated until the seventh week. At this time, in male fetuses the primitive sex cords transform into seminiferous (Gillman, 1948; Van Wagenen and Simpson, 1965). Shortly thereafter, the distal ends of the seminiferous cords interconnect to form a network of solid cords, the 'rete testis'. Since the gonad is situated on the medial side of the urogenital crest, the rete testis is in direct contact with the mesonephric tubules within the crest. During the third month of development, the rete testis connects with the neighboring mesonephric tubules, and by the sixth month of fetal life the cords of the rete testis acquire a lumen which becomes continuous with that of the mesonephric tubules (Narbaitz, 1974).

The fetal testis produces a second hormone 'the Müllerian inhibiting factor'. This hormone is a peptide and also acts locally to suppress the growth of the Müllerian (female) ducts. In certain mammalian species some animals cannot respond to androgens (testicular feminization) or the response can be suppressed by treatment with the anti-androgen cyproterone acetate. Neither Wolffian nor Müllerian ducts develop, because the actions of testosterone are prevented but the Müllerian inhibiting factor is operating normally.

1.4. Urogenital differentiation

The morphogenesis of structures, composed of epithelium and stroma (mesenchyme), depends on an interaction between these tissues (Kratochwil, 1972; Saxen et al., 1976). The stromal or mesenchymal component induces and specifies the developmental fate of the epithelium. Epithelial–mesenchymal analysis of urogenital development has demonstrated that: (a) urogenital mesenchyme from male accessory sex glands (and not that from other organ systems) provides conditions that are permissive for androgenic response of embryonic epithelia from developing prostate or seminal vesicle; (b) urogenital mesenchyme induces specific patterns of urogenital gland morphogenesis and cytodifferentiation in

nontarget epithelia from skin or bladder; (c) these morphogenetic inductive properties depend on the presence of the wild-type allele at the Tfm locus (Cunha and Lung, 1979); and (d) loss of morphogenetic sensitivity of the female urogenital sinus to androgens (i.e., the ability to form prostate) is due to maturational changes in the stroma (Cunha, 1976). The pronephros, a vestigial and transitory structure representing a primitive kidney, consists of a few transient mesenchymal cell aggregates or vesicles derived from the intermediate mesoderm just lateral to the cervical somites (Cunha and Lung, 1979). From these vesicles a duct forms, growing caudally to join the cloaca — the hind caudal portion of the gut. The pronephros, consisting of 7–10 paired segments, appears on day 22 of gestation, but undergoes regression during the fifth week (Hamilton and Mossman, 1972; Vaughan and Middleton, 1975). Although the pronephros degenerates, its duct persists. Once this duct becomes associated with the developing mesonephros its name changes to the Wolffian or mesonephric duct.

1.5. Male accessory organs

Under hormonal influence the mesonephric tubules differentiate into the ductuli efferentes, while the Wolffian ducts give rise to the epididymis, ductus deferens, seminal vesicles and ejaculatory ducts. The urogenital sinus forms the prostate, bulbourethral

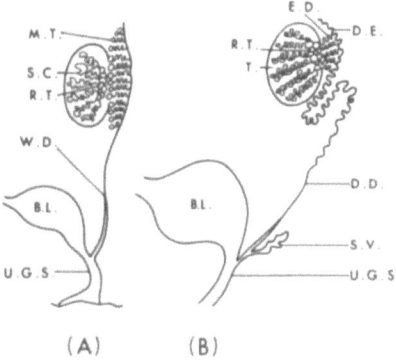

Figure 4. Schematic illustration of the development of the derivatives of the mesonephric apparatus. (A) At the beginning of the third month. (B) After the fourth month (prostatic cords growing from the urogenital sinus have been omitted for the sake of simplicity). B.L., bladder; D.D., deferent duct; D.E., ductus epididymis; E.D., efferent ductules; M.T., mesonephric tubules; S.C., seminiferous cords; S.V., seminal vesicles; U.G.S. urogenital sinus; W.D., Wolffian duct; T., testis; R.T., rete testis (Narbaitz, 1974).

glands and most of the urethra (Fig. 5). The bulbo-urethral glands which arise as paired buds from the endodermal epithelium in the caudal part of the urogenital sinus appear and complete most of their development between the third and fifth months of intrauterine life.

1.6. External genitalia

The sexual differentiation of the external genitalia is shown for the male and female fetus (Fig. 6) (See chapter 2).

2. NEONATAL DEVELOPMENT

At birth, the testes contain considerable numbers of interstitial cells. Seminiferous cords are approximately 75μ in diameter and are lined with several rows of dark-staining nuclei. A few large cells, often referred to as primordial germ cells or gonocytes appear in the central parts of the cords. The Sertoli cells do not fully differentiate until puberty. During the first few months after birth the interstitial cells regress and it is believed that all the large cells in the tubules disappear (Gier and Marion, 1970).

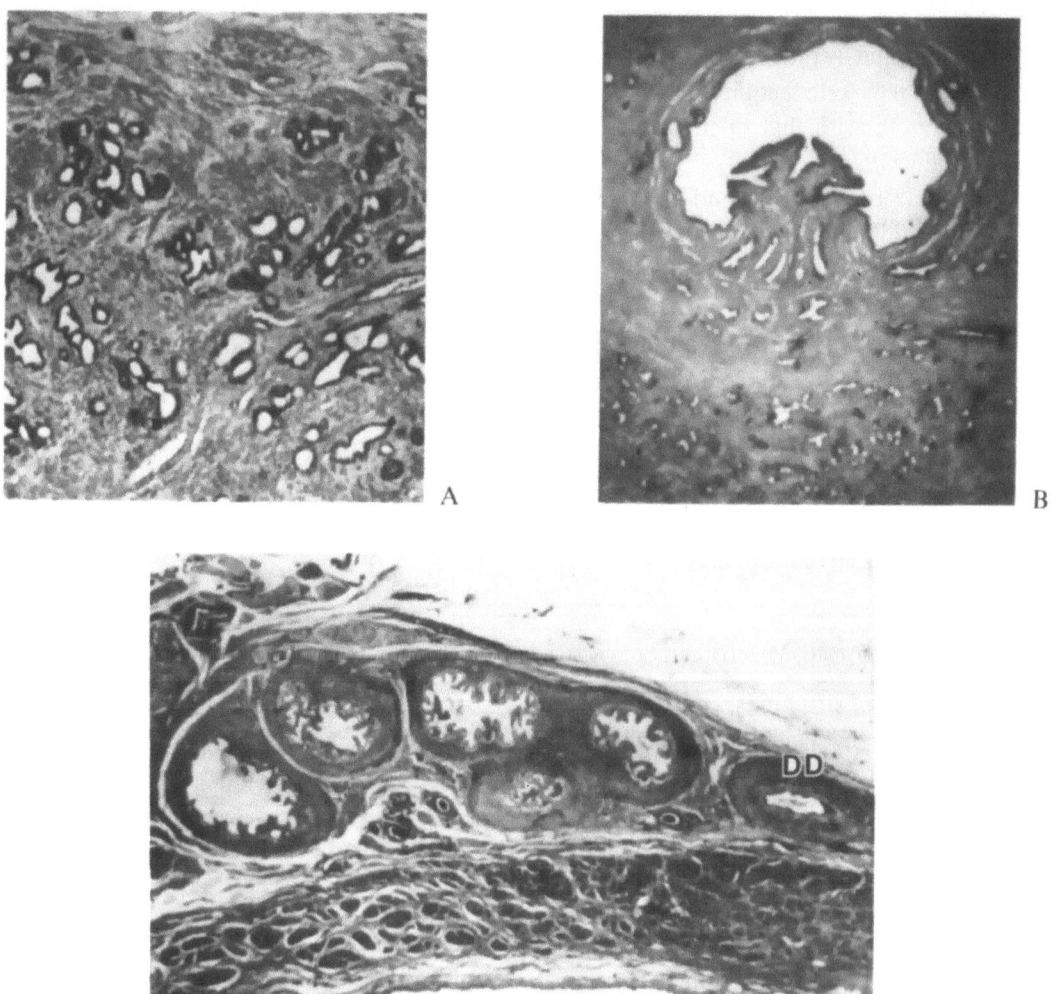

Figure 5. (A) Prostate gland near the area of the capsule (third trimester). (B) Verumontanum of prostate gland in the area where the prostatic utricle and ejaculatory ducts empty into the urethra. (C) Sagittal section of seminal vesicle in third trimester. Note ductus deferens (DD) adjacent to the gland (Carnegie Collection, No. 1172).

The prostate gland of the newborn is about 17 × 14 × 4 mm in size (Peter and Graper, 1938). At this stage the prostatic tubules are incompletely differentiated. Terminal parts are varied histologically; some cords remain solid, while others have developed patent lumens lined by one or more layers of cuboidal cells. In the neonate, the five fetal lobes are no longer separable into discrete anatomical units, and the anterior group is poorly represented (McNeal, 1976). The prostatic utricle in the newborn is quite variable in size, but usually attains a length of a little over 1 mm (Cunha and Lung, 1979). Its lining epithelium is usually nonkeratinized stratified squamous. In some neonates the utricular epithelium may be parakeratotic due to the metaplastic effects of maternal estrogens (Zondek and Zondek, 1975).

Each gland consists of a single tortuously coiled and folded tube with several irregularly placed branches. The glands are about 10 mm in length in the newborn and continue to grow slowly until puberty, when they rapidly reach adult proportions (Cunha and Lung, 1979). The bulbourethral glands are very small in the newborn, but grow to a diameter of 5–15 mm, having ducts up to 40 mm in length in the adult.

It is interesting to note that the weight of fetal organs expressed as a percentage of body weight, shows essentially no change from mid-term to birth and the main change in this parameter occurs after birth.

3. TEMPORAL INTERACTION AND FETAL MALFORMATION

The temporal interaction of acquisition of hormonal sensitivity, secretion of androgenic steroids and the Müllerian Inhibiting Substance, and acquisition of the metabolic pathways for conversion of testosterone to dihydrotestosterone are all important for normal male sex differentiation. Absence of temporal coordination may cause several fetal anomalies. For example, if acquisiton of sensitivity to androgens is delayed or fails to occur, efferent ducts, epididymis, ductus deferens, seminal vesicles, prostate or bulbourethral glands will be malformed or absent (Cunha and Lung, 1979). Expression of such defects is greatest in mutant individuals, who never acquire sensitivity to androgens (testicular feminization syndrome), in which all of the masculine accessory sex structures may fail to develop (Naftolin and Judd, 1973; Ohno, 1977).

Any delay in androgen synthesis and secretion may result in defects or the total absence of mesonephric derivatives (epididymis, ductus deferens and seminal vesicles). Hypoplasia or the failure of morphogenesis of the prostate and bulbourethral glands may also occur under these conditions (Cunha and Lung, 1979). If on the other hand, the adrenal of the female fetus is activated in the synthesis of androgens during early periods before sex determination of accessory sexual structures has taken place, masculinization of both internal and external genitalia occurs.

This adrenogenital syndrome, which results from congenital virilizing adrenal hyperplasia, causes masculinization of the external genitalia and can cause the retention and abnormal development of parts of male internal genitalia (Schlegel and Gardner, 1975). The role of 5α-reductase activity in normal urogenital morphogenesis and pseudohermaphroditism is discussed in chapter 10.

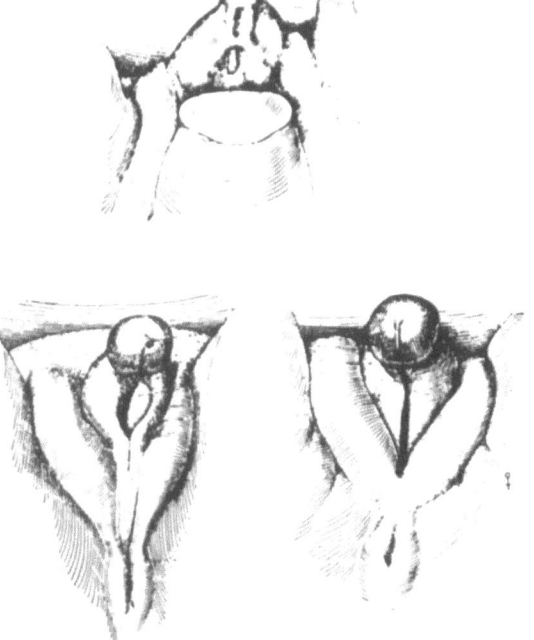

Figure 6. Development of the human external genitalia. (Top) Undifferentiated external genitalia of an embryo of 16.8 mm. (Below) External genitalia during the period of sexual differentiation; (left) Male embryo of 45 mm, (right) female embryo of 49 mm. (Spaulding MH (1921) Contributions to Embryology, Carnegie Institution of Washington, 13: 69).

8

REFERENCES

Arey LB (1965) Developmental anatomy. Philadelphia: W.B. Saunders.

Barnes AC (1968) Intra-uterine development. Philadelphia: Lea & Febiger.

Croisille Y, Gumpel-Pinot M, Martin C (1976) On some aspects of kidney organogenesis in birds. In Balls M, Monnickendom MA, eds. Organ culture in biomedical research, pp 95–109. New York: Cambridge University Press.

Cunha GR (1976) Epithelial–stromal interactions in development of the urogenital tract. Int Rev Cytol 47: 137.

Cunha GR, Lung B (1979) Development of male accessory glands. In Spring-Mills E, Hafez ESE, eds. Accessory glands of the male reproductive trance, Vol 6, pp 1–28. Ann Arbor, Mich: Ann Arbor Science.

Cunha GR, Lung B, Kato K (1977) Role of the epithelial–stromal interaction during the development and expression of ovary-independent vaginal hyperplasia. Dev Biol 56: 52.

Didier E (1968) Données expérimentales sur la formation du canal de Müller chez l'embryon d'oiseau. Ann Embryol Morphogen 1: 341.

Gier HT, Marion GB (1970) Development of mammalian testis. In Johnson AD, Gomes WR, Vandemard NL, eds. The testis, Vol I: Development, anatomy, and physiology. New York: Academic Press.

Gillman J (1948) The development of the gonads in man, with a consideration of the role of fetal endocrines and the histo-genesis of ovarian tumors. Contrib Embryol 32: 81.

Glenister TW (1962) The development of the utricle and the so-called middle or median lobe of the human prostate. J Anat 96: 443.

Gruenwald P (1941) The relation of the growing Müllerian duct to the Wolffian duct and its importance for the genesis of mal-formations. Anat Rec 81: 1.

Hamilton WJ, Mossman HW (1972) Human embryology. Balti-more: Williams & Wilkins.

Kratochwil K (1972) Tissue interaction during embryonic devel-opment. General properties. In Tarin D, ed. Tissue interactions in carcinogenesis, pp 1–47. New York: Academic Press.

McNeal JE (1976) Development and comparative anatomy of the prostate. In Grayhacek JT, Wilson JD, Scherbenske MJ, eds. Benign prostatic hyperplasia Workshop sponsored by Kidney Disease and Urology Program, Bethesda, MD DHEW Pub. No. (NIH) 76–1113.

Moore KL (1977) The developing human. Philadelphia: W.B. Saunders.

Naftolin F, Judd HL (1973) Testicular feminization. In Wynn RW, ed. Obstetrics and gynecology annual, pp 25–53. New York: Appleton-Century-Crofts.

Narbaitz R (1974) Embryology, anatomy and histology of the male sex accessory glands. In Brandes D, ed. Male accessory sex organs, pp 3–15. New York: Academic Press.

Ohno S (1977) Testosterone and cellular response. In Blandau RJ, Bergsma D, eds. Morphogenesis and malformation of the genital system, pp 99–108. New York: A.R. Liss.

O'Rahilly R (1973) The embryology and anatomy of the uterus. In Norris HJ, Hertig AT, Abell MR, eds. The uterus, pp 17–39. Baltimore: Williams & Wilkins.

Peter K, Graper L (1938) Geschlechtsorgane, Organa Genitalia. In Peter K, Wetzel G, Heiderrich F, eds. Handbuch der Ana-tomie des Kindes, Vol 2.

Potter E (1965) Development of the human glomerulus. Arch Pathol 80: 241.

Saxen LM, Karkinen-Jaaskelainen E, Lehtonen S, Nordling, Wartivaaara J (1976) Inductive tissue interactions. In Poste G, Nicholson GL, eds. The cell surface in animal embryogenesis and development, pp 331–408.

Schlegel RL, Gardner LI (1975) Ambiguous and abnormal geni-talia in infants; differential diagnosis and clinical management. In Gardner LI, ed. Endocrine and genetic diseases of childhood and adolescence, pp 571–609. Philadelphia: W.B. Saunders.

Van Wagenen G, Simpson ME (1965) Embryology of the ovary and testis, *Homo sapiens* and *Macaca mulatta*. New Haven: Yale University Press.

Vaughan ED, Middleton GW (1975) Pertinent genitourinary em-bryology; review for the practicing urologist. Urology 6: 139.

Winter JSD, Fairman C, Reyes FI (1977) Sex steroid production by the human fetus: its role in morphogenesis and control by gonadotropins. In Blandau RJ, Bergsma D, eds. Morphog-enesis and malformation of the genital system, pp 41–58. New York: A.R. Liss.

Witschi E (1948) Migrations of the germ cells of human embryos from the yolk sac to the primitive gonadal folds. Contrib Em-bryol Carneg Inst 32: 67.

Zondek T, Zondek LH (1975) The fetal and neonatal prostate. In Goland M, ed. Normal and abnormal growth of the prostate, pp 5–28. Springfield, Ill.: Charles C. Thomas.

2. THE FETAL HORMONAL ENVIRONMENT AND ITS EFFECT ON THE MORPHOGENESIS OF THE GENITAL SYSTEM

P.J. SMAIL, F.I. REYES, J.S.D. WINTER and C. FAIMAN

1. INTRODUCTION

In the normal male fetus a 46XY genotype leads to gonadal male sex; thereafter it is the hormones produced by the fetal testis which imprint a male pattern onto the indifferent embryonic genital precursor (Jost, 1953; Wilson, 1978). This chapter will review the changes in and regulation of fetal hormonal levels and their relation to male genital differentiation.

2. THE MORPHOLOGY OF MALE GENITAL DIFFERENTIATION

2.1. Testis

At about 3 weeks after fertilization the primitive germ cells begin to migrate from the yolk sac to the mesoderm of the gut, and by 7–8 weeks they reach the genital ridges of coelomic epithelium located on the medial aspects of the pronephros (Peters, 1976). Thereafter the testes rapidly differentiate under the organizing influence of the H-Y antigen (see chapter 7). Sex cords containing germ cells and Sertoli cell precursors begin to appear at 7 weeks and by 8 weeks of fetal age Leydig cells are apparent (Fig. 1). These latter proliferate, so that by 14–18 weeks they occupy half the volume of the fetal testes, following which they gradually involute, until term. They disappear in early postnatal life. Fetal Leydig cells show the histological characteristics of steroid producing cells, with abundant smooth endoplasmic reticulum and many large mitochondria (Fig. 1) (Niemi et al., 1967), features which are also observed in the testes of immature animals following stimulation with human chorionic gonadotropin (Merkow et al., 1968). Histochemical evidence of peak ac-

tivity of 3β-hydroxysteroid dehydrogenase and other steroidogenic enzymes is observed at 14–16 weeks, which as will be seen is the time of peak fetal testosterone production (Niemi et al., 1967).

Canalization of the sex cords to form seminiferous tubules occurs at 14–16 weeks when the primitive germ cells are becoming spermatogonia. Development of the seminiferous tubules progresses as the Leydig cells involute; however, unlike the situation in the female gonad, meiosis does not occur until puberty.

2.2. Internal genitalia

Until 8–9 weeks of fetal age genital development is similar in both sexes. Thereafter the internal accessory reproductive organs arise from the Wolffian (mesonephric) and Müllerian (paramesonephric) ducts, while the external genitalia are derived from the genital tubercle and urogenital sinus (Fig. 2). The Wolffian duct appears at the 5–6 week stage as a duct connecting the mesonephric kidney to the urogenital sinus; in the male this becomes modified to form the appendix of the epididymis, rete testes, epididymis, vas deferens, seminal vesicles, ejaculatory duct, and the urethral tubercle (Jirasek, 1971). The lower portion of the urogenital sinus forms the prostatic and membranous urethra (Glenister, 1954). The prostate gland arises from a series of endodermal buds which appear in the urethral lining at the 10 week stage and grow into the surrounding mesenchyme which forms the muscular and connective tissue components (McNeal, 1976).

The Müllerian duct arises shortly after the Wolffian duct and consists of a cephalic portion formed from coelomic epithelium and a caudal portion formed from the mesonephric duct. In the female the cephalic portion forms the Fallopian tubes and

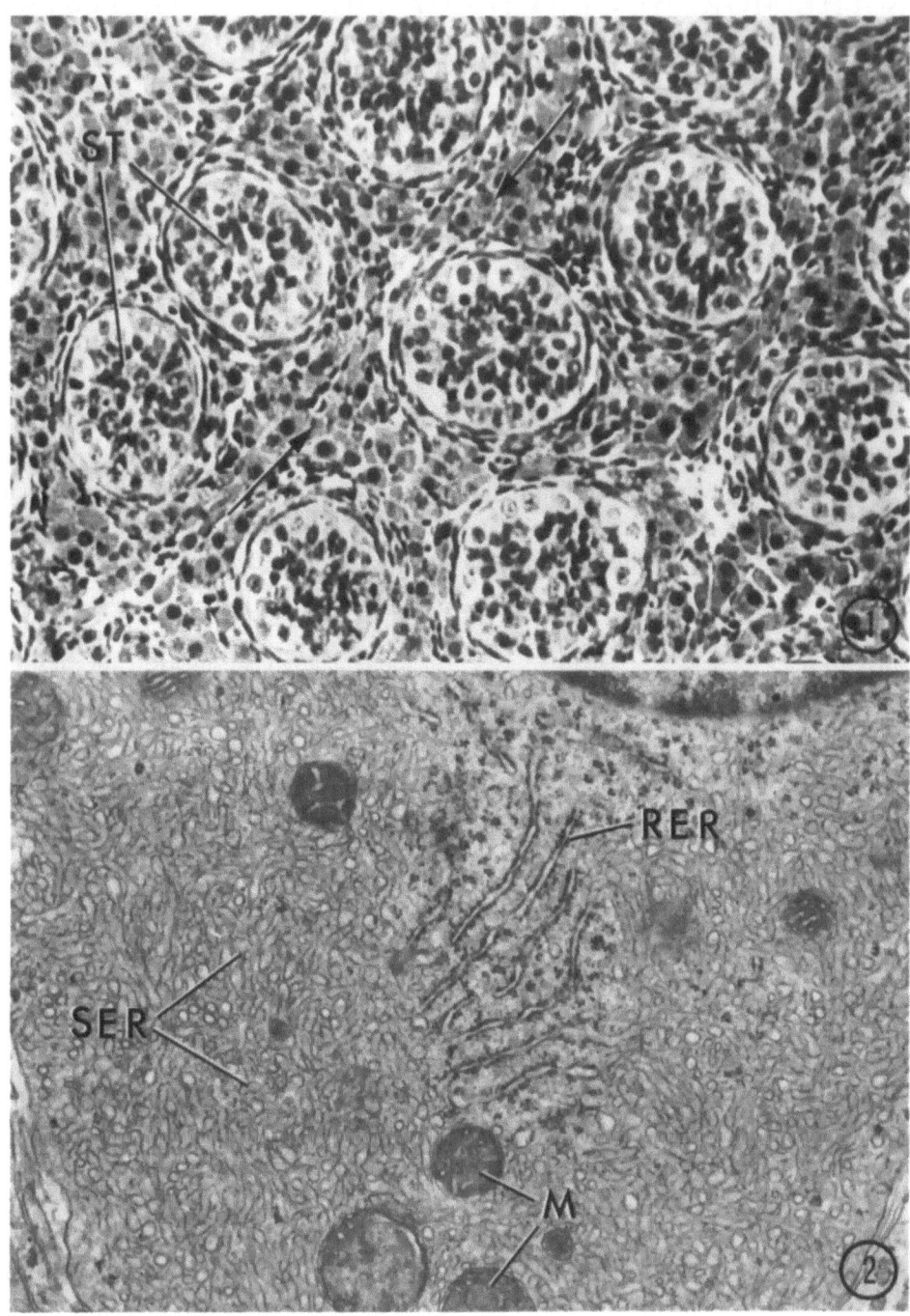

Figure 1. Testis from fetus of 14 weeks gestational age. *(Top)* Light micrograph showing numerous Leydig cells (arrowed) interspersed between developing seminiferous tubules (ST). 910 ×. *(Bottom)* Electron micrograph showing smooth endoplasmic reticulum (SER), rough endoplasmic reticulum (RER) and mitochondria. 19,750 ×. (Courtesy of Dr. J.A. Thliveris.)

the caudal portion of the uterus and upper vagina. In the male the Müllerian ducts regress by 20 weeks, leaving only a remnant as the appendix testis.

2.3. External genitalia

Masculinization of the external genitalia begins with elongation of the genital tubercle to form the penis and ventral fusion of the urethral folds to form the penile urethra (Fig. 3) (Patten, 1953). The line of closure of the urethral groove remains marked by the penile raphe. As the penis develops it migrates anteriorly becoming more distant from the anus. The fetus is recognizable as a male by 9–10 weeks, Masculinization of the external genitalia is complete by 16–20 weeks, at which time the prepuce covers the glans penis and the urogenital swellings on both sides of the urethra have migrated ventrally and anteriorly to form the scrotum.

3. THE HORMONAL ENVIRONMENT IN THE MALE FETUS

3.1. Testosterone

Jost's classical experiments showed that early castration of fetal rabbits of either sex resulted in female internal and external genital differentiation. Local androgen implants could replace most of the masculinizing influences of the fetal testis, but could not bring about regression of the Müllerian ducts (Jost, 1953).

Incubation of the fetal testis in vitro and perfusion studies in vivo have shown that formation of testosterone from acetate or pregnenolone occurs as early as 7–8 weeks of fetal age (Siiteri and Wilson, 1974; Payne and Jaffe, 1975). Direct assays of fetal testes confirm that testosterone is the principal endogenous steroid present with peak concentrations ob-

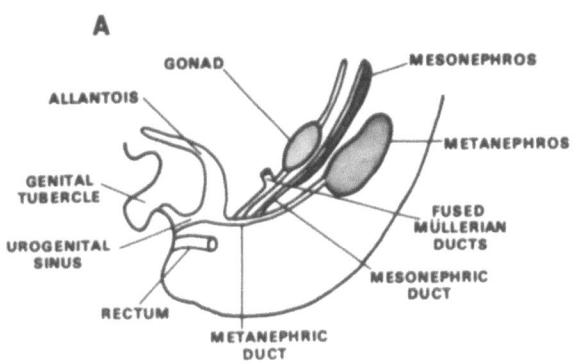

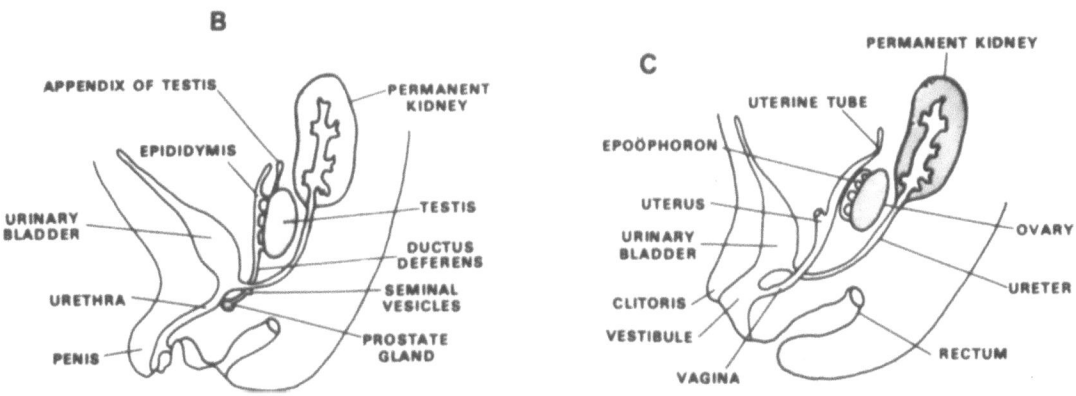

Figure 2. Diagrammatic sagittal sections of the internal genitalia of the 8 week fetus (A) and at 13 weeks fetal age in the male (B) and female (C) fetus.

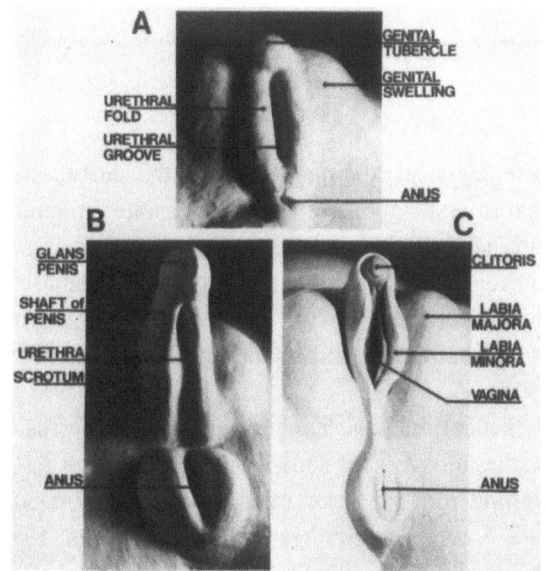

Figure 3. Models of the external genitalia at 8 weeks (A) and at 13 weeks in the male (B) and female (C) fetus. (Originals prepared by Mr. K.J. Butler.)

served at 12–14 weeks (Huhtaniemi et al., 1970; Reyes et al., 1973). Neither ovaries nor adrenal glands contain significant amounts of testosterone.

Serum testosterone levels in the male fetus (Figs. 4 and 5) reach a peak at 14–16 weeks, slightly later than the peak testicular concentration (Fig. 6). At

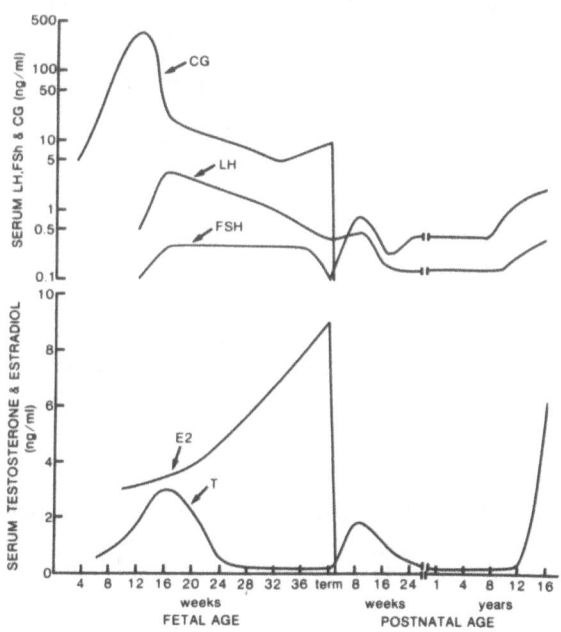

Figure 5. Mean serum levels of testosterone, estradiol, CG, LH and FSH in the male fetus and infant (Abramovich, 1974; Clements et al., 1976; Forest et al., 1973; Huhtaniemi et al., 1970; Reyes et al., 1973; Reyes et al., 1974 and Takagi et al., 1977).

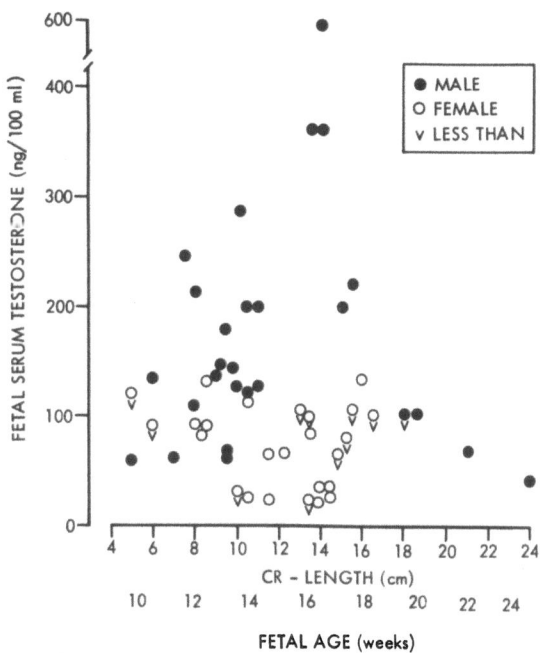

Figure 4. Human fetal serum testosterone concentrations as a function of crown-rump (CR) length and fetal age. (Reproduced with permission from Reyes et al., 1974.)

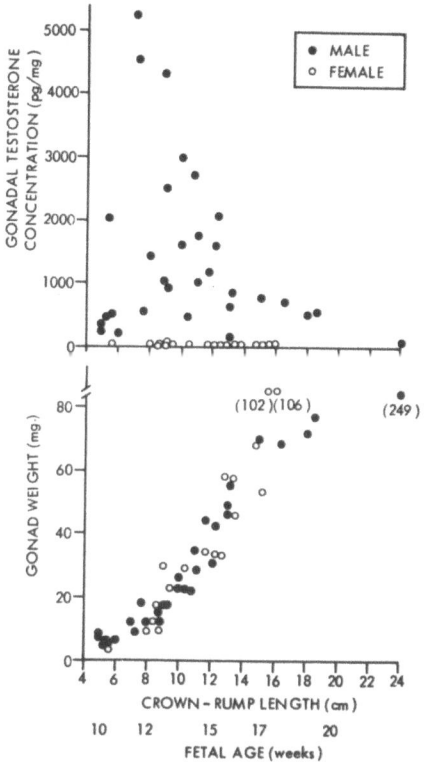

Figure 6. Gonadal testosterone concentrations and total wet weight (organ pairs) in male and female fetuses as a function of crown-rump length and fetal age. (Reproduced with permission from Reyes et al., 1973.)

this time values are within the adult male range (2.3.–10 ng/ml) (Reyes et al., 1974; Abramovich, 1974). After 24 weeks there is no significant sex difference in umbilical arterial serum testosterone (Takagi et al., 1977), although umbilical arterial and peripheral venous levels are slightly higher in male newborns at term (Forest et al., 1973).

Amniotic fluid after 14 weeks of gestation provides a convenient technique for assessing the fetal environment and is in general use for diagnosis of genetic disease and assessment of fetal wellbeing. In view of the many possible factors which could theoretically influence amniotic fluid hormone concentrations, it is remarkable that in many cases changes in these values parallel those in fetal serum levels.

Amniotic fluid testosterone concentrations in male fetuses (Fig. 7) show a peak at 14–16 weeks and until 20 weeks gestation are 3–10 times higher than in female fetuses (Warne et al., 1977). Amniotic fluid levels of testosterone and FSH may prove useful in prenatal diagnosis of fetal sex and also some forms of hypogonadism and pseudohermaphroditism.

In man the principal binding proteins for both androgens and estrogens are sex hormone binding globulin and albumin. In the fetus, sex hormone binding globulin levels are one twentieth of maternal serum levels (Anderson et al., 1976), while albumin levels are only half those at term. It appears that other fetal serum proteins, such as α-fetoprotein, lack sex steroid binding capabilities in man. Thus the

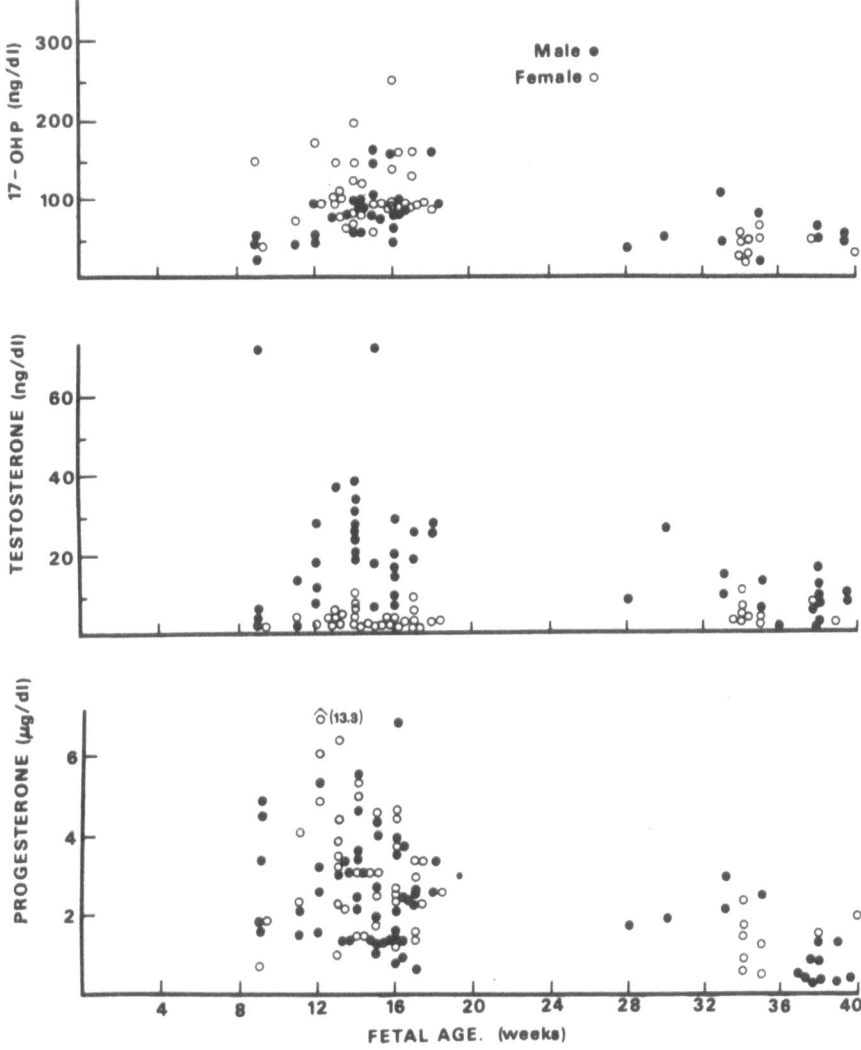

Figure 7. Concentrations of 17–OH progesterone, testosterone and progesterone in human amniotic fluid as a function of fetal age and sex. (From Warne et al. (1977) with permission.)

biologically active free testosterone level in the first trimester male fetus may be considerably higher than that in the adult male.

3.2. Anti-Müllerian hormone (see chapters 4 and 5)

Anti-Müllerian hormone (AMH) appears to be a protein of molecular weight 200,000–320,000 daltons, which appears in the fetal testes at 7–8 weeks of fetal age, just before the commencement of Müllerian duct regression. Even though all duct remnants have disappeared by 20 weeks, Müllerian inhibitory activity persists to 28 weeks when it decreases rapidly, disappearing completely in early neonatal life (Josso et al., 1977). Recent evidence has suggested that this factor may be under direct or indirect control by the fetal pituitary.

3.3. Other hormones

Both male and female fetuses are exposed to very high levels of estrogens. Fetal serum estradiol levels are variable but show no sex difference (Fig. 8) and

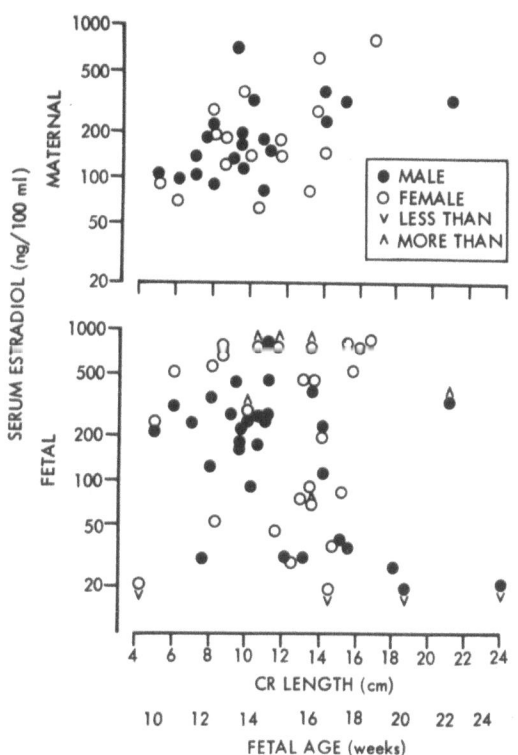

Figure 8. Semi-logarithmic plot of maternal and fetal serum estradiol-17β concentrations as a function of crown-rump (CR) length and fetal age. (From Reyes et al. (1974) with permission.)

are in general well above the maximum non-pregnant female level (30 ng/dl). Also, because of differences in protein binding, the term fetus may have a 100 times greater level of free estradiol than the non-pregnant female. There appears to be a low level of estrogen production by the fetal ovary; nonetheless most of the circulating estradiol in the fetus of both sexes is of placental origin (Reyes et al., 1974).

Circulating fetal progesterone is also primarily of placental origin. Minor sex differences in term umbilical arterial and venous levels have been described but no information is available on serum levels during fetal life.

4. CONTROL OF TESTOSTERONE PRODUCTION

4.1. Chorionic gonadotropin

Indirect evidence suggests that testicular production of androgen during the period of genital differentiation is dependent on placental rather than pituitary gonadotropin. Male anencephalic or hypopituitary fetuses do not show genital ambiguity though they may be cryptorchid or have hypotrophic external genitalia (Fig. 9). Thus pituitary gonadotropin-dependent androgen production does have an influence on genital growth and development in late fetal life. CG levels in fetal serum and amniotic fluid parallel those in maternal serum (Figs 10 and 11) although the fetal serum concentration is only approximately 1/30th the maternal serum level

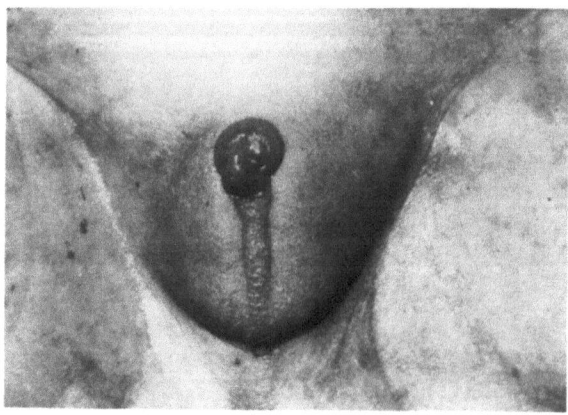

Figure 9. External genitalia of a male infant with hypopituitarism secondary to hydroencephaly (showing micropenis, scrotal hypoplasia and cryptorchidism).

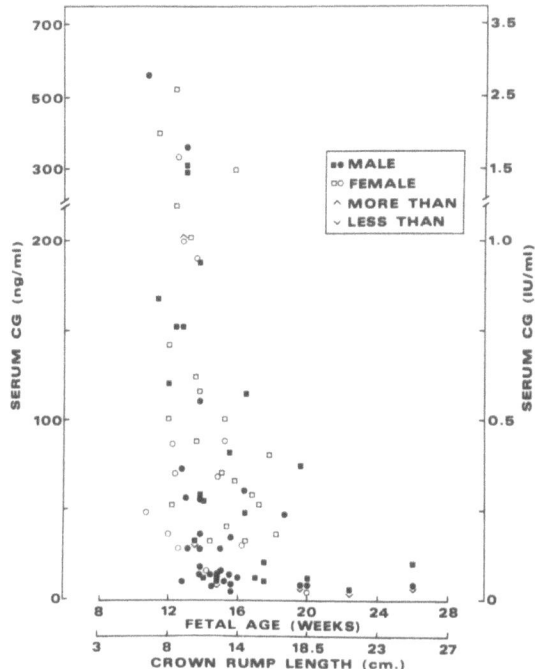

Figure 10. Serum concentrations of human chorionic gonadotropin in male and female fetuses as a function of crown-rump length and fetal age. Values shown by squares were obtained by radioimmunoassay utilizing an anti-HCG antiserum and values shown by circles with an anti-HCG β-subunit antiserum. (From Clements et al. (1976) with permission.)

throughout gestation. CG appears in the circulation between 1 and 2 weeks after ovulation and rises to a peak at 10–12 weeks of gestational age, in parallel with the pattern of testicular testosterone production. Thereafter there is a rapid fall in CG serum levels to about 16 weeks gestation, followed by a more gradual decline to 32 weeks, with a possible slight rise at term (Clements et al., 1976; Takagi et al., 1977). Studies in vivo and in vitro have shown that fetal Leydig cells have receptors for CG/LH and that both can stimulate adenyl cyclase activity and testosterone production (Huhtaniemi et al., 1977; Abramovich et al., 1974; and Ahluwalia et al., 1974).

4.2. LH and FSH

LH and FSH do not appear in the fetal serum or amniotic fluid until 11 weeks of gestation, although the anterior pituitary appears at 4–5 weeks and can synthesize both the α- and β-subunits of LH and FSH by 10 weeks. Both gonadotropins reach peak serum levels at 12–13 weeks (Figs. 12 and 13); thereafter LH levels fall steadily to term while at mid-

gestation FSH levels are strikingly higher in female fetuses than in males, reaching the adult castrate range. This sex difference presumably reflects the negative feedback influence of testicular androgens, since both sexes are exposed to similar amounts of estrogen (Clements et al., 1976; Takagi et al., 1977).

4.3. Luteinizing hormone release hormone (LH-RH)

LH-RH can be detected in the fetal brain by 5–6 weeks of fetal age (Winters et al., 1974) and LH-RH producing neurons can be demonstrated in the hypothalamus by immunocytochemical techniques at 9–11 weeks (Bugnon et al., 1977). The fetal hypothalamic content of LH-RH increases 250-fold between 8 and 18 weeks gestation (Clements et al., 1980) Fig. 14); by 10–13 weeks fetal pituitary cells can respond in vivo and in vitro to LH-RH (Goodyer et al., 1977; Takagi et al., 1977). Recent evidence from this laboratory suggests that capil-

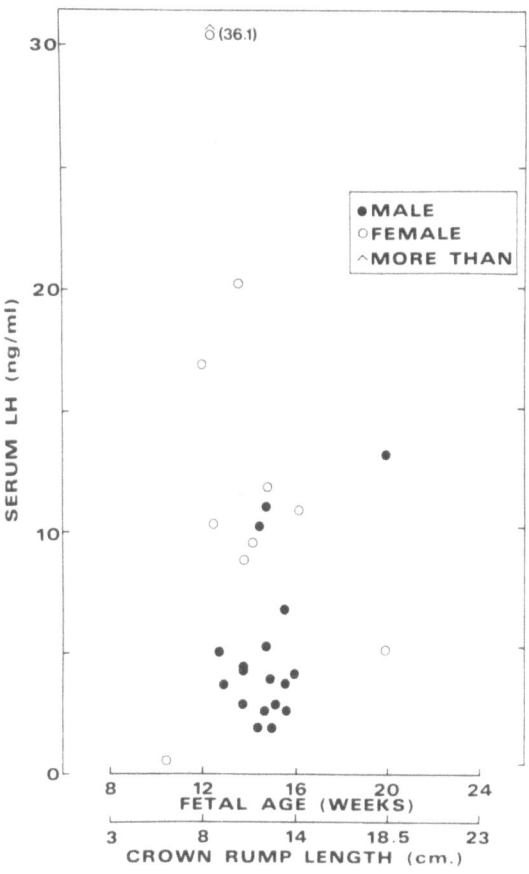

Figure 11. Amniotic fluid concentrations of HCG as a function of fetal age, crown-rump length and sex. (From Clements et al. (1976) with permission.)

16.

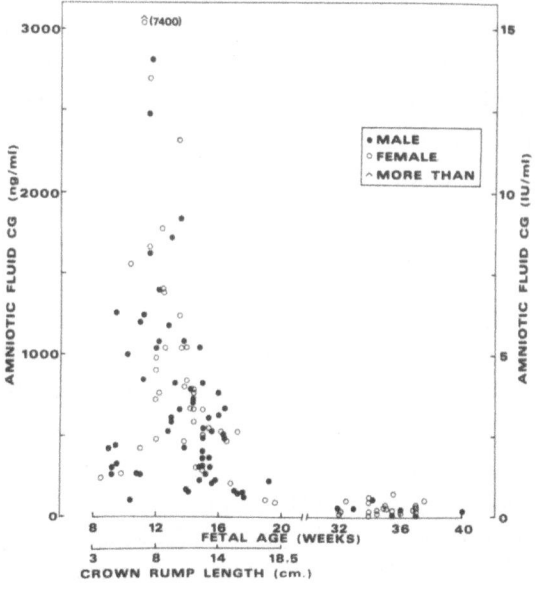

Figure 12. Human fetal serum concentrations of LH measured by βLH assay as a function of fetal age, crown-rump length and sex. (From Clements et al. (1976) with permission.)

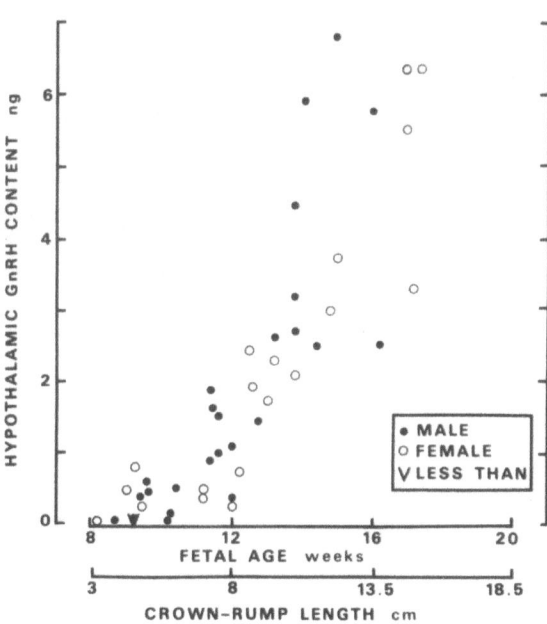

Figure 14. Content of LH-RH in human fetal hypothalami as a function of fetal age and crown-rump length. (From Clements et al. (1980) with permission.)

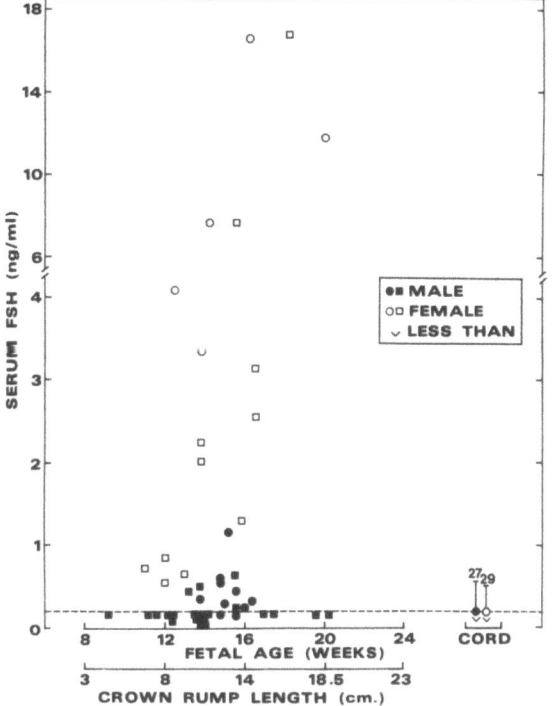

Figure 13. Human fetal concentrations of FSH as a function of fetal age, crown-rump length and sex. Term cord levels are shown (median and range) with the number of samples indicated. The dotted line indicates the detection limit of the assay (0.1 ng/ml). (From Clements et al. (1976) with permission.)

lary connections between the hypothalamus and pituitary may be present by 12 weeks gestation (Thliveris, 1980). It remains unclear whether hypothalamic control of the fetal pituitary occurs solely via such a vascular connection or also by simple diffusion or via the cerebrospinal fluid.

5. THE RELATIONSHIP OF GENITAL DIFFERENTIATION IN THE MALE FETUS TO HORMONAL CHANGES

5.1. *Target organ responses to androgens*

Masculinization of each Wolffian duct appears to be a local effect of testosterone from the ipsilateral testis (Jost, 1953). Thus Wolffian duct differentiation coincides with the peak in testicular testosterone concentration, which occurs 1–2 weeks earlier than that in serum (Reyes et al., 1973, 1974). This explains why in true hermaphrodites male internal genitalia develop only on the side which contains a testis.

Conversely, urogenital sinus and external genital virilization occurs in response to circulating androgen, and requires therefore only one functioning testis. The intracellular effector of this virilization appears to be dihydrotestosterone, which these tissues can form from testosterone by 6 weeks of gestational age. In contrast Wolffian duct structures do not develop 5α-reductase activity until 12 weeks, and thus the effector of internal genital differentiation would seem to be testosterone itself (Siiteri and Wilson, 1974). In the absence of either normal testosterone biosynthesis or normal target cell 5α-reductase activity, masculinization of the external genitalia will be incomplete (Fig. 15).

5.2. *The hypothalamic-pituitary-testicular axis*

Though the fetal Leydig cells contain receptors responding in equivalent fashion to either LH or CG, the temporal relation of Leydig cell growth and testosterone secretion to the rise in CG, prior to the appearance of LH in the fetal serum, suggests that it is CG which is the primary stimulus to testosterone production during the period of male differentiation.

The coincident appearance of FSH in the fetal serum and of spermatogonia and Sertoli cells in the testis suggests that fetal seminiferous tubule maturation may depend on FSH. Thus hypogonadotropic infants and monkeys hypophysectomized in utero show reduced testicular weight and numbers of spermatogonia (Zondek and Zondek, 1965; Gulyas et al., 1977). In the latter half of pregnancy, fetal pituitary LH appears to influence testicular testosterone production, and also the further growth of the male genitalia and descent of the testes (Hadžiselimović and Girard, 1977). It seems likely

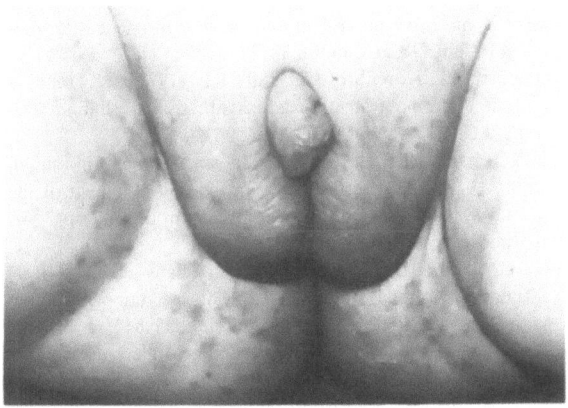

Figure 15. External genitalia of a male infant with 17α-hydroxylase deficiency, a disorder of testosterone synthesis, showing genital ambiguity with a hypospadiac penis and hypotropic bifid scrotum.

that pituitary secretion of LH and FSH is at all times under the control of the hypothalamus through the secretion of LH-RH.

5.3. *Development of feedback*

The sex differences in FSH and to a lesser extent in LH production in mid-gestation fetuses suggest that in the male fetus testicular testosterone suppresses gonadotropin release. However an estrogen-mediated feedback mechanism does not appear to develop in either sex until late gestation, even though estrogen binding cytosol receptors can be found in the pituitary, hypothalamus and other brain tissues of the fetus (Davies et al., 1975)

6. ADAPTATION TO EXTRA-UTERINE LIFE

The hormone environment in the fetus is characterized by very high circulating levels of placental hormones. Serum estradiol levels at term range from 2 to 16 ng/ml and progesterone from 120 to 500 mg/ml. CG rises slightly in the last few weeks of pregnancy to about 10 ng/ml (Takagi et al., 1977). LH and FSH levels in cord serum at term are low, presumably because of the development of feedback inhibition by placental estrogens during late pregnancy (Winter et al., 1975). During labor there is a rise in steroids of adrenal origin (Aria and Yanaihara, 1977).

Immediately after delivery serum concentrations of CG and placental sex steroids fall precipitously, so that CG is no longer detectable and estradiol reaches low levels by 5 days of age. Presumably as a result of the withdrawal of the inhibitory influence of placental estrogens, serum LH and FSH levels in the male infant begin to rise during the second week of life, reach a peak at 4–8 weeks of age, and then decline to the normal low prepubertal level by 4 months of age (Winter et al., 1975). In response to this surge in gonadotropins serum testosterone concentrations rise, so that by 10 weeks of age they reach mean levels of 2 ng/ml; thereafter they decline to prepubertal levels (less than 0.2 ng/ml) by 4–6 months of age (Forest et al., 1973). This testosterone surge is reduced in cryptorchid infants (Gendrel et al., 1978). During infancy the testosterone response of male infants to administered

CG is greater than that seen in older children and of a level nearer to that of adolescents (Job et al., 1977; Winter et al., 1972).

7. CONCLUSION

Recent studies have shown that while the term fetus may show immature function of many organ systems, it has a relatively mature hypothalamic–pituitary-gonadal axis. Active testicular function, with the secretion of Müllerian inhibitory factor and testosterone, is necessary in early fetal life for male differentiation. At first fetal testosterone secretion is mediated by placental CG, but in later fetal life pituitary LH also plays a role. Pituitary FSH and LH also appear to be involved in germ cell and Sertoli cell development and testicular descent. It should be obvious how abnormalities of fetal testicular func-

tion can lead to ambiguous sexual differentiation, while deficiencies of hypothalamic or pituitary function present in the male with normally formed but hypotropic genitalia. It is likely that even more subtle disorders of fetal endocrine function underlie some unexplained problems of postnatal reproductive function. Finally it remains to be defined to what extent during fetal life or infancy exposure to exogenous sex steroids and other environmental agents can interfere with the normal pattern of reproductive endocrine development (Aarskog, 1979).

ACKNOWLEDGEMENTS

The original work which forms the basis for this communication was supported by grants form the Medical Research Council of Canada (PG5), the Winnipeg Children's Hospital Research Foundation and the Richardson Foundation.

REFERENCES

Aarskog D (1979) Maternal progestins as a possible cause of hypospadias. New Engl J Med 300: 75.

Abramovich DR (1974) Human sexual differentiation — in utero influences. J Obstet Gynecol Br Commun 81: 444.

Abramovich DR, Baker TG, Neal P (1974) Effect of human chorionic gonadotrophin on testosterone secretion by the human fetal testes. J Endocrinol 60: 179.

Ahluwalia B, Williams J, Verma P (1974) In vitro testosterone biosynthesis in the human fetal testes: II. Stimulation by cyclic AMP and human chorionic gonadotropin (hCG) Endocrinology 95: 1411.

Anderson DC, Lasley BL, Fisher RA, Shepherd JH, Newman L, Hendrickxx AG (1976) Transplacental gradients of sex hormone-binding globulin in human and simian pregnancy. Clin Endocrinol 5: 657.

Arai K, Yanaihara T (1977) Steroid hormone changes in fetal blood during labor. Am J Obstet Gynecol 127: 879.

Bugnon C, Bloch B, Fellman D (1977) Cyto-immunological study of the ontogenesis of the gonadotropic hypothalamo-pituitary axis in the human fetus. J Steroid Biochem 8: 565.

Clements JA, Reyes F, Winter JSD, Faiman C. (1976) Studies on human sexual development: III. Fetal pituitary, serum and amniotic fluid concentrations of LH, CG and FSH. J Clin Endocrinol Metab 42: 9.

Clements JA, Reyes FI, Winter JSD, Faiman C. (1980) Ontogenesis of gonadotropin releasing hormone in the human fetal hypothalamus. Proc Soc Exp Biol Med (in press).

Davies IJ, Naftolin F, Ryan KJ, Sui V. (1975) A specific high affinity, limited-capacity estrogen binding component in the cytosol of human fetal pituitary and brain tissues. J Clin Endocrinol Metab 40: 909.

Forest MG, Cathiard AM, Bertrand JA. (1973) Total and unbound testosterone levels in the newborn and in normal and hypogonadal children. J Clin Endocrinol Metab 36: 1132.

Gendrel D, Job J-C, Roger M. (1978) Reduced postnatal rise of testosterone in plasma of cryptorchid infants. Acta Endocrinol 89: 372.

Glenister TW (1954) The origin and fate of the urethral plate in man. Anat 88: 413.

Goodyer CG, St. George Hall C, Guyda H, Robert F, Giroud CJ-P. (1977) Human fetal pituitary in culture: hormone secretion and response to somatostatin, luteinizing hormone releasing factor, thyrotropin releasing factor and dibutyryl cyclic AMP. J Clin Endocrinol Metab 45: 73 (1977).

Gulyas BJ, Tullner WW, Hodgen GD. (1977) Fetal or maternal hypophysectomy in rhesus monkeys (Macaca mulatta): effects on the development of testes and other endocrine organs. Biol Reprod 17: 650.

Hadžiselimović F, Girard J. (1977) Pathogenesis of cryptorchidism. Horm Res 8: 76.

Huhtaniemi IT, Ikonen M, Vikho R. (1970) Presence of testosterone and other neutral steroids in human fetal testes. Biochem Biophys Res Commun 38: 715.

Huhtaniemi IT, Korenbrot CC, Jaffe RB. (1977) hCG binding and stimulation of testosterone biosynthesis in the human fetal testis. J Clin Endocrinol Metab 44: 963.

Jirasek JE (1971) Development of the genital system in human embryos and fetuses. In: Cohen Jr., ed. Development of the genital system and male pseudohermaphroditism, pp 3–41. Baltimore: Johns Hopkins Press.

Job J-C, Gendrel D, Safar A, Roger M, Chaussain J-L. (1977) Pituitary LH and FSH and testosterone secretion in infants with undescended testes. Acta Endocrinol 85: 644.

Josso N, Picard JY, Tran D. (1977) The anti-Müllerian hormone. In: Blandau RJ, Bergsma D, eds. Birth defects: original article series Vol 13, No. 2: Morphogenesis and malformation of the genital systems, pp 59–84. New York: Alan R. Liss.

Jost A (1953) Problems of fetal endocrinology. Recent Progr Horm Res 8: 379.

McNeal JE (1976) Developmental and comparative anatomy of

the prostate. In Grayhack JT, Wilson JD, Scherbenske MJ, eds. Benign prostate hyperplasia, pp 1–9. Bethesda: National Institutes of Health.

Merkow L, Acevedo HF, Stefkin M, Caito BJ (1968) Studies on the interstitial cells of the testis. Am J Pathol 53: 47.

Niemi M, Ikonen M, Hervonen A. (1967) Histochemistry and fine structure of the interstitial tissues in the human fetal testis. In Wolstenholme GEW, ed. Ciba Foundation Colloquia on Endocrinology, Vol 16: The testis, pp 31–53. London: Churchill.

Patten BM (1953) Human embryology, 2nd edn, pp 549–607. New York: McGraw-Hill.

Payne AH, Jaffe RB (1975) Androgen formation from pregnenolone sulfate by fetal, neonatal and adult human testes. J Clin Endocrinol Metab 40: 102.

Peters H (1976) Intrauterine gonadal development. Fertil Steril 27: 493.

Reyes FI, Winter JSD, Faiman C (1973) Studies on human sexual development: I. Fetal gonadal and adrenal sex steroids. J Clin Endocrinol Metab 37: 74.

Reyes FI, Boroditsky RJ, Winter JSD, Faiman C (1974) Studies on human sexual development: II. Fetal and maternal serum gonadotropin and sex steroid concentration. J Clin Endocrinol Metab 38: 612.

Siiteri PK, Wilson JD (1974) Testosterone formation and metabolism during male sexual differentiation in the human embryo. J Clin Endocrinol Metab 38: 113.

Takagi S, Yoshida T, Tsubata K, Ozaki H, Fujü TK, Nomura Y, Sawada M (1977) Sex differences in fetal gonadotropins and androgens. J Steroid Biochem 8; 609.

Thliveris JA (1980) Personal communication.

Warne GL, Faiman C, Reyes FI, Winter JSD (1977) Studies on human sexual development: V. Concentrations of testosterone, 17-hydroxyprogesterone and progesterone in human amniotic fluid throughout gestation. J Clin Endocrinol Metab 44: 934.

Wilson JD (1978) Sexual differentiation. Ann Rev Physiol 40: 279.

Winter JSD, Taraska S, Faiman C (1972) The hormonal response to HCG stimulation in male children and adolescents. J Clin Endocrinol Metab 34: 348.

Winter JSD, Faiman C, Hobson WC, Prasad AV, Reyes FI (1975) Pituitary-gonadal relations in infancy; I. Patterns of serum gonadotropin concentrations from birth to four years of age in man and chimpanzee. J Clin Endocrinol Metab 40: 545.

Winters AJ, Eskay RL, Porter JC (1974) Concentrations and distribution of TRH and LRH in the human fetal brain. J Clin Endocrinol Metab 39: 960.

Zondek LH, Zondek T (1965) Observations on the testis in anencephaly with special reference to the Leydig cells. Biol Neonate 8: 329.

3. STROMAL INFLUENCE ON EXPRESSION OF MORPHOLOGICAL AND FUNCTIONAL CHARACTERISTICS OF UROGENITAL EPITHELIA

GERALD R. CUNHA, HIROHIKO FUJII, BLAKE L. NEUBAUER, JOHN M. SHANNON and BETH A. REESE

1. INTRODUCTION

The etiology of malformations of the genital system is based upon knowledge of normal urogenital morphogenesis, genetics, fetal endocrinology, and molecular biology. From these studies it is known that gonadal sex is determined following fertilization through expression of the H-Y antigen, which induces testicular development in the gonadal anlage (Ohno, 1979; Wachtel, 1980) (Fig. 1). Ovarian development occurs in the absence of the H-Y antigen. Once the gonadal sex is specified, subsequent development of internal and external genitalia, as well as sexual differentiation of certain neural centers within the brain, is determined by hormonal conditions within the fetus (Jost et al., 1977; Price and Ortiz, 1965; Wilson et al., 1980). The fetal testes produce androgens that induce masculine development of the internal and external genitalia (Price and Ortiz, 1965; Jost et al., 1977; Winter et al., 1977). The Müllerian Inhibiting Substance, also produced by the fetal testes, causes regression of the Müllerian ducts in male fetuses (see Donohoe et al., 1976, and chapter 9). The fetal ovaries produce estrogenic steroids during early phases of sex development (Wilson et al., 1980), and at later fetal periods apparently produce androgens (Price et al., 1971). These ovarian hormones do not appear to be required for feminization of the urogenital tract, since the female phenotype is expressed in the absence of ovaries (Price and Ortiz, 1965; Jost et al., 1977). However, this does not imply that developing male or female reproductive tracts are insensitive to pharmacological doses of exogenous estrogens. In fact, a variety of teratogenic and possibly carcinogenic effects may be elicited in developing urogenital tracts by exogenous estrogen (Bern et al., 1976; Takasugi, 1976, 1979; McLachlan and Dixon, 1977;

Kohrman, 1978; McLachlan et al., in press).

At the molecular level, it is known that the masculinizing effects of androgens are mediated during development by androgen receptor proteins (see Ohno, 1979; Wilson et al., 1980, and chapter 16). Testosterone is the effective intracellular androgen for masculine development of the Wolffian ducts, whereas dihydrotestosterone, produced from testosterone by 5α reductase, is the hormone responsible for masculinization of the urogenital sinus and external genitalia (see Wilson et al., 1980).

From this body of experimental data several genital malformations have been explained in terms of 5α reductase deficiency (Imperato-McGinley et al., 1974), absence of androgen receptors (Ohno, 1979), abnormal production or absence of H-Y antigen (Wachtel, 1980), or excessive androgen

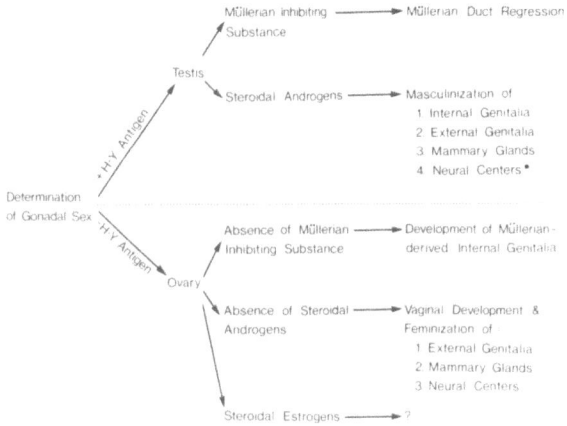

Figure 1. A summary of sex differentiation in mammals. The key events are (1) determination of gonadal sex by the H-Y antigen or its absence, (2) determination of Müllerian development by the Müllerian Inhibiting Substance, and (3) determination of sexual differentiation of the internal and external genitalia, mammary glands, and neural centers by sex steroids produced by the gonads. * Masculinization of the brain by androgens may be mediated through their metabolic conversion to estrogens.

S.J. Kogan and E.S.E. Hafez (eds.), Pediatric andrology, 21–36. All rights reserved.
Copyright © 1981, Martinus Nijhoff Publishers bv, The Hague/Boston/London.

production by the fetal adrenals (Schlegel and Gardner, 1969).

An additional level of complexity of urogenital development is introduced when it is realized that all glandular accessory sexual organs are composed of two fundamental tissues, epithelium and mesenchyme (stroma). Since development of glandular urogenital organs is dependent upon interactions between these tissues, we have attempted to elucidate the relationship between hormonal effects and epithelial–stromal interactions during urogenital development. The major findings of these studies are described below.

2. DEFINITIONS AND METHODOLOGY

Epithelium, the primary parenchymal (functional) element of accessory sexual glands, is a tissue organized into sheets or tubules composed of cells closely apposed over a large part of their surface. This tissue typically forms a fluid-tight barrier between the tissue fluid compartment (interstitial space) and the external environment or glandular lumina by virtue of the presence of tight junctions between adjacent cells. The stroma is separated and demarcated from the epithelium by a distinct, ultrastructurally defined entity, the basal lamina, which is composed of finely fibrillar collagen and glycoprotein (Kefalides, 1973). While the predominant cells within the stromal compartment are fibroblasts and smooth muscle cells, other cell types such as wandering blood cells, adipose cells, macrophages, and ganglion cells may also be present. Most resident (non-wandering) stromal cells are derived from undifferentiated loose embryonic connective tissue called mesenchyme. This compartment also contains variable amounts of extracellular materials, primarily collagen.

Analysis of epithelial–mesenchymal interactions during urogenital development involves enzymatic separation of organs into their epithelial and stromal (mesenchymal) elements. Separated stroma may be reassociated with its native epithelium (homotypic recombination) or with epithelium derived from other organ (heterotypic recombination) (Fig. 2). Recombinants can be grown under a variety of in vivo or in vitro conditions, in the presence or absence of hormonal stimuli. Hormonal effects can

be evaluated through a variety of experimental criteria: morphological, biochemical, autoradiographic, histochemical, or immunocytochemical.

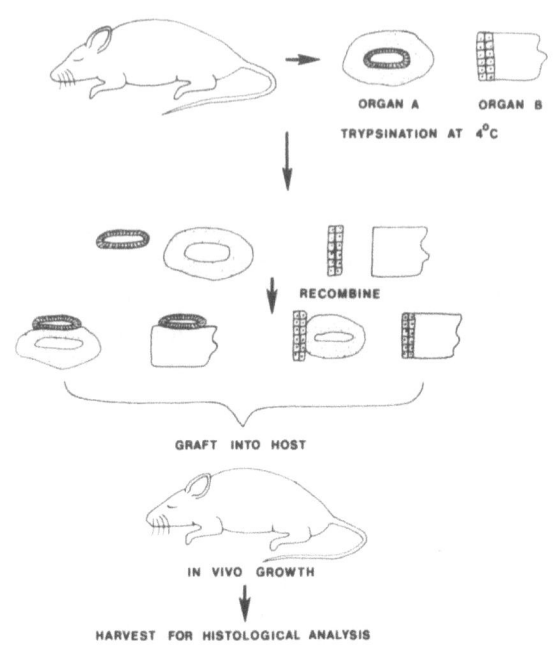

Figure 2. The methodology of tissue separation and recombination. Organs are excised from the animal, and incubated for 2–3 hours in 1% trypsin in Tyrode's solution at 4°C and separated into their mesenchymal (stromal) and epithelial components. Tissues are then recombined (homo- or heterotypically) and grown in vivo in male or female hosts. Following the in vivo growth, the recombinants are harvested for histological or other types of analysis. (From Cunha et al. 1980.)

3. HORMONE-INDUCED MORPHOGENESIS OF ACCESSORY SEXUAL STRUCTURES REQUIRES AN INTERACTION BETWEEN EPITHELIUM AND MESENCHYME

Although morphogenesis of male and female accessory sexual glands is directed by hormonal signals (the presence or absence of fetal testicular androgen), the development of these glands requires an interaction between epithelium and mesenchyme. Isolated epithelium usually does not survive when grown in vitro or in vivo, with or without hormonal stimulation. Conversely, isolated mesenchyme will survive under these conditions, but merely differentiates into a mass of fibroblasts and smooth muscle cells (Cunha, 1976a; Cunha and Lung, 1979). In contrast, if isolated epithelium and mesenchyme are reassociated following tryptic-separation, morphogenesis of both components proceeds normally, and after four weeks of growth in the appropriate adult host (male or female) morphogenesis is advanced, and in many cases functional (secretory) activity may be expressed (Cunha, 1976a; Cunha and Lung, 1979). These observations have been made for developing prostate, seminal vesicle, uterus, and vagina, and are in agreement with similar studies utilizing organs whose morphogenesis is not dependent upon sex hormones (Grobstein, 1967; Saxen et al., 1976).

4. MESENCHYME MEDIATES THE EFFECTS OF ANDROGENS DURING PRENATAL MASCULINE MORPHOGENESIS OF ACCESSORY SEX GLANDS

The embryonic urogenital sinus, when grown in the presence of androgens, gives rise to the elaborately branched ductal-acinar network of the prostate. Homotypic recombinants of this genital anlagen grown under androgenic conditions also form glandular acini virtually identical to those of the host's prostate. However, when epithelium of the urogenital sinus is associated with mesenchyme from the embryonic integument and grown under identical conditions, androgenic stimulation has no apparent effect (Fig. 3). The epithelium of the urogenital sinus, instead of forming prostate, differentiates into a stratified squamous epithelium (Cunha, 1972a, b). Likewise, epithelium of the embryonic seminal vesicle (Wolffian duct epithelium) expresses androgen-induced morphogenesis only when associated with mesenchyme of the seminal vesicle or urogenital sinus, and not with non-target integumental mesenchyme. Although the absence of glandular development in these recombinants may be interpreted as an "epidermalization" of the urogenital epithelia, the consistent absence of specific integumental derivatives such as hair or integumental glands suggest that the integumental inductors were not eliciting epidermalization of the urogenital epithelia. Thus, the morphogenetic effects of androgen upon developing urogenital epithelium are apparently mediated through relatively specific properties of urogenital mesenchyme that are not expressed in mesenchyme from other, non-target organ systems such as the integument (Cunha,

1972a, b, c, 1976a; Cunha and Lung, 1979). A corollary to this observation is that the presence of androgen per se is not sufficient to permit masculine morphogenesis, but instead certain mesenchymal requirements are of utmost importance. Similar studies of in vitro prostatic development in rats have led Lasnitzki and Mizuno (1979) to similar conclusions.

The concept that mesenchyme is the prime mediator of the morphogenetic effects of androgens upon target epithelium is further strengthened by tissue recombination experiments utilizing wild-type and Tfm (testicular feminization syndrome) tissues. Due to the relative or complete absence of functional androgen receptor activity within cells of Tfm/Y males, androgen target organs of these mice are insensitive to endogenous testicular androgen, resulting in the absence of masculine development (Bardin and Bullock, 1974; Bardin et al., 1978); for example, the urogenital sinus of Tfm/Y males forms a vagina instead of differentiating as prostate. How-

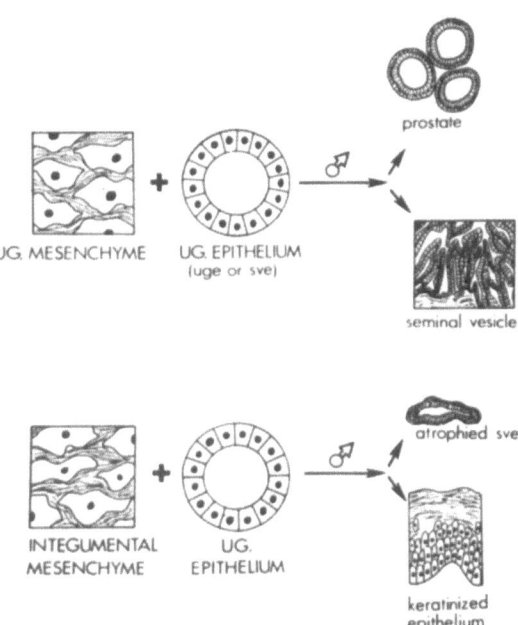

Figure 3. A summary of recombination experiments with urogenital and integumental tissues. Urogenital epithelia from embryonic urogenital sinus (UGE) or seminal vesicle (SVE) exhibit androgen-induced glandular morphogenesis when grown for 4 weeks in male hosts. By contrast, these urogenital epithelia fail to express glandular development when grown under identical conditions, but instead associated with integumental mesenchyme. In the presence of this nonurogenital mesenchyme, UGE forms a stratified squamous vagina-like epithelium, while SVE forms narrow unbranched tubules of atrophied epithelium. (From Cunha et al., 1980.)

ever, if epithelium of the urogenital sinus of embryonic Tfm/Y mice is associated with wild-type urogenital sinus mesenchyme, the Tfm/Y epithelium participates in androgen-induced prostatic morphogenesis (Fig. 4). In contrast, the reciprocal recombinant composed of Tfm/Y urogenital sinus mesenchyme and wild-type epithelium differentiates as a vaginal mucosa when grown under androgenic conditions (Cunha and Lung, 1978). Thus, the androgenic response of urogenital sinus epithelium is strictly dependent upon the presence of androgen-sensitive, wild-type mesenchyme. These observations, taken together with the results of recombination experiments employing urogenital and integumental tissues, suggest that *urogenital mesenchyme is the primary, essential target of androgenic stimulation and the mediator of morphogenetic effects of androgen upon the epithelium* (Cunha and Lung, 1978, 1979). These concepts are further strengthened by similar tissue separation–recombination experiments on the developing mammary gland (Kratochwil and Schwartz, 1976; Drews and Drews, 1977; Durnberger et al., 1978), and additional studies by Ohno (1979) and Drews and Dietrich (1978) on the Tfm and sex reversed mutations in mice.

A possible mechanism accounting for mesenchymal primacy during embryonic genital development can be proposed from autoradiographic studies of estradiol binding sites in the urogenital tract of the embryonic chick (Gasc et al., 1978). Development of the cloacal–anal region of the chick embryo is under hormonal control. In contrast to mammalian sexual development, castration of the chick produces masculine development, while administration of exogenous estrogen produces the female phenotype. Steroid autoradiography utilizing ^{3}H-estradiol demonstrates that nuclear estrogen binding sites are localized exclusively to the cloacal mesenchyme of the embryonic chick, adjacent epithelial cells being devoid of estrogen binding sites. In the developing mammalian genital system, nuclear estrogen binding sites are also restricted to the mesenchymal component of the mammary gland, urogenital sinus, and gonoducts (Stumpf et al., 1980; Narbaitz et al., 1980). Therefore, the primacy of mesenchyme as the target and mediator of hormonal effects may be due to the fact that it is the mesenchyme alone which possesses hormone receptors during *developmental* periods. At later, post-hatching or postnatal stages, the epithelia of accessory sexual glands acquire androgen, estrogen, and/or progestin receptor activities, which presumably are strict requirements for functional activity of the organ (see Stumpf and Sar, 1976).

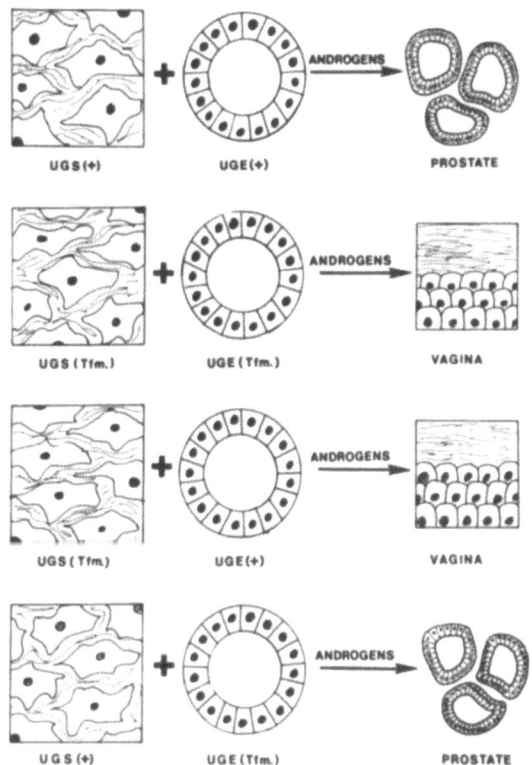

Figure 4. A summary of the developmental response of recombinants prepared with urogenital sinus components from Tfm/Y and wild-type embryos. Prostatic morphogenesis, a positive androgenic response, occurs in all recombinants in which wild-type mesenchyme is utilized (top and bottom recombinants). Conversely, vaginal differentiation occurs in all (middle) recombinants prepared with Tfm/Y mesenchyme. Therefore, androgen-induced morphogenesis requires the presence of the wild-type allele at the Tfm locus within the mesenchymal component. (From Cunha et al., 1980.)

5. UROGENITAL MESENCHYME INDUCES AND SPECIFIES THE MORPHOLOGICAL ORGANIZATION OF EMBRYONIC UROGENITAL EPITHELIUM

In the previous section the ability of urogenital mesenchyme to mediate the morphogenetic effects of androgens upon the epithelium can be characterized as a permissive induction; that is, mesenchyme acts upon epithelium by providing conditions that are permissive for normal epithelial development and expression of epithelial hormonal responsiveness. This type of inductive influence is contrasted by the directive (instructive) induction, in which the mesenchyme actively reprograms the developmental fate of the responding epithelium. This latter type of inductive influence has been demonstrated in a variety of urogenital mesenchymes (Table 1). In males, mesenchyme of the embryonic seminal vesicle, urogenital sinus (a prostatic inductor), and neonatal bulbourethral gland can elicit glandular development (Fig. 5) from a variety of non-glandular epithelia derived from embryonic epidermis and urinary bladder. Epithelia from neonatal and adult urinary bladder and vagina are also responsive to these urogenital inductors (Table 1) (Cunha, 1972b, 1975a; Cunha and Lung, 1978; Cunha et al., 1979, 1980; Fujii and Cunha, in preparation). Similarly, vaginal, cervical, and uterine morphogenesis in females is mediated by stromas that function as directive inductors (Cunha, 1976b; Cunha and Lung, 1979).

The fact that development of vaginal, cervical, and uterine epithelium is induced and determined by the subadjacent stroma provides an explanation for the development of the marked regional differences in morphology and function of Müllerian epithelium. For instance, the oviducts, uterus, cervix, and upper portion of the vagina share a common developmental origin from the epithelium of the Müllerian ducts (Forsberg, 1973; Cunha, 1975b). The regional differences in morphogenesis and cytodifferentiation of this common population of Müllerian epithelial cells appear to be determined by regional differences in stromal induction, since uterine stroma elicits uterine differentiation from

vaginal epithelium (Fig. 6), and vaginal and cervical stroma elicits the differentiation of a stratified mucosa from uterine epithelium (Fig. 7). Thus, stroma is the regional determinant for Müllerian differentiation in the female urogenital tract.

Lastly, several morphological observations suggest the possibility that the directive inductive activities of mesenchyme of the urogenital sinus, cervix, and vagina may be eliciting both a morphological reorganization of the epithelium as well as the expression of a new functional epithelial phenotype. This is suggested in recombinants composed of urogenital sinus mesenchyme and embryonic bladder epithelium, in which putative secretory product appears within the induced acini (Fig. 5a). Another observation consistent with this idea comes from analysis of recombinants composed of uterine epithelium associated with either vaginal or cervical stroma; under these conditions the uterine epithelium is induced to differentiate as a stratified vaginal or cervical epithelium. The alternating phases of epithelial differentiation (Fig. 8) in these recombinants from the cornified to the mucified state (which parallel similar changes during the estrous cycle in the host's vaginal and cervical epithelium) provide morphological evidence suggestive of the expression of a new epithelial function in the induced uterine epithelium (see Cunha et al., 1980).

6. UROGENITAL SINUS MESENCHYME ELICITS EXPRESSION OF A NEW FUNCTIONAL PHENOTYPE FROM EMBRYONIC BLADDER EPITHELIUM

To determine the extent to which epithelium of the

Table 1. Mesenchyme (stroma)-induced alteration of epithelial differentiation in accessory sexual structures.

Mesenchymal inductor	Responding epithelium	Epithelial response	Reference
Uterus (neonatal)	Vagina (neonatal)	Uterine	Cunha (1976b)
Vagina (neonatal and adult)	Uterus (neonatal)	Vaginal	Cunha (1976b)
Cervix (neonatal and adult)	Uterus (neonatal)	Cervical	Cunha and Lung (1979)
Seminal vesicle (embryonic)	Epidermis (embryonic)	Glandular	Cunha (1972a)
Seminal vesicle (neonatal)	Bladder (neonatal and adult)	Glandular	Fujii and Cunha (unpublished)
Urogenital sinus (embryonic)	Bladder (neonatal and adult)	Prostatic	Cunha and Lung (1978) Cunha et al. (1979a)
Bulbourethral (neonatal)	Bladder (neonatal)	Bulbourethral gland	Fujii and Cunha (unpublished)
Urogenital sinus (embryonic)	Vagina (neonatal and adult)	Prostatic	Cunha (1975b)
Urogenital sinus (embryonic)	Skin (embryonic)	Glandular	Cunha (1972a)

From Cunha et al. (1980).

embryonic urinary bladder is altered in a functional (biochemical) sense by inductive influences from mesenchyme of the urogenital sinus, three histochemical tests were performed upon adult bladder, prostate, and recombinants prepared with embryonic urogenital sinus mesenchyme and epithelium of embryonic urinary bladder (UGM +

BLE → prostate-like acini). As indicated in Table 2, markers indicative of urinary bladder disappeared while prostate-like markers were expressed by the induced bladder epithelium (Lung et al., 1979a).

Ultrastructural evidence also demonstrates a profound change in epithelial phenotype in the UGM + BLE recombinants (Fig. 9); for example,

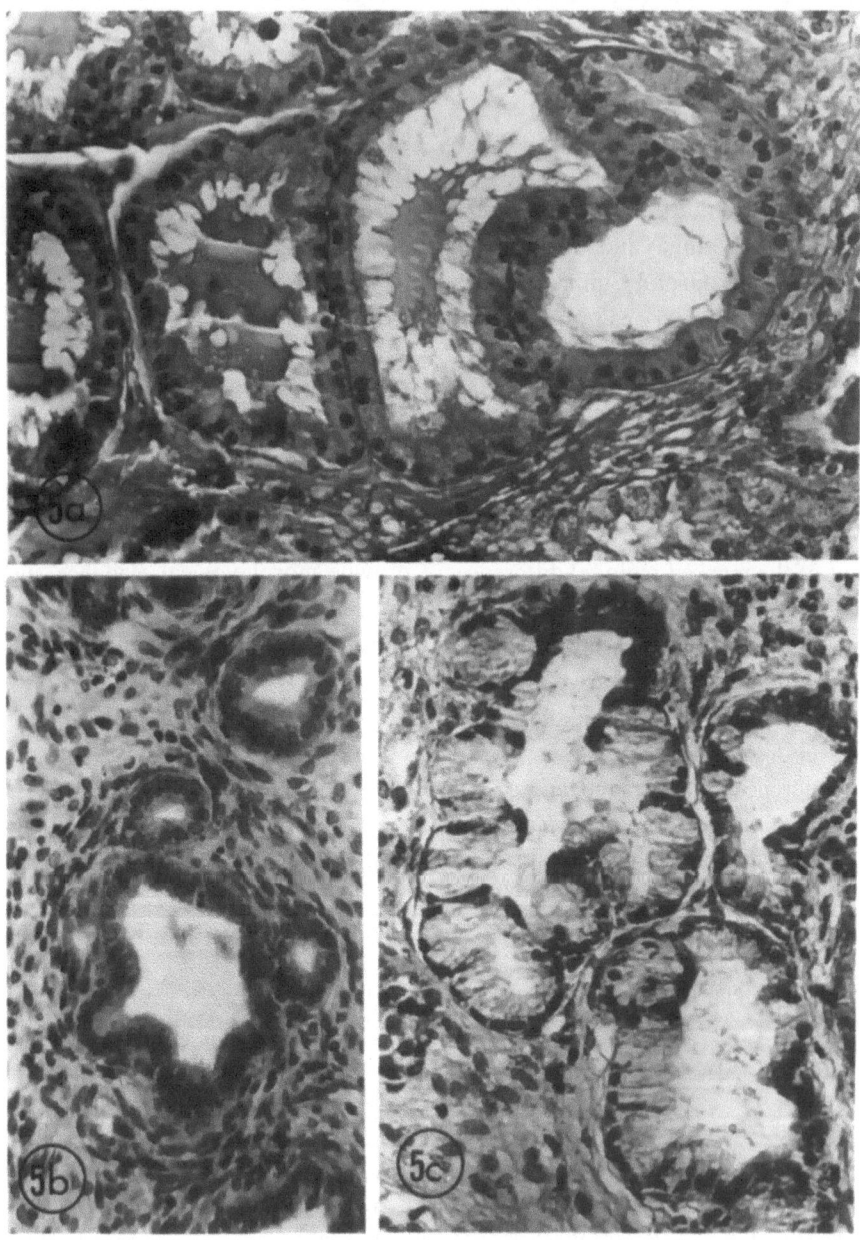

Figure 5. Recombinations illustrating the ability of mesenchyme of the urogenital sinus, seminal vesicle, and bulbourethral gland to function as directive glandular inductors. (a) Urogenital sinus mesenchyme elicits prostatic morphogenesis from epithelium from the embryonic urinary bladder. (b) Mesenchyme of the seminal vesicle induces glandular development from embryonic bladder epithelium. (c) Stroma from the neonatal bulbourethral gland induces bladder epithelium to form structures resembling the bulbourethral gland. (5a, from Cunha et al., 1980.)

the highly specialized ultrastructural features of urothelium (the asymmetric unit membrane and fusiform vesicles (Hicks, 1975; Hicks and Chowaniec, 1978) were absent in the epithelium of UGM + BLE recombinants, which instead develop an epithelium resembling that of prostatic acini containing arrays of RER, Golgi, and secretory granules (Lung et al.,

1979b). Furthermore, the epithelial response to exogenous estradiol of UGM + BLE recombinants is similar to that of the host's prostate, in that the epithelia in both instances become hyperplastic and may exhibit squamous metaplasia (Lung et al., 1979a).

More compelling evidence for an alteration of bio-

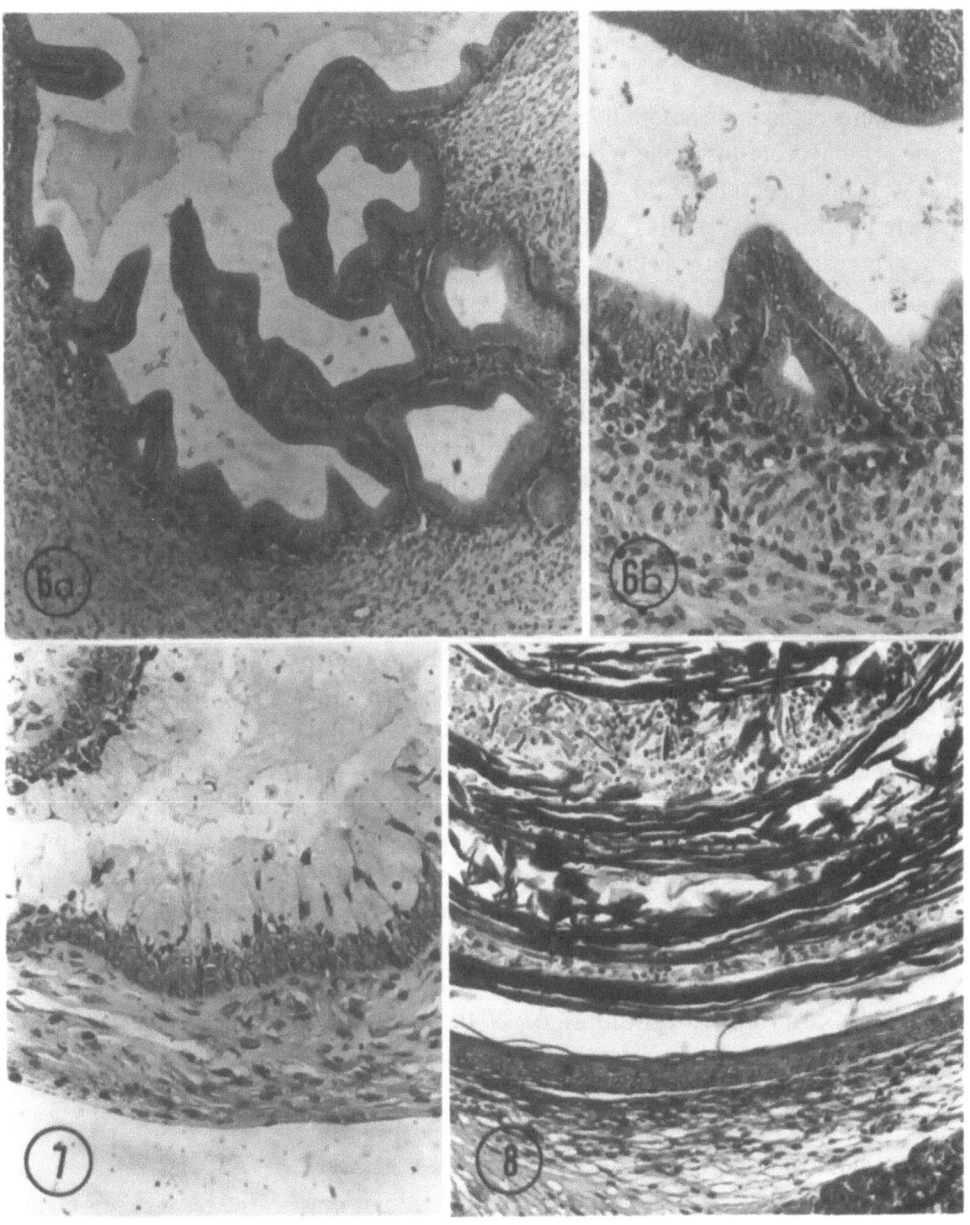

Figure 6. Vaginal epithelium differentiates as a simple columnar uterine epithelium when experimentally associated with uterine stroma. The recombinant was grown in a female host for 4 weeks. a: 200×; b: 500×. (From Cunha, 1976b.)

Figure 7. Uterine epithelium differentiates as a stratified vaginal epithelium when grown in association with vaginal stroma. Since the female host was sacrificed during diestrus, the epithelium is mucified. Note the tall mucous cells. (From Cunha, 1976b.)

Figure 8. Uterine epithelium differentiates as a stratified squamous cervical epithelium when associated with cervical stroma. Note the alternating layers of cornified and mucified cells indicating that the epithelium has cycled with the changing hormonal titers during the host's estrous cycles. 320×. (From Cunha and Lung, 1979.)

Table 2. Histochemical analysis of prostate, bladder, and tissue recombinants prepared with urogenital sinus mesenchyme (UGM) and epithelia from urinary bladder from embryonic mice.

Specimen	Epithelial morphology	Histochemical characteristics of epithelia		
		Alcian blue	Nonspecific esterase	Alkaline phosphatase
Adult prostate	Glandular	+	+	−
Adult urinary bladder	Transitional	−	− or ±	+
UGM + embryonic bladder epithelium	Glandular	+	+	−

From Cunha et al. (1980).

chemical expression is based upon autoradiographic localization of ^{3}H-dihydrotestosterone (^{3}H-DHT) binding sites. Male hosts bearing UGM + BLE recombinants were injected with ^{3}H-DHT, and autoradiograms were prepared utilizing the thaw–mount method of Stumpf and Sar (1975). As expected for non-target organs, host urothelium has a random distribution of silver grains without preferential localization over nuclei (Cunha et al., 1980). Conversely, silver grains were preferentially localized over the nuclei of epithelial cells of the host's prostate and the UGM + BLE recombinants (Fig. 10). Since there appears to be a relationship between hormone action and nuclear uptake of hormone [both of which are mediated by specific hormone receptors (Liao, 1977)], it is likely that nuclear concentration of ^{3}H-labelled steroids as visualized autoradiographically is related to the quantity of available receptor molecules (Stumpf and Sar, 1976). Therefore the inductive influence of mesenchyme of the urogenital sinus elicits a morphological as well as a fundamental biochemical reprogramming of embryonic bladder epithelium.

7. STROMAL (MESENCHYMAL) INFLUENCE ON HORMONAL RESPONSIVENESS OF THE FEMALE UROGENITAL SINUS

The female urogenital sinus has two primary developmental options: vaginal or prostatic morphogenesis. Under the influence of exogenous androgen, prostatic morphogenesis can be elicited in the urogenital sinus of fetal and early neonatal females. However, by 5 days postpartum the sinus vagina (the lower portion of the vagina derived from the urogenital sinus) mucifies in response to androgen,

but does not form prostate. To determine which tissue (stroma or epithelium) accounts for this age-dependent loss in morphogenetic responsiveness to androgens, epithelial and stromal tissues from the sinus vagina of 1- to 20-day-old mice were associated with epithelium or mesenchyme from urogenital sinuses of 16-day-old embryonic mice as depicted in Fig. 11. Vaginal epithelium from mice of all ages (1 to 20 days postpartum) was able to form prostatic acini when combined with embryonic urogenital sinus mesenchyme (Cunha, 1975a). Conversely, when urogenital sinus epithelium was associated with vaginal stroma from 1- to 20-day-old mice, a progressive, age-dependent decrease was observed in the incidence of prostatic morphogenesis. In fact, at 20 days postpartum vaginal stroma was incapable of participating in prostatic morphogenesis with epithelium of the embryonic urogenital sinus. These observations indicate that maturational changes within vaginal stroma are responsible for the age-dependent loss of the ability of this organ to form prostatic acini in response to androgenic stimulation (Cunha, 1975a). The molecular basis of this alteration is not known, but may be related to changes within vaginal stroma in the levels of 5α reductase, the ability to metabolize androgen, or the level or type of androgen receptor proteins.

8. SUMMARY

Development of glandular accessory sexual glands in both males and females is dependent upon interactions between epithelium and mesenchyme. The mesenchyme (specifically urogenital mesenchyme) appears to be the actual target of androgenic steroids and mediates the morphogenetic effects of hormones

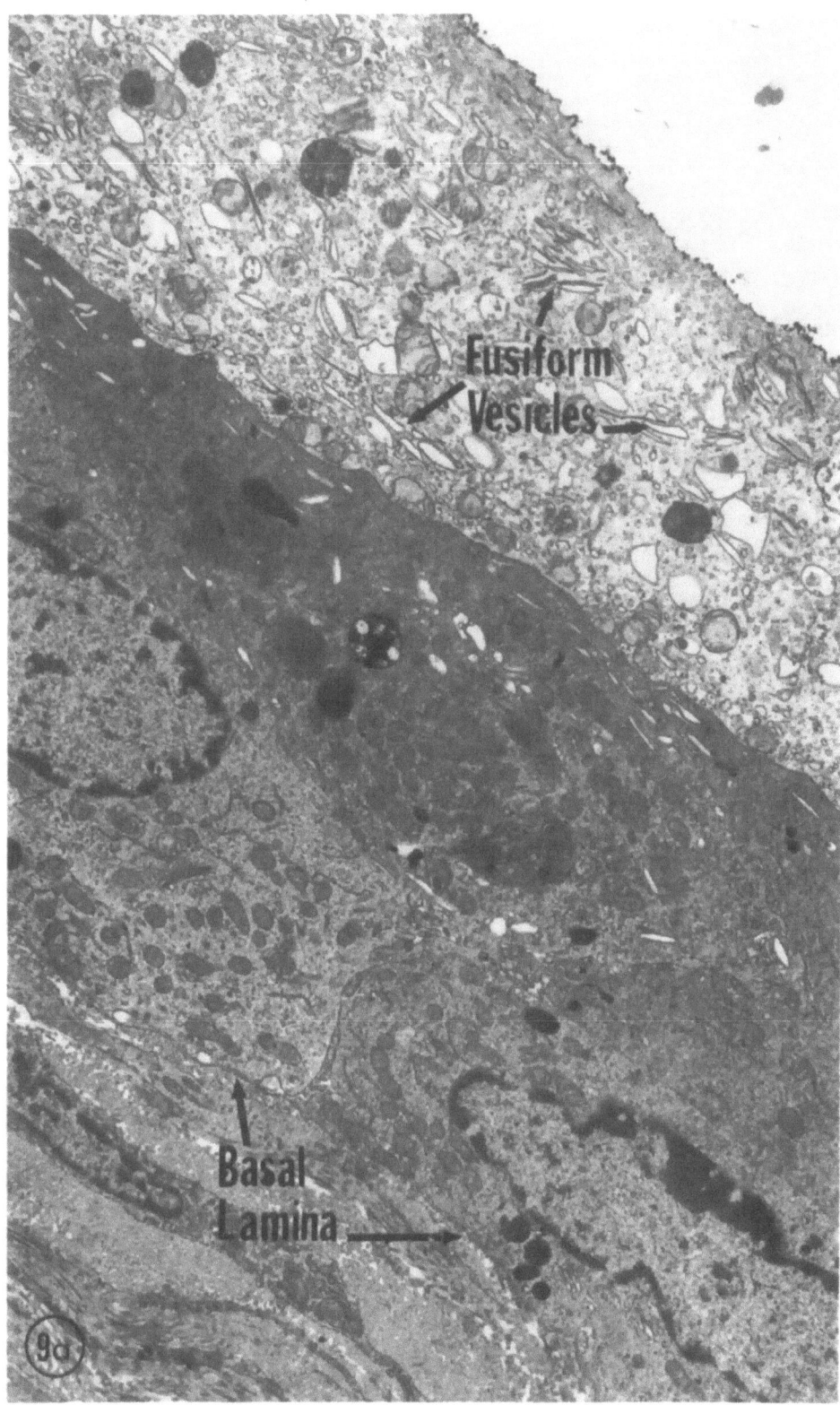

Figure 9. Ultrastructural analysis of glandular induction of epithelium from embryonic urinary bladder by mesenchyme of the urogenital sinus (UGM + BLE). The morphological alterations of BLE by the prostatic inductor (UGM) depicted in Fig. 5a are accompanied by marked ultrastructural changes. (a) Normal differentiation of epithelium of the urinary bladder results in the development of a stratified urothelium 3–4 layers in thickness. Basal cells rest upon the basal lamina and are relatively undifferentiated. Differentiation occurs progressively in intermediate and apical layers resulting in fully mature apical cells having the unique asymmetric apical plasma membrane and containing an abundance of the characteristic fusiform vesicles. 9500 ×. For (b) and (c) see following pages.

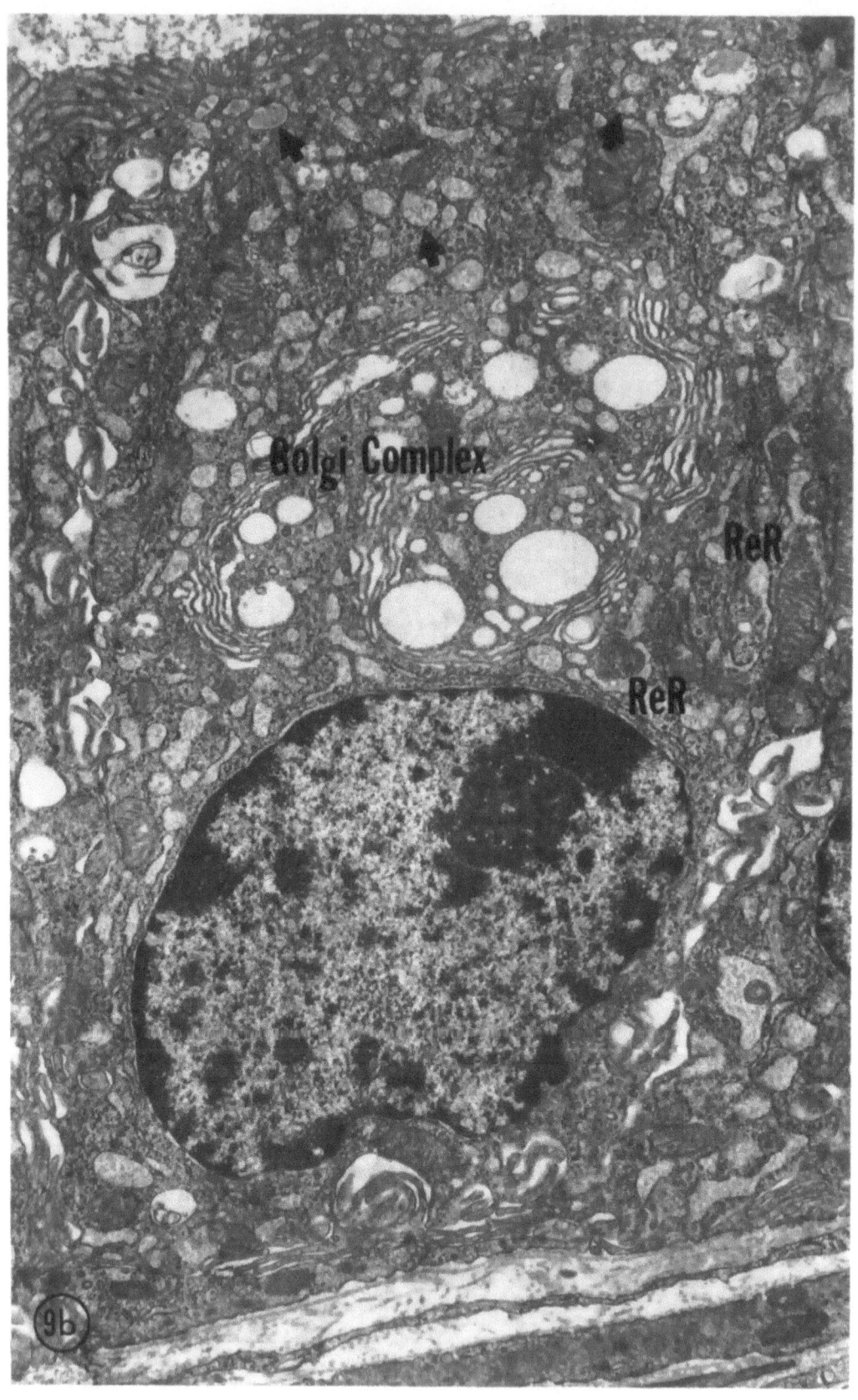

Figure 9(b) In contrast, prostatic epithelial cells are specialized for secretion and exhibit organelles indicative of that function: rough endoplasmic reticulum (RER), Golgi, and secretory granules (arrows). 13,500×.

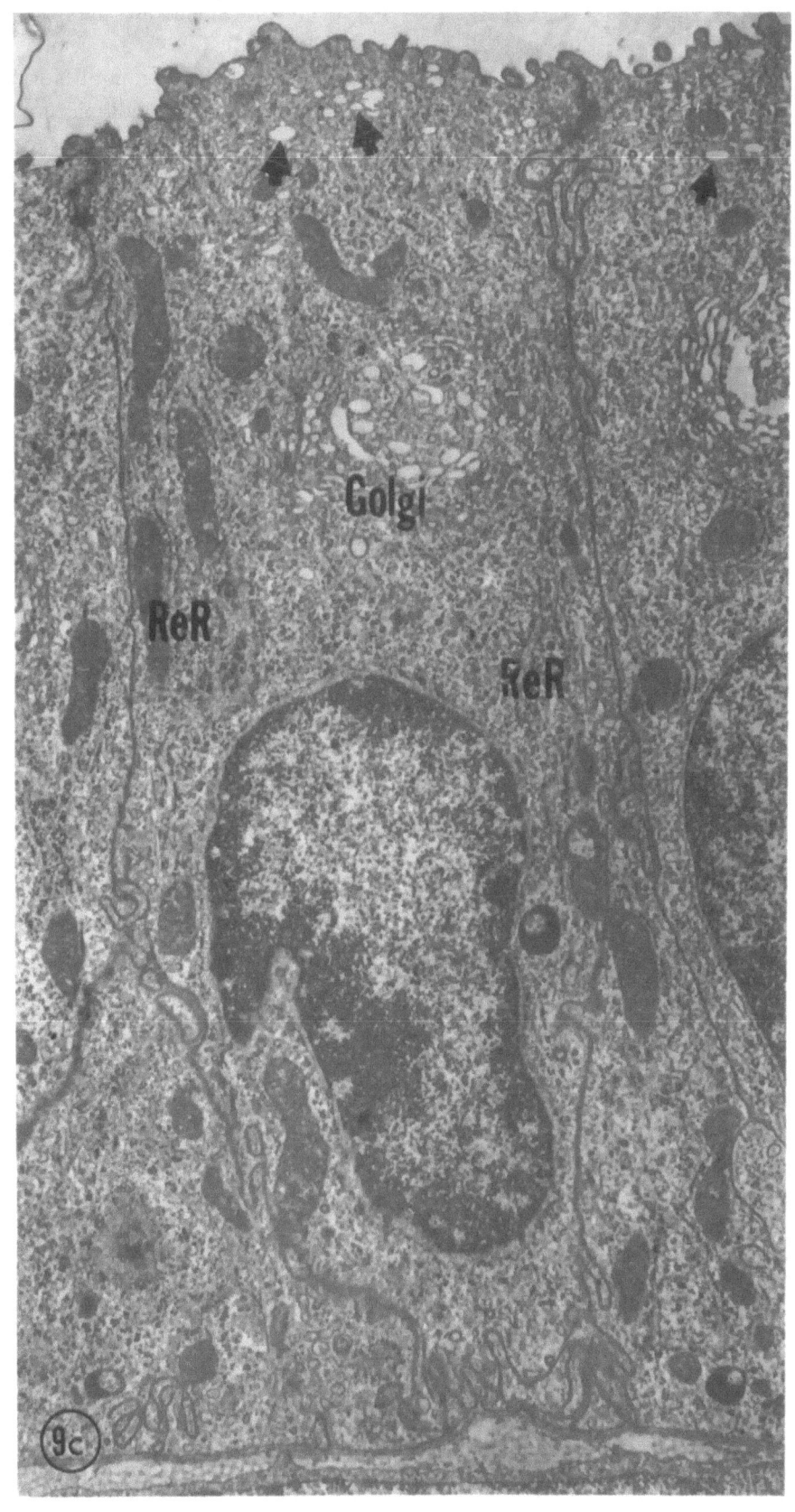

Figure 9(c) In UGM + BLE recombinants, the epithelial cells, like those of prostate, also appear to be specialized for secretion. The cells in this field resemble immature secretory cells, having sparse RER, a supranuclear Golgi complex, and a few apically-located secretory granules (arrows). 13,500 ×. (From Cunha et al., 1980.)

upon the epithelium, thus allowing or permitting (permissive induction) a urogenital epithelium to express its normal program of morphogenesis and cytodifferentiation. In addition, urogenital mesenchyme from both male and female genital rudiments can induce and specify the developmental fate of a heterotypic epithelium: this type of induction is designated as directive. Both permissive and directive inductive influences have been detected during embryonic, neonatal, and adult periods. The directive inductive influences, which have been observed to play an important role in development of the prostate, bulbourethral gland, seminal vesicle, uterus, cervix, and vagina, appear to be involved in generating specific morphological patterns within the epithelium, as well as apparently eliciting the ex-

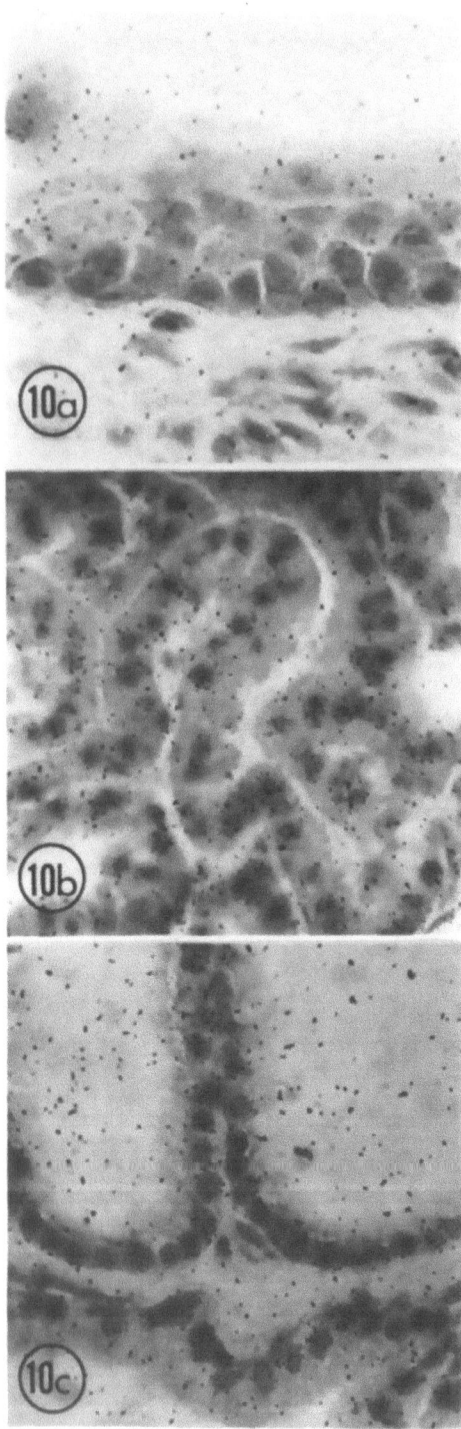

Figure 10. Steroid autoradiograms of ^{3}H-dihydrotestosterone (^{3}H-DHT) localization prepared by the thaw-mount method of Stumpf and Sar (1975). (a) Host urinary bladder. Silver grains are randomly distributed over the entire field. 1000×. (b) Host coagulating gland, a lobe of the prostate, exhibiting the characteristic nuclear uptake of ^{3}H-DHT. 1600×. (c) UGM + BLE recombinant. Note the preferential nuclear uptake of ^{3}H-DHT indicative of nuclear androgen binding sites. 1000×. (From Cunha et al., 1980.)

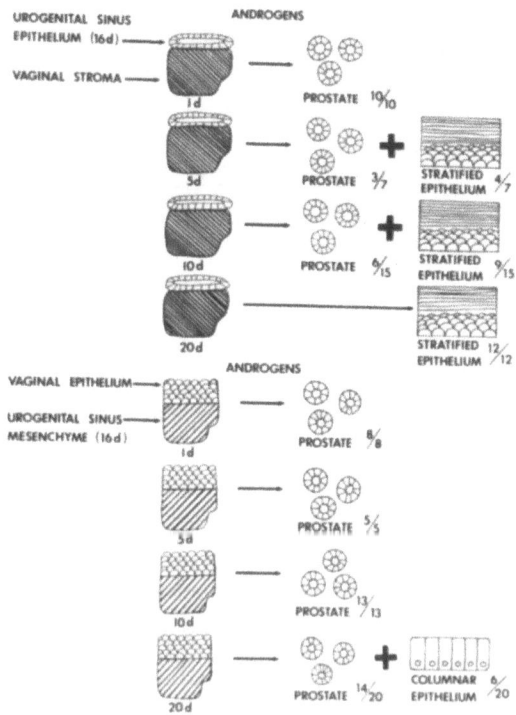

Figure 11. A summary of epithelial–mesenchymal recombination experiments between postnatal vagina and embryonic urogenital sinus. Vaginal epithelium from all ages (1–20 days postpartum) is able to participate in prostatic morphogenesis when associated with mesenchyme of the embryonic urogenital sinus. Conversely, when vaginal stroma from 1- to 20-day-old neonates is recombined with urogenital sinus epithelium, there is progressive, age-dependent decline in the ability of vaginal stroma to induce prostatic morphogenesis. Therefore, the age-dependent loss of the ability of the sinus vagina to form prostate in response to steroidal androgens is due to maturational changes within the stroma. (From Cunha et al., 1980.)

pression of specific functional (biochemical) phenotypes. For example, in the induction of prostate from epithelium of embryonic urinary bladder, the urothelium is induced to form glandular acini that resemble prostate as judged histologically, ultrastructurally, and histochemically. In addition, the bladder epithelium, normally considered to be a nontarget tissue that lacks androgen receptor activity, is induced to express nuclear androgen binding sites. Thus, mesenchymal (stromal) influences appear to be involved in the control of epithelial morphogenesis and the establishment of specific types of epithelial cytodifferentiation. Moreover, several lines of evidence suggest that continued maintenance of adult epithelial morphology and function is also controlled via continued inductive influences from adult stromal cells (Cunha et al. 1979, 1980). Implicit, in the idea that stroma (mesenchyme) induces, specifies, and maintains epithelial morphology and functional activity is the concept that perturbation of stromal–epithelial interactions may lead to the pathogenesis of disorders involving growth or differentiation. Several lines of evidence concerning abnormal vaginal differentiation (Cunha et al., 1977), benign prostatic hyperplasia (McNeal, 1978), and mammary pathogenesis (De Cosse et al., 1973; Sakakura et al., 1979) support this concept (see Cunha et al., 1980, for review).

9. POSSIBLE RELEVANCE OF EPITHELIAL-MESENCHYMAL INTERACTIONS TO CONGENITAL BIRTH DEFECTS

Attempts to relate congenital birth defects of the urogenital system with epithelial–mesenchymal interactions is, at this time, largely speculative. For the Tfm syndrome (testicular feminization) the failure of prostatic development appears to be related to the inability of Tfm urogenital sinus mesenchyme to function as a prostatic inductor (Cunha and Lung, 1978; Cunha et al., 1980). Similarly, failure of androgen-induced regression of male mammary rudiments in Tfm mice is due to an inability of the mammary mesenchyme to mediate the effect of androgen upon the epithelial anlagen (Kratochwil and Schwartz, 1976; Drews and Drews, 1977; Durnberger et al., 1978).

Agenesis of the kidney, vas deferens, and seminal vesicles [a relatively common spectrum of malformations (Marshall, 1978)] is probably a fundamental mesonephric abnormality. This spectrum of malformations may be related to epithelial–mesenchymal interactions, since morphogenesis and cytodifferentiation of both the mesonephros, Wolffian duct, metanephric kidney, and seminal vesicle are dependent upon epithelio-mesenchymal interactions (Wolff, 1968; Croisille et al., 1976; Cunha, 1976c; Saxen, 1977; Cunha, 1972a, b, c; Cunha et al., 1980).

The inductive influence of mesenchyme upon epithelium presupposes the presence of adequate numbers of mesenchymal cells for this process to occur. Therefore, abnormalities in morphogenetic movements that bring the interacting tissues into proximity may also generate a spectrum of congenital malformations. The constellation of malformations associated with exstrophy of the bladder and epispadias appears to involve a failure of the mesenchyme to migrate into the zone initially occupied by the cloacal membrane (Muecke, 1964). This may result in a massive defect in the anterior abdominal wall, suprapubic communication of the bladder with the outside (exstrophy of the bladder), separation (nonfusion) of the pubic symphysis, and a urethral gutter on the dorsum of the penis (epispadias). These defects may be caused by a failure of mesenchymal migration, or alternatively by cell death within the mesenchymal cell population.

The prune belly syndrome, which is characterized by a deficiency of abdominal wall musculature, ureteral dilation, a dilated bladder, urethral stenosis, and hypoplasia of the prostate, may have an etiology similar to that described above for exstrophy and epispadias, owing to a relative deficiency of musculature of mesenchymal origin (Nunn and Stephens, 1961; Williams and Burkholder, 1967). Hypoplasia of the prostate in this syndrome has been suggested by DeKlerk and Scott (1978) to be due to a lack of normal epithelial–stromal interactions during prostatic morphogenesis.

Another spectrum of malformations that certainly are related to mesenchymal function are those induced within animals and humans by prenatal or early neonatal exposure to exogenous estrogen. The morphological changes reported in human females exposed in utero to diethylstilbestrol include vaginal adenosis, vaginal ridges, cervical erosion, T-shaped uterus, as well as clear cell adenocarcinoma of the vagina (Robboy et al., 1977; Herbst et al., 1979; Kaufman et al., 1977). Many of these same lesions have also been reported in laboratory animals, but additional findings in female mice and hamsters exposed during the perinatal period include ovary independent persistent vaginal cornification (Takasugi, 1976, 1979), squamous metaplasia and cystic hyperplasia of the uterus, stromal hyperplasia of the cervix, hypospadias, and polycystic ovaries (Rustia, 1979; McLachlan et al., in press; Cunha, unpublished). Since normal development of the female genital tract is dependent upon directive inductive influences from stroma, it is likely that the pathogenesis of many of the above malformations may be related to estrogen-induced alterations in stromal function. Direct evidence for such an effect upon the developmental properties of vaginal stroma has been demonstrated for the induction and continued expression of ovary-independent persistent vaginal hyperplasia (Cunha et al., 1977). Vaginal epithelium is normally dependent upon estrogens for proliferation and cornification. Mice neonatally injected with estradiol-17β (20 μg per day on days 1 to 5 postpartum) develop a vaginal epithelium that is independent of estrogen for its proliferation and cornification, a condition called ovary-independent persistent vaginal cornification or hyperplasia. Induction of this condition with exogenous estradiol is facilitated by maintenance of the normal association between vaginal epithelium and stroma during the period of estrogen exposure. Furthermore, the perpetuation of ovary-independent persistent hyperplasia in adult mice neonatally treated with estradiol-17β, is mediated in part by the estrogenized stroma, which can induce or elicit an ovary-independent hyperplasia and parakeratosis in normal, untreated vaginal epithelium (Cunha et al., 1977).

Finally, hypospadias in the male is a condition which may also be related to epithelial–mesenchymal interactions. Normal morphogenesis of the penile urethra results from fusion of the epithelium of the urogenital folds which bound the urethral groove on the ventral aspect of the penis. Following fusion of the epithelium, the epithelial seam breaks down resulting in the establishment of mesenchymal

confluence ventral to the urethra. This process of epithelial fusion followed by breakdown of the epithelial seam is very similar to the process of secondary palate formation. In the palate, the fusion potential of the epithelium is related to the type of subadjacent supporting mesenchyme, since epidermis from tail (a non-fusing epithelium) can be induced to fuse with another epithelial layer when both epithelia are experimentally associated with palatal mesenchyme (Pourtois, 1972). The similarities between hypospadias and cleft palate suggest the possibility that certain concepts developed for the morphogenesis of the palate may aid our understanding of development and malformation of the penile urethra.

Until recently those studying the development of the urogenital tract have focused upon the endocrinological and genetic aspects of this process. We have added additional perspective by focusing upon the interaction between epithelium and mesenchyme during development and function of urogenital organs. Full comprehension of the mechanisms of urogenital morphogenesis will require the application of a variety of approaches focused upon the role of the extracellular matrix, the cytoskeleton, the nuclear matrix, and the metabolic processes involved in the intracellular processing of sex steroids. Progress in this exciting area of cell and organismal biology will undoubtedly have important application to clinically important human diseases such as benign prostatic hyperplasia, diethylstilbestrol-induced lesions of the male and female genital tracts, carcinogenesis of the prostate, cervix, endometrium and mammary gland, and development of congenital birth defects of the genital system.

ACKNOWLEDGEMENTS

Thanks are due to Marnie Sekkingstad and Caroline Damian for their technical assistance; Dr. Ben Lung for his assistance in preparation of the electron micrographs; and Betty Aguilar and Sharon Ferdinandsen for typing the manuscript. The authors also are grateful to Dr. L.W.K. Chung for critically reading the manuscript.

This paper was supported by the following grants: Contract Grants #N0-1-CP-55649 and #N0-1-CP-75875 fom NCI; Grants PDT-8 and PDT-139 from the American Cancer Society; Grant #1-670 from the National Foundation; and Grants AM25266, CA24718, and HD12116 from NIH.

REFERENCES

Bardin CW, Bullock LP (1974) Testicular feminization: studies of the molecular bases of a genetic defect. J Invest Dermatol 63: 75.

Bardin CW, Bullock LP, Mills NC, Lin Y-C, Jacob ST (1978) The role of receptors in the anabolic action of androgens. In O'Malley BW, Birnbaumer L, eds. Receptors and hormone action, Vol II, pp 83–104. New York: Academic Press.

Bern HA, Jones LA, Mills KT (1976) Use of the neonatal mouse in studying long-term effects of early exposure to hormones and other agents. J Toxicol Environ Health, Suppl 1: 103.

Croisille Y, Gumpel-Pinot M, Martin C (1976) On some aspects of kidney organogenesis in birds. In Balls M, Monnickendon MA, eds. Organ culture in biomedical research. New York: Cambridge University Press.

Cunha GR (1972a) Tissue interactions between epithelium and mesenchyme of urogenital and integumental origin. Anat Rec 172: 529.

Cunha GR (1972b) Epithelio-mesenchymal interactions in primordial gland structures which become responsive to androgenic stimulation. Anat Rec 172: 179.

Cunha GR (1972c) Support of normal salivary gland morphogenesis by mesenchyme derived from accessory sexual glands of embryonic mice. Anat Rec 173: 205.

Cunha GR (1975a) Age-dependent loss of sensitivity of female urogenital sinus to androgenic conditions as a function of the epithelial–stromal interaction in mice. Endocrinology 95: 665.

Cunha GR (1975b) The dual origin of vaginal epithelium. Am J Anat 143: 387.

Cunha GR (1976a) Epithelial–stromal interactions in development of the urogenital tract. Int Rev Cytol 47: 137.

Cunha GR (1976b) Stromal induction and specification of morphogenesis and cytodifferentiation of the epithelia of the Müllerian ducts and urogenital sinus during development of the uterus and vagina in mice. J Exp Zool 196: 361.

Cunha GR (1976c) Alterations in the developmental properties of stroma during the development of the urogenital ridge into ductus deferens and uterus in embryonic and neonatal mice. J Exp Zool 197: 375.

Cunha GR, Lung B (1978) The possible influences of temporal factors in androgenic responsiveness of urogenital tissue recombinants from wild-type and androgen-insensitive (Tfm) mice. J Exp Zool 205: 181.

Cunha GR, Lung B (1979) The importance of stroma in morphogenesis and functional activity of urogenital epithelium. In Vitro 15: 50.

Cunha GR, Lung B, Kato K (1977) Role of the epithelial–stromal interaction during the development and expression of ovary-independent vaginal hyperplasia. Dev Biol 56: 52.

Cunha GR, Lung B, Reese B (1979) Induction of glandular differentiation in adult urinary bladder epithelium by mesenchyme of the urogenital sinus. J Cell Biol 83: 399a.

Cunha GR, Chung LWK, Shannon JM, Reese BA (1980) Stromal–epithelial interactions in sex differentiation. Biol Reprod 22: 19.

DeCosse JJ, Gossens CL, Kuzma JF (1973) Breast cancer: induction of differentiation by embryonic tissue. Science 181: 1057.

DeKlerk DP, Scott WW (1978) Prostatic maldevelopment in the prune belly syndrome: a defect in prostatic stromal–epithelial interaction. J Urol 120. 341.

Donohoe PK, Ito Y, Marfatia S, Henderson WH (1976) The production of Müllerian inhibiting substance by the fetal, neonatal and adult rat. Biol Reprod 15: 329.

Drews U, Dietrich HJ (1978) Cell death in the mosaic epididymis of sex reversed mice, heterozygous for testicular feminization. Anat Embryol 152: 193.

Drews U, Drews U (1977) Regression of mouse mammary gland anlagen in recombinants of Tfm and wild-type tissues: testosterone acts via the mesenchyme. Cell 10: 401.

Durnberger H, Heuberger B, Schwartz P, Wanser G, Kratochwil K (1978) Mesenchyme-mediated effect of testosterone on embryonic mammary epithelium. Cancer Res 38: 4066.

Forsberg JG (1973) Cervicovaginal epithelium: its origin and development. Am J Obstet Gynecol 115: 1025.

Gasc J-M, Stumpf WE, Sar M (1978) Estrogen target sites in the cloacal region of female and male chick embryos. Cell Tiss Res 193: 457.

Grobstein C (1967) Mechanisms of organogenetic tissue interactions. Natl Cancer Inst Monogr 26: 279.

Herbst AL, Scully RE, Robboy SJ (1979) Prenatal diethylstilbestrol exposure and human genital tract abnormalities. In Rice JM, ed. Perinatal carcinogenesis, pp 25–35. Washington, D.C.: U.S. Government Printing Office.

Hicks RM (1975) The mammalian urinary bladder: an accommodating organ. Biol Rev 50: 215.

Hicks RM, Chowaniec J (1978) Experimental induction, histology, and ultrastructure of hyperplasia and neoplasia of the urinary bladder epithelium. Int Rev Exp Pathol 18: 199.

Imperato-McGinley J, Guerrero L, Gautier T, Peterson RE (1974) Steroid 5α-reductase deficiency in man: an inherited form of male pseudohermaphroditism. Science 186: 1213.

Jost A, Prepin J, Vigier B (1977) Hormones in the morphogenesis of the genital system. In Blandau RJ, Bergsma D, eds. Morphogenesis and malformation of the genital system, pp 85–98. New York: A.R. Liss.

Kaufman RH, Binder GL, Gray PM, Adam E (1977) Upper genital tract changes associated with exposure in utero to diethylstilbestrol. Am J Obstet Gynecol 128: 51.

Kefalides NA (1973) Structure and biosynthesis of basement membranes. Int Rev Connective Tiss Res 6: 63.

Kohrman AF (1978) The newborn mouse as a model for study of the effects of hormonal steroids in the young. Pediatrics 62: 1143.

Kratochwil K, Schwartz P (1976) Tissue interaction in androgen response of embryonic mammary rudiment of mouse: identification of target tissue of testosterone. Proc Natl Acad Sci USA 73: 4041.

Lasnitzki I, Mizuno T (1979) The role of the mesenchyme in the induction of the rat prostate gland by androgens in organ culture. J Endocrinol, 82: 171.

Liao S (1977) Molecular actions of androgen. In Litvak G, ed. Biochemical actions of hormones, Vol 4, pp 351–405. New York: Academic Pess.

Lung B, Cunha GR, Reese BA (1979a) Prostatic induction of mouse urinary bladder epithelium by urogenital sinus mesenchyme. Anat Rec 193: 607, Abst.

Lung G, Cunha GR, Frank VE (1979b) Ultrastructural analysis of prostatic induction of embryonic mouse urinary bladder. J Cell Biol 83: 16a.

Marshall FF (1978) Embryology of the lower genitourinary tract. Urol Clin N Am 5: 3.

McLachlan JA, Dixon RL (1977) Toxicologic comparisons of experimental and clinical exposure to diethylstilbestrol during gestation. Adv Sex Horm Res 3: 309.

McLachlan JA, Newbold RR, Bullock BL (1980) Prenatal exposure to diethylstilbestrol in mice: long term effects on the female genital tract. Cancer Res, in press.

McNeal JE (1978) Origina and evolution of benign prostatic enlargement. Invest Urol 15: 340.

Muecke EC (1964) The role of the cloacal membrane in exstrophy: the first successful experimental study. J Urol 92: 659.

Narbaitz R, Stumpf WE, Sar M (1980) Estrogen receptors in mammary gland primordia of fetal mouse. Anat Embryol 158: 161.

Nunn IN, Stephens FD (1961) The triad syndrome: a composite anomaly of the abdominal wall, urinary system and testes. J Urol 86: 782.

Ohno S (1979) Major sex determining genes, pp 1–140. New York: Springer-Verlag.

Pourtois M (1972) Morphogenesis of the primary and secondary palate. In Slavkin HC, Bavetta LA, eds. Developmental aspects of oral biology, pp 81–108. New York: Academic Press.

Price D, Ortiz E (1965) The role of fetal androgens in sex differentiation in mammals. In DeHaan RL, Ursprung H, eds. Organogenesis, pp 629–652. New York: Holt, Rinehart & Winston.

Price D, Ortiz E, Zaaijer JJP (1971) In vitro studies of the relation of fetal sex hormones to sex differentiation in the guinea pig. In Hamburgh M, Barrington EJW, eds. Hormones in development, pp 631–643. New York: Appleton-Century-Crofts.

Robboy SJ, Scully RE, Welch WR, Herbst AL (1977) Intrauterine diethystilbestrol exposure and its consequences. Arch. Pathol Lab Med 101: 1.

Rustia M (1979) Role of hormone imbalance in transplacental carcinogenesis induced in Syrian golden hamsters by sex hormones. In Rice JM, ed. Perinatal carcinogenesis, pp 77–88. Washington, D.C.: U.S. Government Printing Office.

Sakakura T, Nishizuka Y. Sakagami Y (1979) A new system for experimental mammary tumorigenesis in C3H mice. Gann 70: 459.

Saxen L (1977) Directive versus permissive induction: a working hypothesis. In Lash JW, Burger MM, eds. Cell and tissue interactions, pp 1–10. New York: Raven Press.

Saxen L, Karkinen-Jaaskelainen M, Lehtonen E, Nordling S, Wartiovaara J (1976) Inductive tissue interactions. In Poste G, Nicholson GL, eds. The cell surface in animal embryogenesis and development, pp 331–408. New York: North-Holland.

Schlegel RL, Gardner LI (1969) Ambiguous and abnormal genitalia in infants: differential diagnosis and clinical management. In Gardner LI, ed. Endocrine and genetic diseases of childhood and adolescence, pp 571–609. Philadelphia: W.B. Saunders.

Stumpf WE, Sar M (1975) Autoradiographic techniques for localizing steroid hormones. Meth Enzymol 36: 135.

Stumpf WE, Sar M (1976) Autoradiographic localization of estrogen, androgen, progestin, and glucocorticosteroid in "target tissues" and "nontarget tissues". In Pasqualini JR, ed. Receptors and mechanism of action of steroid hormones, pp 41–84. New York: Marcell Dekker.

Stumpf WE, Narbaitz R, Sar M (1980) Estrogen receptors in the fetal mouse. J. Steroid Biochem 12: 55.

Takasugi N (1976) Cytological basis for permanent vaginal changes in mice treated neonatally with steroid hormones. Int Rev Cytol 44: 193.

Takasugi N (1979) Development of permanently proliferated and cornified vaginal epithelium in mice treated neonatally with steroid hormones and the implication in tumorigenesis. In Rice JM, ed. Perinatal carcinogenesis, pp 57–66. Washington, D.C.: U.S. Government Printing Office.

Wachtel SS (1980) The dysgenetic gonad: a study of aberrant testicular differentiation. Biol Reprod 22: 1.

Williams DI, Burkholder GV (1967) The prune belly syndrome. J Urol 98: 244.

Wilson JD, Griffin JE. George FW (1980) Sexual differentiation: early hormone synthesis and action. Biol Reprod 22: 9.

Winter JSD, Faiman C, Reyes FI (1977) Sex steroid production by the human fetus: its role in morphogenesis and control by gonadotropins. In Blandau RJ, Bergsma D, eds. Morphogenesis and malformation of the genital system, pp 41–58. New York: A.R. Liss.

Wolff E (1968) Specific interactions between tissues during organogenesis. Curr Top Dev Biol 3: 65.

4. THE BIOCHEMISTRY AND BIOLOGY OF MÜLLERIAN INHIBITING SUBSTANCE

PATRICIA K. DONAHOE, GERALD P. BUDZIK and DAVID A. SWANN

1. INTRODUCTION

Müllerian Inhibiting Substance, a fetal testicular product, acts upon the ductal elements of the urogenital ridge, causing regression of both the epithelial Mullerian duct and its surrounding mesenchyme. Early in regression, mesenchymal cells align with their long axes tangential to the basement membrane of the duct, and interstitial spaces are lost as the cells condense toward the basement membrane. Sequentially, the basement membrane is broken down and cell migration occurs across the eroded boundary, macrophages in and epithelial cells out. Subsequently, the lateral tip of the ductal portion of the urogenital ridge disappears. Whether the testicular product (MIS) acts upon the epithelial cells directly or upon the mesenchymal cells which in turn interact with the epithelium is not certain.

Epithelial–mesenchymal interactions are a prominent feature of developing tissues but the mechanisms which mediate these interactions at the molecular level are not understood. The isolation of molecular signals between interacting embryonic tissues has met with little success. Müllerian Inhibiting Substance from the nearby embryonic testis appears to interact with the urogenital ridge, initiating a mesenchymal–epithelial interaction, resulting in eventual disappearance of the entire system. Since this effect can be reproduced in vitro in a biological assay system, it provides a unique opportunity to study the interactions at the molecular level.

The existence of Müllerian Inhibiting Substance was first proposed by Jost (1946a, b, 1947) after a series of in vivo rabbit embryonic experiments in which he established the autonomy of the development of the uterus, Fallopian tubes, and vagina from the embryonic Müllerian ducts unless a testicular substance was present to prevent their development.

Jost gonadectomized fetuses at the sexually indifferent stage, i.e., when Wolffian and Müllerian ducts were both present, and before the gonad had differentiated (Fig. 1). If the indifferent gonad was replaced with ovary or with no gonad, then the Müllerian ducts persisted and developed into uterus, vagina, and Fallopian tubes, and the Wolffian ducts regressed. If the indifferent gonad was replaced with testis, then the Wolffian duct developed into seminal vesicles, vas deferens, and epididymis, and the Müllerian ducts regressed ipsilaterally. If testis were replaced with testosterone alone then the Wolffian duct was stimulated but the Müllerian ducts did not regress. This lack of regression after implantation of testosterone led Jost to suggest the existence of a nonsteroidal testicular substance, Müllerian Inhibiting Substance (Jost, 1953), which was responsible for the active regression of an embryonic Müllerian duct system.

Picon (1969) devised a method for detecting Müllerian Inhibiting Substance in vitro and demonstrated that the Müllerian duct of the 14 day rat embryo regressed when cultured with rat fetal testis in organ culture. Müllerian Inhibiting Substance could be detected invariably throughout gestation in the rat and intermittently for three weeks after birth. This work was confirmed by Constantinople and Walsh (1973). Using the same organ culture technique, Josso demonstrated that Müllerian Inhibiting Substance was present in human (Josso, 1972) and bovine (Josso, 1973) testis during mid and late gestation, and that activity was limited to the seminiferous tubules and most probably to the Sertoli cell (Blanchard and Josso, 1974).

The endocrinologic phenomena that control Müllerian Inhibiting Substance are not yet established, but its early appearance embryologically before Leydig cell differentiation occurs in the calf testis

S.J. Kogan and E.S.E. Hafez (eds.), Pediatric andrology, 37–46. All rights reserved.

38

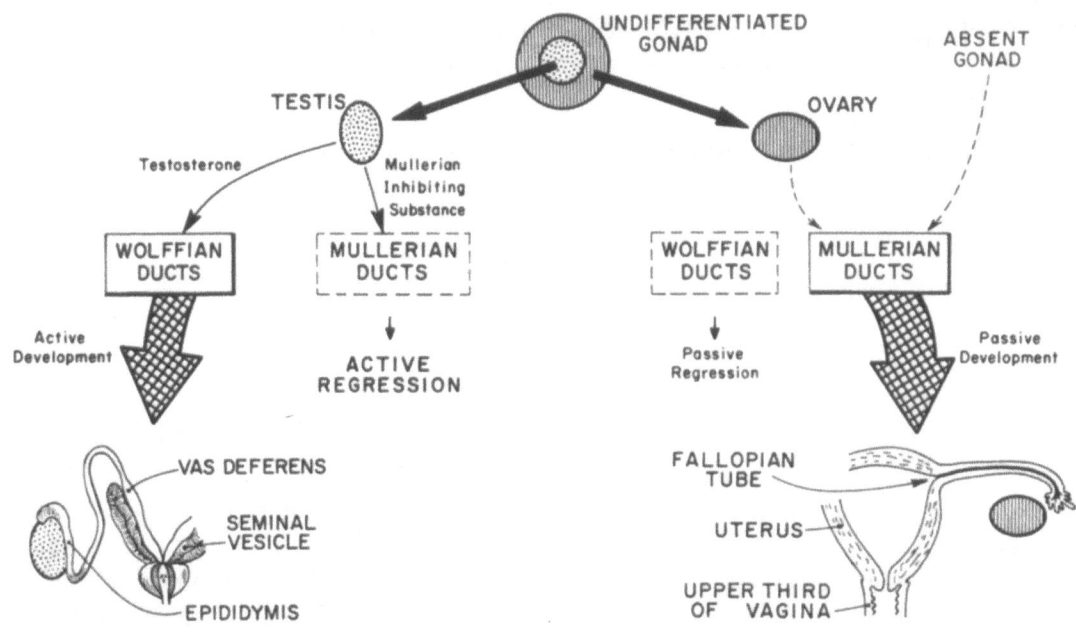

Figure 1. Diagram of Jost's early experiments of effects of in vivo gonadectomy and gonadal replacement on the ductal development of the fetal rabbit. These experiments established the role of Müllerian Inhibiting Substance as an obligate fetal regressor in the developing male mammalian genital tract.

(Jost, 1972) and in the pig testis (Pellinieme, 1976), and its failure to respond to either the addition of testosterone or to treatment with cyanoketone, an inhibitor of hydroxysteroid dehydrogenase (Josso, 1970), indicates that the Leydig cell is not the cell from which Müllerian Inhibiting Substance orirginates.

To investigate this question further, Blanchard and Josso (1974) treated separated seminiferous tubule cells with trypsin. After centrifugation, the cell pellet was plated in monolayer culture since it is known that Sertoli cells preferentially adhere to the monolayer (Kodani and Kodani, 1966). One week later the cultures were washed, treated with trypsin, washed again, centrifuged, and the cell pellet placed on a fragment of vitelline membrane adjacent to the reproductive ducts of the 14 day rat embryo. These cells, which were morphologically indistinct from Sertoli cells when studied on stained Leighton tube cover slips, produced Müllerian duct regression. The seminiferous tubules were again washed and the interstitial or Leydig cell harvested. However, co-culture of Leydig cells with the indifferent sex ducts caused no regression. Picon (1976) measured Müllerian Inhibiting Substance activity in the presence of dibutyryl cyclic AMP, a competitive analogue of cyclic AMP. Müllerian Inhibiting Sub-

stance activity was decreased, implicating cyclic AMP as a possible inhibitor of Müllerian duct regression. Media concentrated after incubating fetal bovine testes for 4 hours produced Müllerian duct regression (Josso et al., 1975). Activity was destroyed by heat and by treatment with iodoacetic acid, and diminished by treatment with cycloheximide. The presence of activity in the media was thought to be due to the de novo synthesis of a macromolecular protein. Column chromatography of the media indicated that the macromolecule was of the order of 200 to 250,000 MW (Picard and Josso, 1976; Josso et al., 1977). The active media labelled with ^{3}H-fucose was then subjected to sucrose density gradient and gel electrophoresis. ^{3}H-fucose uptake into a presumed glycoprotein correlated with bioactivity. Although biological activity could not be recovered after preparative isoelectric focusing, the radioactive moiety focused in a broad peak at pH 6 (Picard et al., 1978).

2. ORGAN CULTURE ASSAY

A graded organ culture bioassay for the semi-quantitative detection of Müllerian Inhibiting Substance has been established (Donahoe et al., 1977b) after the method of Picon (1969). Sterile urogenital ridges containing Müllerian duct, Wolffian duct, surrounding mesenchyme, and adjacent ovary were dissected from the retroperitoneum of the 14 day female rat embryo and placed on a stainless steel grid thinly coated with agar (Fig. 2). One to two millimeter tissue fragments to be assayed for the presence of Müllerian Inhibiting Substance were placed adjacent to the ducts. A perpendicular suture was placed to mark the cephalic end of the duct and the coculture incubated for three days at 37°C in 5% CO_2, 95% air and high humidity. Specimens were fixed, embedded in paraffin, cut in serial cross section, and stained with hematoxylin and eosin. Regression of the cephalic end of the duct was graded from 0 to 5+ by two independent, experienced observers. This meticulous assay was adapted for the detection of Müllerian Inhibiting Substance in soluble extracts (Fig. 3). Using this assay, this laboratory confirmed the findings of Picon (1969) and Constantinople and Walsh (1973) in the postnatal rat, and demonstrated a gradually diminished production of Müllerian Inhibiting Substance until 20 days after birth (Donahoe et al., 1976) (Fig. 4), after which it can no longer be detected by organ culture methodology. We demonstrated that Müllerian duct regression could be elicited by fetal testis placed at

a distance from the ducts without requiring direct tissue contact, thereby documenting the humoral action of Müllerian Inhibiting Substance and establishing the potential for isolating an active hormone in solution.

After standardizing methods of handling, transporting, and freezing (Donahoe et al., 1977c) fetal testis which maintained Müllerian Inhibiting Substance activity, we discovered that the bovine testis continued to produce Müllerian Inhibiting Substance after birth for 8–10 weeks (Donahoe et al., 1977e) (Fig. 5), after which activity could no longer be detected in the organ culture system. The bovine neonatal testis now provides an excellent source for

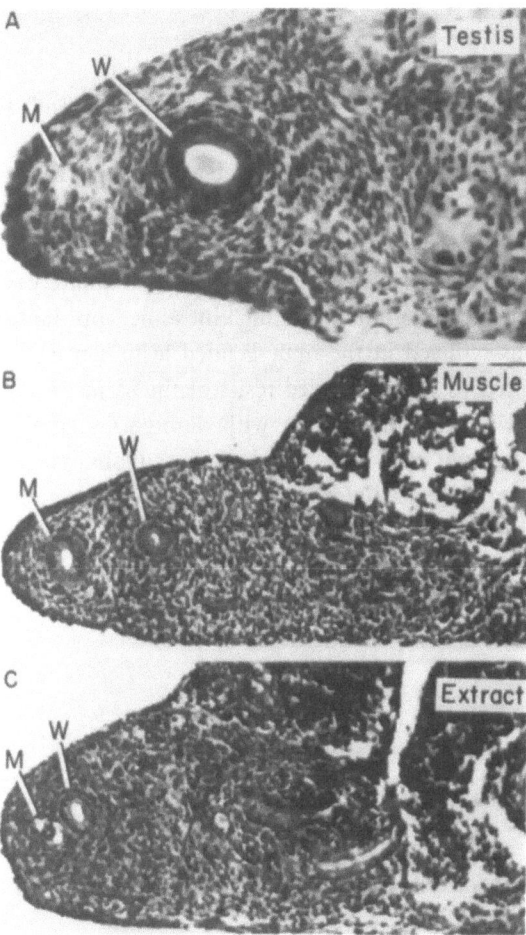

Figure 3. (A) Newborn calf testis cocultured with the urogenital ridge of the 14½ day female fetal rat caused almost complete regression (grade IV) of the Müllerian duct (M). The Wolffian duct (W) by comparison is stimulated. (B) Muscle cocultured with the female fetal urogenital ridge caused no regression (grade 0) of the Müllerian duct (M). (C) Concentrated and dialyzed supernatant after guanidine extraction of newborn calf testis caused grade IV regression when added to the media beneath the female fetal urogenital ridge.

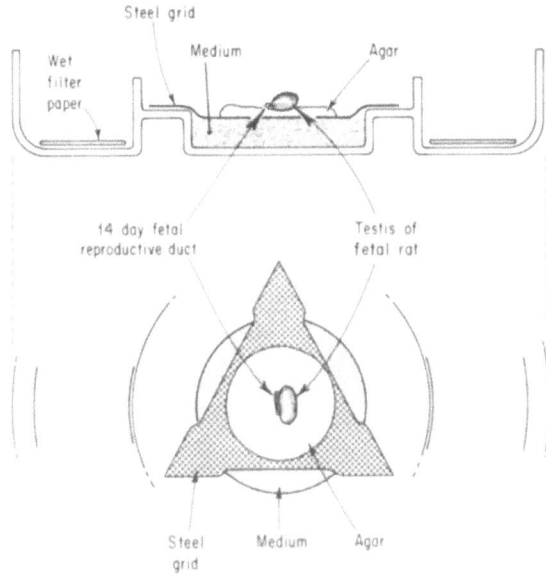

Figure 2. In vitro culture of urogenital ridge of 14½ day old female rat fetus adjacent to tissue to be assayed. Soluble extracts or fractions of extracts can be added to the media and regression observed in the Müllerian duct of the urogenital ridge placed in agar at the airmedia interface.

40

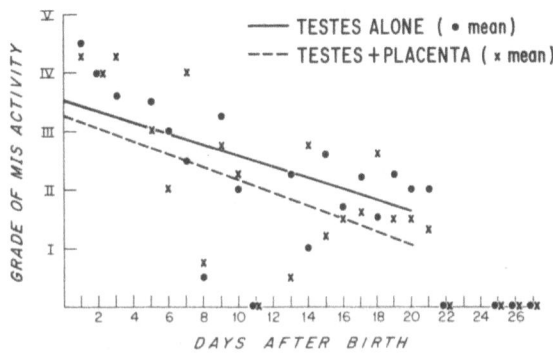

Figure 4. Müllerian Inhibiting Substance levels detected in testis of newborn rats from birth to 28 days gestation. There is a linear regression from birth to 20 days of age. Each point represents mean of four experiments.

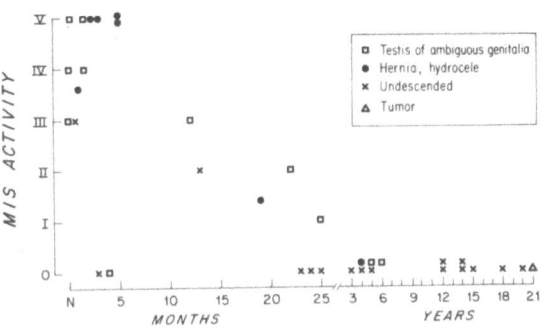

Figure 6. Müllerian Inhibiting Substance levels in the human testis after birth. Activity declines during the first 2 years of life. A dysgenetic testis (at 3 months) has no activity, and undescended testes have less Müllerian Inhibiting Substance activity when compared to descended testes at each age.

the isolation and characterization of Müllerian Inhibiting Substance.

Human testis (Donahoe et al., 1977d) (Fig. 6), biopsied during the investigation of newborn infants with ambiguous genitalia, produced Müllerian Inhibiting Substance after birth for approximately two years. Müllerian Inhibiting Substance production was reduced in the undescended testis when compared to the descended testis of the same age. All newborns and children with ambiguous genitalia (Hendren and Crawford, 1972; Donahoe and Hendren, 1976) including Male Pseudohermaphroditism (Donahoe et al., 1977a), True Hermaphroditism (Donahoe et al., 1978), Mixed Gonadal

Dysgenesis (Donahoe et al., 1979a), and pure gonadal dysgenesis, who have been diagnostically and therapeutically managed at the Massachusetts General Hospital, have had diagnostic gonadal biopsy. Müllerian Inhibiting Substance assay was performed on a portion of the gonadal tissue and the results correlated with anatomic findings (Fig. 7) and the age of the child. The assay has been helpful in establishing the diagnosis in these conditions. Human Müllerian Inhibiting Substance appears to be active only ipsilaterally. Its productivity, which is inversely related to the degree of dysgenesis of the testis, ceases after two years of age. Undescended testes produce less Müllerian Inhibiting Substance then descended

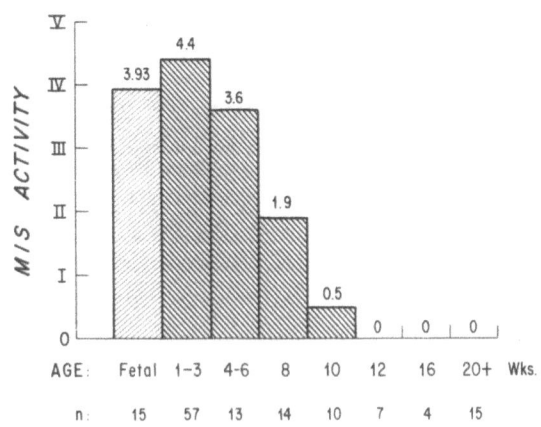

Figure 5. Müllerian Inhibiting Substance levels detected in the testis of fetal and postnatal calf (the number at the top of the bar graph is the average of regressive activity for N assays).

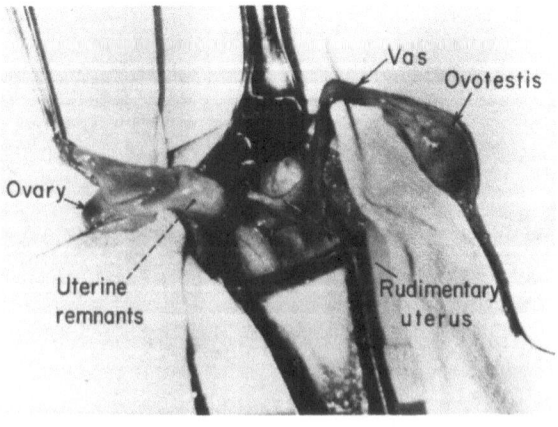

Figure 7. True hermaphrodite intraoperative findings. Müllerian Inhibiting Substance activity is ipsilaterally localized in the human to the side of the ovatestis where the Müllerian duct has regressed and the vas persists. Müllerian derivatives (uterus and Fallopian tubes) persist on the side of the ovary.

testes at the same age. Speculation has been raised that Müllerian Inhibiting Substance may influence descent of the testis (Donahoe et al., 1977d; Radhakrishnan et al., 1979).

3. PRELIMINARY PURIFICATION OF TESTIS EXTRACTS

The analytical approach adopted in the biochemical studies carried out thus far in this laboratory has been based upon the observation that Müllerian Inhibiting Substance is a testicular macromolecular constituent (Josso et al., 1975) that can act at a distance from its source of synthesis (Donahoe et al., 1976). It should, therefore, be possible to isolate and characterize this tissue "hormone". Initial efforts at isolation were hampered by the limited quantities of biologically active tissue available, but were later simplified by the finding that newborn calf testes possess high Müllerian Inhibiting Substance activity (Donahoe et al., 1977d). Our efforts, therefore, were concentrated on developing procedures to obtain biologically active extracts from this tissue (Swann et al., 1979) (Fig. 8). Extration with 1 M guanidine-HCl yielded a biologically active supernatant. Consistently active extracts were not obtained until benzamidine, a protease inhibitor, was added to the extracting solution. The extract, at the proper concentrations, caused morphological regression of the Müllerian ducts quite similar to that observed when testicular fragments were cocultured with the Müllerian duct, and provided a suitable dose-response curve. The presence of DNA caused the extracts to be very viscous and hampered further fractionation by column procedures. To circumvent this problem, density sedimentation in cesium chloride solutions (Fig. 9) was used to separate the DNA and protein fractions. Gel filtration chromatography of the biologically active density gradient protein fraction on a Bio-Gel A 0.5 M column (Fig. 10) yielded an active protein fraction which eluted between Kav values of 0.19 and 0.38. Ion exchange chromatography on a DEAE Bio-Gel A column (Fig. 11) (20 × 2 cm) gave an active fraction which eluted at concentrations between 0.1 and 0.15 M sodium chloride.

Amino acid analysis of the gel chromatography fraction B showed that the biologically active con-

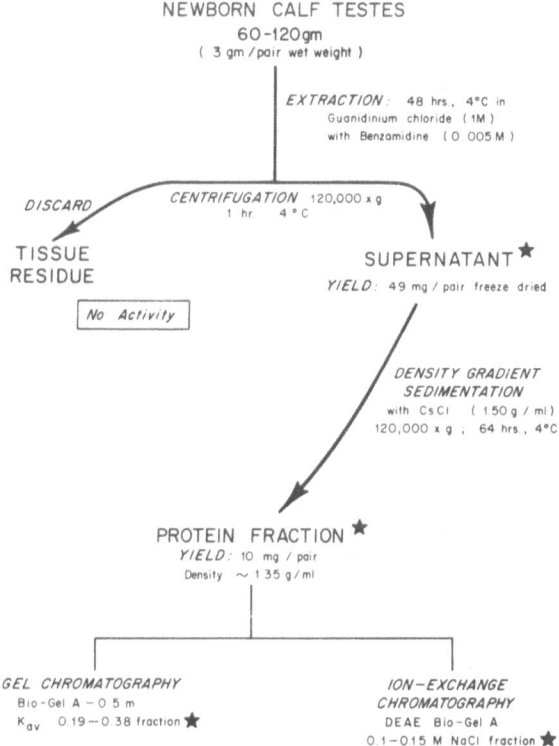

Figure 8. Early purification scheme after extraction of newborn calf testes using ultrafiltration, density gradient sedimentation, gel chromatography and ion exchange chromatography, Gel chromatography and ion exchange chromatography could not be done sequentially without loss of biological activity. Total protein yields of freeze dried samples are indicated at each step.

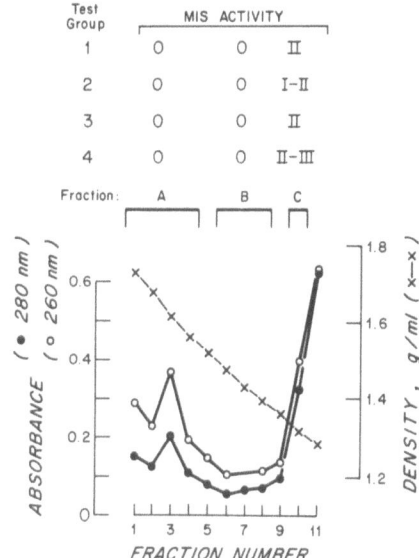

Figure 9. Density sedimentation with supernatant density adjusted to 1.5 g/ml by addition of cesium chloride and centrifuged at 120,000 g for 64 hours at 4°C. Nucleic acids were detected by measuring the absorbance at 260 nm at 280 nm. Biological activity for Müllerian Inhibiting Substance (nearest number to the mean of >10 assays) was always found in protein fraction 11.

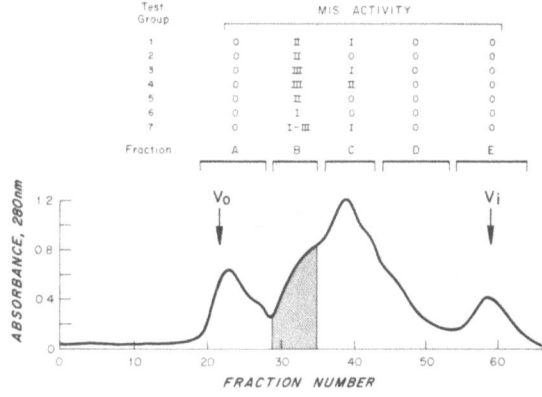

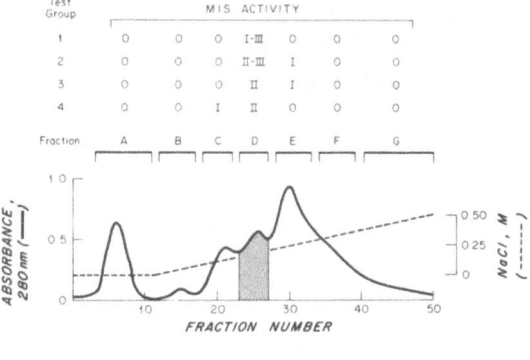

Figure 10. Protein fraction 11 was collected after density sedimentation, dialyzed against the column eluant, applied to a 200×2 cm column packed with Bio-Gel A–0.5 M, eluted with 1 M guanidine, 0.05 M Tris–HCl, pH 7.2 at a flow rate of 20 ml/hr, and 11 ml fractions collected. V_o = blue dextran. V_i = ^3H_2O. Fractions for bioactivity testing were obtained by pooling the column fractions as shown. Active fractions are shaded. Each test group represents the mean of > 10 assays.

Figure 11. Protein fraction 11 was dialyzed against 0.05 M Tris–HCl, pH 7.2 and applied to a column (20×2 cm) containing DEAE Bio-Gel which was washed with buffer until a stable baseline was re-established. The column was eluted with a linear NaCl gradient, monitored by conductivity, at a flow rate of 16 ml/hr, and 8 ml fractions obtained. Fractions were pooled as indicated. Active fractions are shaded.

stituents contained between 82 and 89% protein. Gas liquid chromatography showed that these fractions also contained glucosamine, mannose, galactose, and N-acetylneuraminic acid (Table 1).

After streamlining the previous purification scheme (Fig. 8) by shortening both the extraction and density sedimentation times to 24 hours, and buffering all solutions at pH 7 with 10 mM sodium phosphate, we found that we could sequentially perform extraction, density gradient sedimentation, gel filtration, and ion exchange chromatography and

still maintain high biological activity (Fig. 12). The ion exchange chromatography conditions were further modified in order to better preserve biological activity (Fig. 13). Active material was dialyzed back to 0.05 M NaCl, 10 mM sodium phosphate (pH 7) rather than only phosphate buffer, and the gradient run from 0.05 M NaCl to 0.5 M NaCl. Subsequently, the column was buffered at pH 8 to completely eliminate albumin. Biological activity under these conditions was found in the unbound fraction, and albumin was eluted by the higher salt

Table 1. Chemical composition of the active Bio-Gel fraction (Fig. 10).

Amino acids (residues/thousand residues)		Carbohydrate composition, % wet weigth	
Lysine	65	Mannose	1.5
Histidine	20	Galactose	4.5
Arginine	34	Glucosamine	1.0
Asparitic acid	102	N-acetylneuraminic acid	2.0
Threonine	75		
Serine	98	Total	9.0
Glutamic acid	120		
Proline	62		
Glycine	75		
Alanine	67		
Cystine/2	19		
Valine	73		
Methionine	12		
Isoleucine	31		
Leucine	81		
Tyrosine	31		
Phenylalanine	36		
Total amino acids % wet weight	84.0		

gradient. Using this purification scheme (Fig. 12) we were able to achieve approximately a 200-fold purification.

4. ELECTROPHORETIC ANALYSIS OF SEMI-PURIFIED FRACTIONS

The electrophorectic mobilities of nondialyzable macromolecular components were compared at each sequential step of purification using SDS-polyacrylamide gels (Laemmli, 1970). Simultaneous vertical slab gel electrophoresis of sequentially purified newborn calf testicular macromolecules, with high and low molecular weight standards (Fig. 14) for comparison, demonstrated comigration of bands

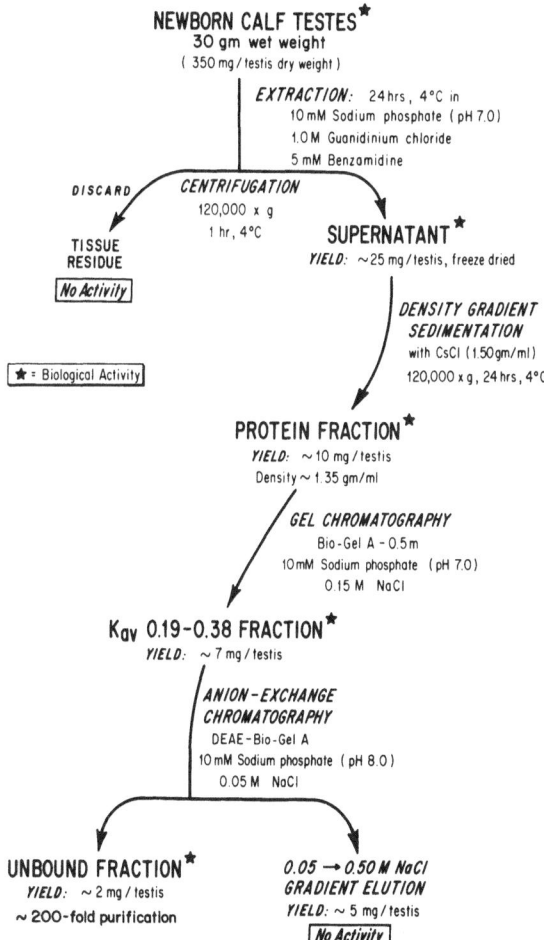

Figure 12. Modified fractionation procedure for Müllerian Inhibiting Substance with anion exchange chromatography run sequentially after Bio-Gel chromatography. Biologically active fractions are indicated by the stars. Protein yields per testis of starting material are noted at each step of purification and an approximate 200-fold purification estimated.

with molecular weights of approximately 50,000 and 70,000 that persist in fractions which demonstrate biological activity in the organ culture assay.

Another slab gel was run under the same conditions and using the same standards, except that the crude testicular extract was fractionated first by ion exchange chromatography on DEAE Bio-Gel A. The unbound biologically active fraction from this step was then concentrated and loaded on the Bio-Gel A 0.5 m column. As before, the biologically active material was found in fraction B. These two columns are identical to those described earlier, however, it should be noted that the order of their use here has been reversed compared to that described earlier (Fig. 12). The slab gel containing the fractions from this reversed fractionation procedure is shown in Fig. 15. Only track 1 (testicular extract), track 5 (DEAE fraction 1), and track 3 (Bio-Gel fraction B) contain biologically active material. Of particular interest is the Bio-Gel fraction B which shows a highly purified MIS fraction that now contains only the 50,000 molecular weight monomer with the complete absence of any material around 70,000, the latter now found in Bio-Gel fraction C (track 4). Though the 50,000 molecular weight species by far the predominant band in Bio-Gel fraction B, trace amounts of several other moieties can be seen. Further purification steps are proceeding to unequivocally verify the exact identity of Müllerian Inhibiting Substance.

5. CYTOTOXICITY AGAINST CULTURED HUMAN OVARIAN CANCER

In 1974, this laboratory proposed the hypothesis that a fetal regressor such as Müllerian Inhibiting Substance might cause regression of tumors derived from the anlagen which undergoes regression in the fetus. We chose to study Müllerian Inhibiting Substance since it was and still is the only fetal regressor capable of being studied in vitro; moreover, it can serve as a probe to understand the morphogenic mechanisms associated with programmed cell death in embryonic remodeling, in the hopes of harnessing these mechanisms for potential chemotherapeutic use.

Tumors have many characteristics of fetality. They are known to express fetal antigens, receptors, enzymes, isoenzymes, proteins, and hormones. For example α-fetoprotein, carcinoembryonic antigen, and galactosyltransferase are known to occur spontaneously in adult tumors. Our hypothesis is that tumors from cell lines which are known to respond to fetal regressors in embryonic life, may respond in the defifferentiated state by retaining or reactivating receptors or gene promotors for the regressor.

A significant cytotoxicity index was obtained when human ovarian cancer cells were exposed

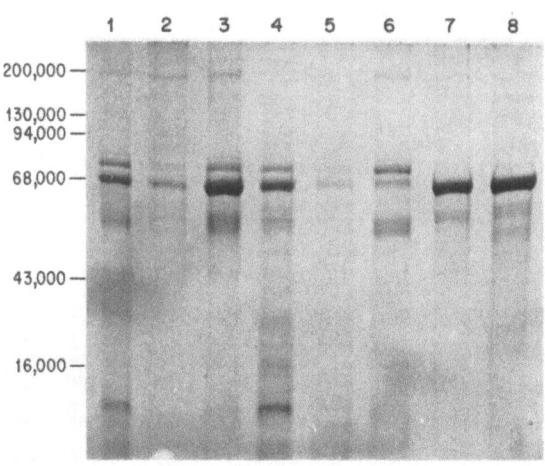

Figure 14. Polyacrylamide-SDS vertical slab gel electrophoresis. The gel consists of a 10%-acrylamide fractionating gel (10 cm) topped by a 3%-stacking gel (2 cm) (not shown), both containing sodium dodecylsulfate as a denaturant. Samples were taken from fractions at each step of a single fractionation procedure from the same starting batch and reduced with 2-mercaptoethanol before loading. The gels from left to right are 1) cesium chloride sedimentation fraction 11; 2) Bio-Gel fraction A; 3) Bio-Gel fraction B; 4) Bio-Gel fraction C; 5) Bio-Gel fraction D; 6) DEAE fraction I; 7) DEAE fraction II; and 8) DEAE fraction III. Approximately 20 μg of each sample was applied and protein bands were detected by staining with Coomassie blue. The mobilities and molecular weights of a set simultaneously electrophoresed standards are shown: myosin, 200,000; β-galactosidase, 130,000; phosphorylase B, 94,000; bovine serum albumin, 68,000; ovalbumin, 43,000; hemaglobin, 16,000.

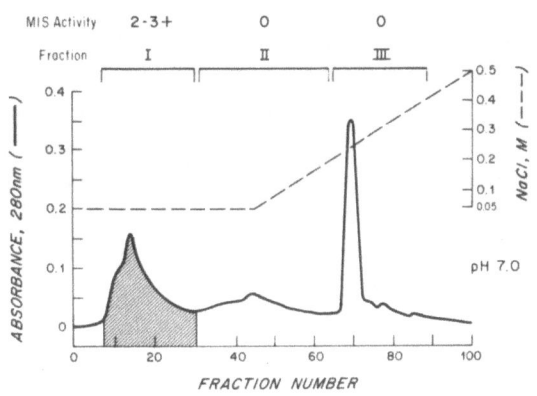

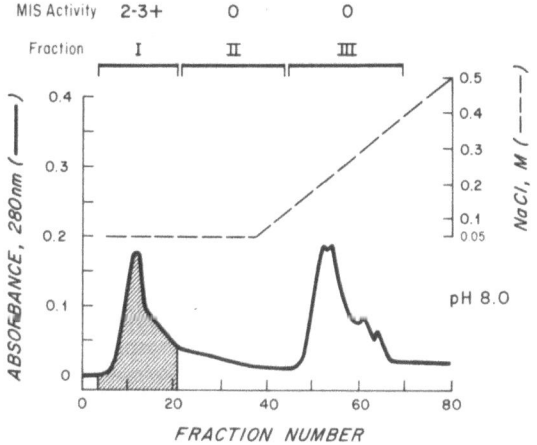

Figure 13. Anion exchange chromatography of Bio-Gel column fraction B. A DEAE Bio-Gel A column (20 × 2 cm) was poured and equilibrated with 0.05 M NaCl, 10 mM sodium phosphate (pH 7.0 or 8.0, as indicated). Fraction B from the Bio-Gel column (Fig. 10) was pooled, concentrated, and dialyzed against the appropriate DEAE column buffer. The dialyzed fraction was loaded on the column at a flow rate of 50 ml/hr and 9 ml fractions collected. The column was washed with low salt buffer until the effluent absorbance approached baseline, at which point a linear gradient of 0.05 M to 0.50 M NaCl was begun. The column effluents were monitored for protein by measuring the absorbance at 280 nm. Fractions for testing in the organ culture assay system were obtained by pooling column fractions as indicated. Active fractions are shaded.

during the S phase of the cell cycle to purified fractions of testis exhibiting high Müllerian Inhibiting Substance biological activity (Donahoe et al., 1979b). The ovarian tumor was surgically removed from a 56 year old woman in 1971 and has since been serially subcultured. Histologically, the tumor is described as a moderately well differentiated papillary serous cystadenoma. The same cytotoxic effect was not observed when Müllerian Inhibiting Substance active fractions were tested against human glioblastoma or fibroblast lines. The epithelial morphology of earlier Müllerian duct structures predominates in ovarian tumors (Scully, 1970). For example, in well differentiated types, serous tumors are characterized by papillary ciliated cells of Fallopian tube character; mucinous tumors have epithelium that resembles the lining of endometrial glands. Clear cell tumors of the ovary (Scully and Barlow, 1967) and the vagina (Herbst and Scully, 1970) are related to an endometrial type of epithelium. Most of the poorly differentiated adenocarcinomas and undifferentiated carcinomas are thought to arise from the same coelomic surface epithelium.

Using methods adapted from those of Wood and Morton (1970) monolayers of the above cell lines were delivered to each well of a Falcon 3034 microtest plate in a 0.01 ml volume and incubated overnight. The following morning, new media and testis and control fractions were added to each well for 24

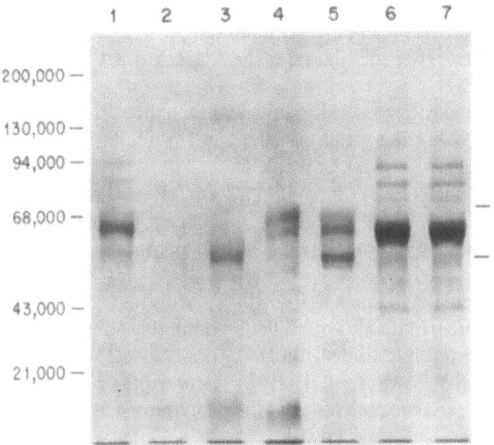

Figure 15. 10% acrylamide-SDS slab gel with 3% stacking gel. A polyacrylamide slab gel was prepared in the same manner as that shown in Fig. 14. Identical standards as described earlier were again electrophoresed simultaneously with samples and their molecular weights are indicated. The samples are taken from a fractionation procedure (see text) in which anion exchange chromatography was run first followed by gel filtration. The gel from left to right includes: 1) crude testis extract; 2) Bio-Gel fraction A; 3) Bio-Gel fraction B; 4) Bio-Gel fraction C; 5) DEAE fraction I; 6) DEAE fraction II; 7) DEAE fraction III. The marks directly adjacent to track 7 localize regions of 70,000 and 50,000 molecular weight, the importance of which is discussed in the text.

hours of incubation. Newborn calf testis or heart fragments were extracted with guanidine, subjected to density gradient sedimentation, and then gel chromatography. Dialyzed and concentrated fractions were then assayed for Müllerian duct regression. Fractions with positive and negative biological activity were mixed with media and added to wells of the microtest plates in which cells of appropriate density were synchronized in the S phase of the cell cycle. After 24 hours incubation, the wells were stained and counted. The counts of the control wells were averaged and compared with the average of the replicate wells of each fraction tested, and a cytotoxicity index (CI = control wells – test wells/ control well counts) calculated. Biologically active fractions in the organ culture assay demonstrated a significant cytotoxicity index against human ovarian cancer. Similar but inactive fractions from heart had no cytotoxicity against the human ovarian cancer. Active fractions had no cytotoxic effect against human glioblastoma or human fibroblast lines.

The finding that a human ovarian cancer can respond to fractions that cause Müllerian duct regression in the embryo implies the presence of Müllerian Inhibiting Substance receptors on the tumor. Continued pursuit of isolation, purification, and synthesis of the fetal regressor seems warranted. Not only will its elucidation bring some understanding of the congenital anomalies associated with ambiguous genitalia, but the purified substance may have potential value as a chemotherapeutic agent for tumors of Müllerian duct origin.

REFERENCES

Blanchard M, Josso N (1974) Sources of the anti-Müllerian hormone synthesized by the fetal testis: Müllerian inhibiting activity of fetal bovine Sertoli cells in tissue culture. Pediat Res 8: 968.

Constantinople N, Walsh P (1973) Activity of Müllerian Inhibiting Substance in postnatal testes. Surg Forum 24: 538.

Donahoe PK, Hendren WH (1976) Evaluation of the newborn with ambiguous genitalia. Pediat Clin N Am 23: 361.

Donahoe PK, Ito Y, Marfatia S, Hendren WH (1976) The production of Müllerian Inhibiting Substance by the fetal, neonatal and adult rat. Biol Reprod 15: 329.

Donahoe PK, Crawford JD, Hendren WH (1977a) Management of the neonate with male pseudohermaphroditism. J Pediat Surg 12: 1045.

Donahoe PK, Ito Y, Hendren WH (1977b) A graded organ culture assay for the detection of Müllerian Inhibiting Substance. J Surg Res 23: 141.

Donahoe PK, Ito Y, Hendren WH (1977c) The preservation of

Müllerian Inhibiting Substance during long-term freezing of testicular fragments. Cryobiology 14: 534.

Donahoe PK, Ito Y, Morikawa Y, Hendren WH (1977d) Müllerian Inhibiting Substance in human testes after birth. J Pediat Surg 12: 322.

Donahoe PK, Ito Y, Price JM, Hendren WH (1977e) Müllerian Inhibiting Substance activity in bovine fetal, newborn, and prepubertal testes. Biol Reprod 16: 238.

Donahoe PK, Crawford JD, Hendren WH (1978) True hermaphroditism – a clinical description and a proposed function for the long arm of the Y chromosome. J Pediat Surg 13: 293.

Donahoe PK, Crawford JD, Hendren WH (1979a) Mixed gonadal dysgenesis, pathogenesis, and management. J Pediat Surg 14: 287.

Donahoe PK, Swann DA, Hayashi A, Sullivan MD (1979b) Müllerian duct regression in the embryo is correlated with cytotoxic activity against a human ovarian cancer. Science 205: 913.

Hendren WH, Crawford JD (1972) The child with ambiguous genitalia. Curr Prob Surg.

46

Herbst AL, Scully RE (1970) Adenocarcinoma of the vagina in adolescence. A report of 7 cases including 6 clear-cell carcinomas (so-called mesonephromas). Cancer 25: 745.

Josso N (1970) Effect of cyanoketone, an inhibitor of hydroxysteroid dehydrogenase, on the reproductive tracts of male fetal rats, in organ culture. Biol Reprod 2: 85.

Josso N (1972) Evaluation of the Müllerian Inhibiting Substance synthesized by the human testis. Effect of fetal, perinatal and postnatal human testicular tissue on the Müllerian duct of the fetal rat in organ culture. Biol Neonate 20: 368.

Josso N (1973) In vitro synthesis of Müllerian Inhibiting Substance hormone by seminiferous tubules isolated from the calf testis. Endocrinology 93: 829.

Josso N, Forrest M, Picard JY (1975) Müllerian Inhibiting Activity of calf testes: relationship to testosterone and protein synthesis. Biol Reprod 13: 163.

Josso N, Picard JY, Tran D (1977) The anti-Müllerian hormone. Rec Prog Horm Res 33: 117.

Jost A (1946a) Sur la differenciation sexuelle de l'embryon de lapin experiences de paraboise. CR Soc Biol 140: 463.

Jost A (1946b) Sur la differenciation sexuelle de l'embryon de lapin remarques au sujet de certaines operations chirurgical. CR Soc Biol 140:

Jost A (1947) Sur les derives mulleriens d'embryons de lapin des deus sexes castres a 21 jours. CR Soc Biol 141: 135.

Jost A (1953) Problems of fetal endocrinology: the gonadal and hypophyseal hormones. Rec Prog Horm Res 8: 379.

Jost A (1972) A new look at the mechanisms controlling sex differentiation in mammal. J Hopkins Med J 130: 38.

Kodani M, Kodani K (1966) The in vitro cultivation of mammalian Sertoli cells. Proc Natl Acad Sci 56: 1200.

Laemmli UK (1970) Cleavage of structural proteins during the assembly of the head of bacteriophage T4. Nature 222: 680.

Pellinieme LJ (1976) Ultrastructure of the indifferent gonad in male and female pig embryos. Tissue Cell 8: 163.

Picard JY, Josso N (1976) Anti-Müllerian hormone: estimation of molecular weight by gel filtration. Biomedicine 25: 147.

Picard JY, Tran D, Josso N (1978) Biosynthesis of labelled anti-Müllerian hormone by fetal testes: evidence for the glycoprotein nature of the hormone and for its disulfide-bonded structure. Molec Cell Endocrinol 12: 17.

Picon R (1969) Action due testicule foeatal sur le development in vitro des canaux de Müller le rat. Arch Anat Micro Exp 58: 1.

Picon R (1976) Testicular inhibition of fetal Müllerian ducts in vitro: effect of dibutryl cyclic AMP. Molec Cell Endocrinol 4: 35.

Radhakrishnan J, Morikawa Y, Donahoe PH, Hendren WH (1979) Observations on the gubernaculum during descent of the testis. Invest Urol 16: 365.

Scully RE (1970) Recent progress in ovarian cancer. Hum Pathol 1: 73.

Scully RE, Barlow JF (1967) "Mesonephroma" of ovary. Cancer 20: 1405.

Swann DA, Donahoe PK, Ito Y, Morikawa Y, Hendren WH (1979) Extraction of Müllerian Inhibiting Substance from newborn calf testis. Dev Biol 69: 73.

Wood WC, Morton DL (1970) Microcytotoxicity test: detection in sarcoma patients of antibody cytotoxic to human sarcoma cells. Science 170: 1318.

5. CONTROL OF MÜLLERIAN INHIBITING SUBSTANCE

Barry B. Bercu, Yasuhide Morikawa and Patricia K. Donahoe

1. INTRODUCTION

It is uncertain whether Müllerian Inhibiting Substance (MIS) is secreted autonomously or under extragonadal influences. Studies of the pituitary control of MIS have been inconclusive and conflicting. Maraud and his colleagues (1969, 1970) demonstrated an increase in MIS activity of the 2-month-old chick testes after hypophysectomy at 1 month of age. However, Groenendijk-Huijbers and Burggraaff (1974) noted a spontaneous return of MIS activity in the testes of the 4-month-old chick. Rats hypophysectomized at 20 days of age failed subsequently to demonstrate an elevation of MIS secretion (Donahoe et al., 1976). Neither prolactin (Donahoe et al., unpublished data) nor placental fragments added to the in vitro culture influenced MIS secretion from the testis (Donahoe et al., 1976).

Previously, we demonstrated that an antiserum to luteinizing hormone releasing hormone (LH-RH-AS) blocked endogenous LH-RH secretion in the neonatal rat (Bercu et al., 1976a, b, 1977). FSH and LH concentrations in serum (Arimura et al., 1976; Koch et al., 1973; Bercu et al., 1980) were likewise reduced after injection of LH-RH antiserum. LH-RH antiserum during pregnancy, with and without gonadotropin replacement and late gestational irradiation, were used to study the hypothalamic–pituitary–gonadal axis in the control of MIS secretion.

2. GONADOTROPIN CONTROL OF MIS

In order to block endogenous secretion of fetal gonadotropins, LH-RH antiserum was given to pregnant rats. Antiserum to LH-RH was generated in rabbits as described previously for thyrotropin releasing hormone (Jackson and Reichlin, 1974) and its specificity previously determined (Bercu et al., 1977). The presence of MIS was assayed by a graded organ culture method (Donahoe et al., 1977a).

Thirteen-day pregnant females were chosen for injection because LH-RH antiserum did not interfere with normal continuation of pregnancy (Arimura, 1976) and Müllerian duct regression had not begun in normal male fetuses (Donahoe et al., 1977a). In an in vitro study (Fig. 1), ten 13-day-old pregnant rats were given 1 ml of LH-RH antiserum i.p., and another ten rats were treated with an equal volume of normal rabbit serum (NRS). At 17 days gestational age, male fetuses were removed from each of two experimental and two control mothers. One testis from each male fetus was removed and a small fragment placed aseptically on an agar coated stainless steel grid adjacent to the urogenital ridge of a $14\frac{1}{2}$-day female rat embryo for MIS assay. The remaining pregnant females were injected i.p. with another dose of 1 ml LH-RH antiserum or NRS on the 20th day of pregnancy. After delivery, the males were carefully marked as LH-RH antiserum or control pups, then were randomly assigned to either experimental or control mothers in equal numbers. At 6 days of age, five experimental and five control animals were killed. The animals were weighed, killed, and the testes removed. One testis was weighed and duplicate 1–2 mm fragments of the other evaluated for MIS assay. The penis was also removed and measured under a Nikon dissecting microscope.

The remaining 6-day-old male pups from a mother treated with LH-RH antiserum were given 0.25 ml LH-RH antiserum i.p., and similarly, the remaining equal number of male pups from a mother which had received NRS were given 0.25 ml NRS i.p.

S.J. Kogan and E.S.E. Hafez (eds.), Pediatric andrology, 47–52. All rights reserved.
Copyright © 1981, Martinus Nijhoff Publishers bv, The Hague/Boston/London.

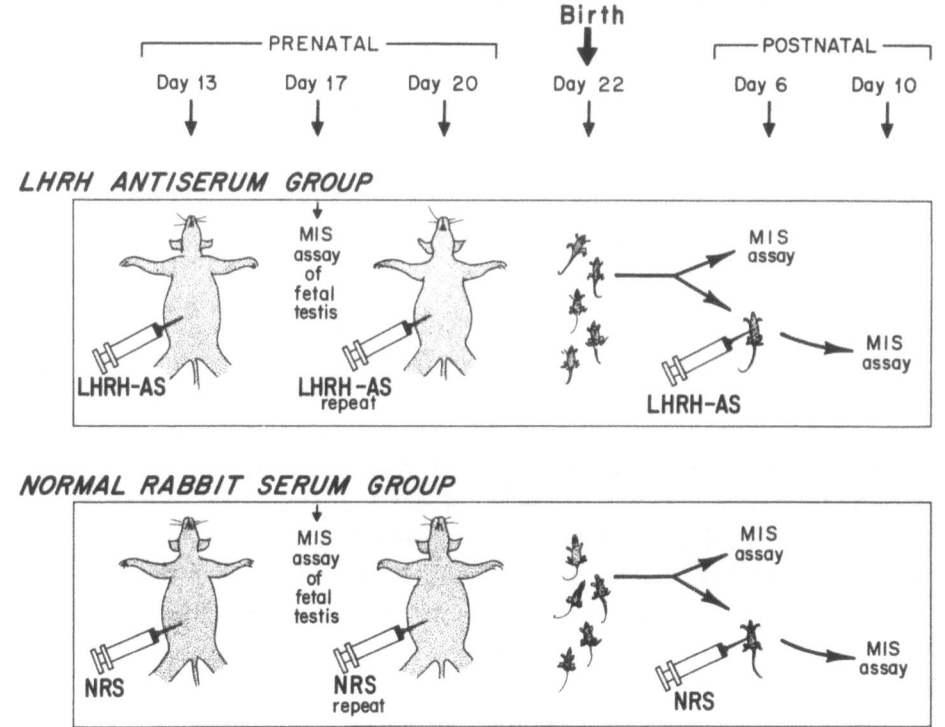

Figure 1. Schematic representation of experimental protocol. Luteinizing hormone releasing hormone antisera (LH-RH-AS) or normal rabbit serum (NRS) were injected into pregnant dams at gestational ages 13 and 20 days, and into pups at 6 days postnatal life. Groups of rat testes from fetuses were assayed for Müllerian Inhibiting Substance (MIS) activity at 17 days fetal age and from pups at 6 and 10 days postnatal life.

At 10 days of age these pups were weighed and their testes and penises removed.

MIS activity after immunological blockade of LH-RH is summarized in Fig. 2. Organ culture of testes from 17-day-old male fetuses from dams treated with LH-RH-antiserum at 13 days fetal age had significantly increased Müllerian duct regression (Grade 4.9 ± 0.1 vs 3.8 ± 0.5, $p < 0.05$). Similarly, the testes from 6-day-old pups from mothers which had received LH-RH antiserum at fetal ages of 13 and 20 days had increased MIS activity (Grade 4.7 ± 0.1 vs 3.6 ± 0.4, $p < 0.01$). Testes from animals 10 days of age did not differ between treatment and control pups (Grade 2.8 ± 0.4 vs 2.1 ± 0.3).

Testicular weights and penis size are summarized in Table 1. Testicular weight was reduced in pups from dams injected with LH-RH antiserum vs that from dams given NRS. Similarly, the penis length was reduced in the same experimental groups.

In order to show that LH-RH-AS crossed the placenta, we measured gonadotropins in the post-natal pups. The female pups were killed at 2 days of age and serum pooled (one value per 12 pups) for measurement of LH and FSH. LH-RH-AS appeared to cross the maternal–placental barrier. Gonadotropins were decreased in the 2 day postnatal female

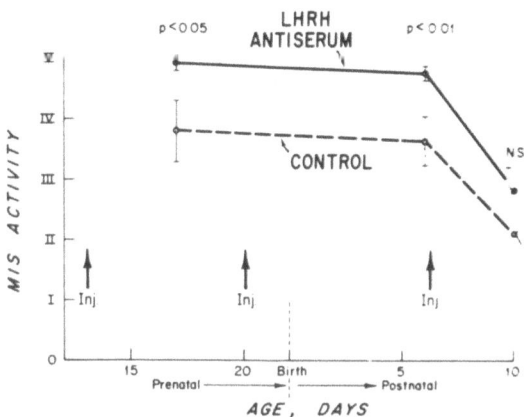

Figure 2. Müllerian Inhibiting Substance activity of testes of fetuses of dams treated with either luteinizing hormone releasing hormone (LH-RH) antiserum or normal rabbit serum. The means ± SE of the graded organ culture assay are compared in 17-day fetuses, 6- and 10-day-old rats.

Table 1. Testis weight, penis length, and body weight in rats born to dams treated with luteinizing hormone releasing hormone antiserum (LH-RH-AS) or normal rabbit serum (NRS).

Treatment	Testis weight (mg)	Penis length (mm)	Body weight (g)
6 days old:			
LHRH-AS	5.8 ± 0.3 *	5.69 ± 0.17 **	10.1 ± 0.3
NRS	7.0 ± 0.3	6.50 ± 0.16	10.0 ± 0.4
10 days old:			
LHRH-As	7.9 ± 0.3 **	5.93 ± 0.07 ***	10.9 ± 0.4
NRS	10.9 ± 0.7	6.84 ± 0.05	11.4 ± 0.4

Each mean ± SE represents 5 to 9 animals; * $p < 0.05$, ** $p < 0.01$, *** $p < 0.001$.

pups (Table 2). In addition, the 6-day-old male pups of LH-RH-AS injected mothers had smaller testes than those pups of control dams (Table 1).

Furthermore, the testes of pups whose mothers had been injected with LH-RH-AS had increased secretion of MIS in the organ culture assay. These studies suggest that one or both fetal gonadotropins inhibit the secretion of MIS in late fetal life. The gonadotropin most likely to be responsible is FSH since there is evidence that the Sertoli cell is the source of MIS (Blanchard and Josso, 1974; Josso, 1973; Donahoe et al., 1977b) and FSH is known to control certain functions of the Sertoli cell (Hansson et al., 1975). The content or release of MIS from the testis is increased in animals whose endogenous serum gonadotropins are reduced. This study indicates that normal MIS secretion is dependent on hypothalamic function through LH-RH regulation of gonadotropin release.

3. POSTNATAL FSH CONTROL OF MIS

In order to determine which of the pituitary gonadotropins influenced MIS secretion, we treated pregnant rats with LH-RH-AS and their male pups postnatally with FSH or HCG. Pregnant dams were in-

Table 2. Serum gonadotropin concentrations in 2-day postnatal rats treated during gestational life (day 13 and 20) with LH-RH-AS or NRS.

	LH ng/ml	FSH ng/ml
LH-RH-AS (60) *	12.2 ± 3.9	621 ± 34
NRS (35) *	33.4 ± 5.0	911 ± 103
p value	$p < 0.02$	$p < 0.05$

* Pooled samples of 11–15 for each point. Statistics using Student's *t* test.

jected with LH-RH-AS or NRS on gestational days 13 and 20, as before, and postnatally, the male pups were given pharmacologic doses of FSH or HCG (Fig. 3).

Twenty 13-day-old pregnant rats were given 1 ml of LH-RH-AS i.p., and another eight rats were treated with an equal volume of NRS. On the 20th day of pregnancy, the females were again injected i.p. with another 1 ml of LH-RH-AS or NRS. After delivery the males were carefully marked as LH-RH-AS or control pups, then they were randomly assigned to six other dams who delivered the same day. Each new mother was assigned randomly coded pups from the following groups: Pups from LH-RH antiserum treated mothers which were subsequently given one of the following treatments, 1) 100 mIU FSH; 2) 60 mIU FSH; 3) 20 mIU FSH; 4) 5 IU HCG; and 5) water (postnatal control); pups from mothers treated with NRS which were given 6) water (pregnancy control). All injections were given daily s.c. for the first 5 days of postnatal life. Testes from pups 6 days of age were studied for MIS activity as before. The animals were weighed and then decapitated. One testis was removed for MIS assay.

Organ culture from testes of 6 day old pups treated from birth with vehicle showed higher MIS activity (Grade 3.4 ± 0.3) if the dam had received LH-RH-AS at 13 and 20 days gestational age rather than NRS (pregnancy control) (Grade 2.3 ± 0.2, $p < 0.01$) (Fig. 4). FSH (100 mIU) given after birth to pups from mothers treated with LH-RH-AS antiserum reduced MIS secretion (Grade 2.3 ± 0.2 vs 3.4 ± 0.3, $p < 0.01$). These FSH treated pups from LH-RH-AS treated mothers had MIS activity similar to that of control pups from mothers treated with NRS (Grade 2.3 ± 0.2 vs 2.3 ± 0.2). Pups from mothers treated with LH-RH-AS given HCG

50

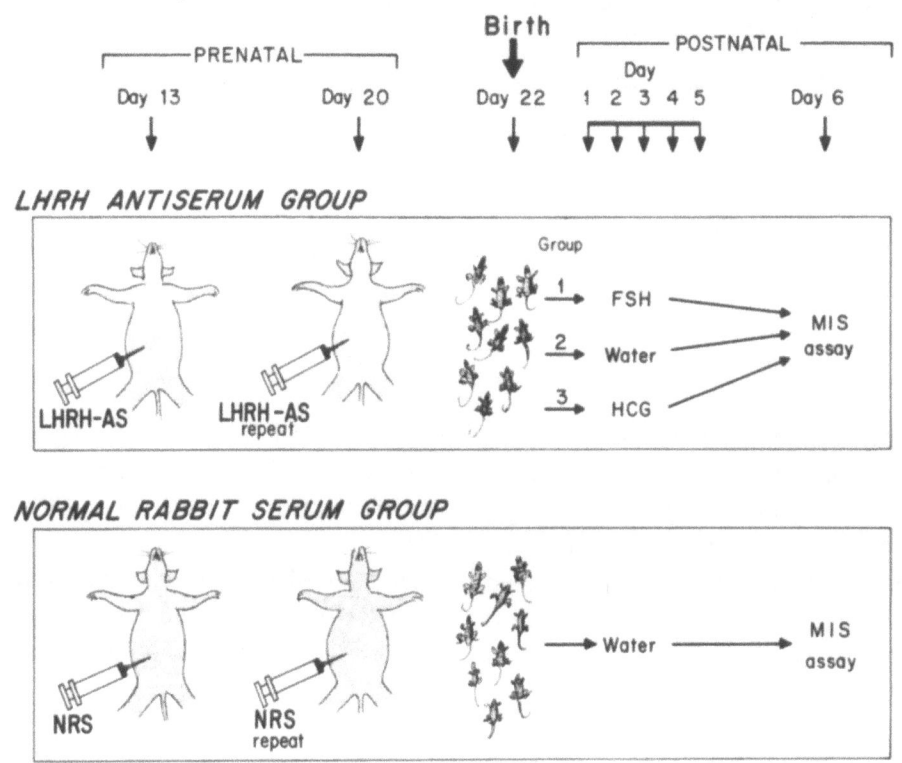

Figure 3. LH-RH-AS or normal rabbit serum (NRS) was injected into pregnant dams at gestational ages 13 and 20 days. After birth, pups from LH-RH-AS treated mothers received various doses of FSH or HCG. Testes from 6-day-old pups were assayed for MIS activity.

failed to alter the increased testicular MIS activity resulting from the LH-RH antiserum treatment of their dams (Grade 3.4 ± 0.4 vs 3.4 ± 0.3). These studies suggest that MIS secretion may be dependent on hypothalamic function through LH-RH regulation of FSH release.

4. SERTOLI CELL PRODUCTION OF MIS

FSH is known to control certain functions of the Sertoli cell (Hansson et al., 1975). Because of the above observation of FSH inhibition of Müllerian Inhibiting Substance secretion, we studied "Sertoli cell only" preparations created in vivo by irradiation to determine if MIS production could be maintained. Blanchard and Josso presented evidence that the Sertoli cell is responsible for MIS production (Josso, 1973; Blanchard and Josso, 1974). They stripped bovine fetal testes, isolated the seminiferous tubules by washing off the interstitial cells, and cultured the remaining seminiferous tubules with Müllerian ducts, causing regression. They then

irradiated the seminiferous tubules in vitro but the ability to cause Müllerian duct regression (Josso, 1974) was retained. An irradiation experiment was designed in vivo to confirm these findings and further document that the Sertoli cell secreted Müllerian Inhibiting Substance. Means and Huckins (1974) have shown that low dose radiation therapy to 20-day pregnant rats produced a "Sertoli cell only" preparation in the seminiferous tubules of the male pups, since the germ cells of the male fetus were exquisitely sensitive to low dose x-radiation. In the present study, pregnant rats were treated with low dose radiation therapy and their postnatal pups' testes examined for the production of MIS. Based on the previous model, 6-day-old postnatal pups were chosen to evaluate the testicular secretion of MIS.

Fifty-six experimental pregnant animals were irradiated with 125 rads at 20 days of gestation. An equal number of controls were studied. The remainder of the male pups were allowed to grow to adulthood (110 days of age).

MIS activity of the testes from 6-day-old postnatal pups was the same in both the treatment and

PREGNANT MOTHER TREATMENT	PUPS TREATMENT		MIS ASSAY	n=	p VALUES
NRS	Water		2.3 ± 0.2	10	
LHRH-AS	Water		3.4 ± 0.3	12	p<0.01
LHRH-AS	FSH	100mIU	2.3 ± 0.2	8	p < 0.001
		60mIU	2.4 ± 0.6	5	N.S
		20mIU	2.9 ± 0.6	6	N.S
LHRH-AS	HCG	5 IU	3.4 ± 0.4	6	p < 0.02

Figure 4. MIS activity (mean) of testes from 6-day-old pups whose mothers were treated with 1 ml LH-RH-AS or normal rabbit serum (NRS). Pups from LH-RH-AS treated mothers were given various doses of FSH or HCG daily s.c. for 5 days. Pups from NRS treated mothers were given an equal volume of water. The means ± SE of the graded organ culture assay are compared.

control groups when the mothers were irradiated on day 20 (3.6 ± 0.2 vs 3.0 ± 0.3; 4.3 ± 0.1 vs 4.2 ± 0.1, treatment vs control in separate studies assayed at two different times). Irradiated animals weighed less and had smaller testes (5.5 ± 4 μg vs 7.9 ± 0.6, $p < 0.05$). The histology of the testis of adult animals treated in utero showed absence of germ cells in the seminiferous tubules (Fig. 5). Six-day-old animals had no differences in circulating FSH, LH, testosterone and dihydro-testosterone. The hormonal values were as follows: FSH, 215 ± 26 vs 172 ± 22 ng/ml; LH, <50 vs <50 ng/ml; testosterone, 44.3 ± 2.0 vs 36.3 ± 5.0 ng/ml; dihydrotestosterone, <10 vs <10 ng/dl, treatment vs control, respectively).

Since testicular MIS activity of 6-day-old pups was the same in all groups, the data suggest that the Sertoli cells produce MIS. Germ cells were destroyed but Leydig and Sertoli cells were intact. The lack of change in the serum concentrations of T and DHT and LH suggest that the hypothalamic–pituitary–Leydig cell axis was intact as is usually the case at this age (Goldman et al., 1975). These data also suggest that the negative feedback axis from the Sertoli cell to the portion of the hypothalamic–pituitary axis responsible for FSH secretion, was also intact.

These data do not exclude completely that the Leydig cells make Müllerian Inhibiting Substance. However, previous experiments by Josso, in which she separated interstitial cells from seminiferous tubules and demonstrated MIS activity in the latter,

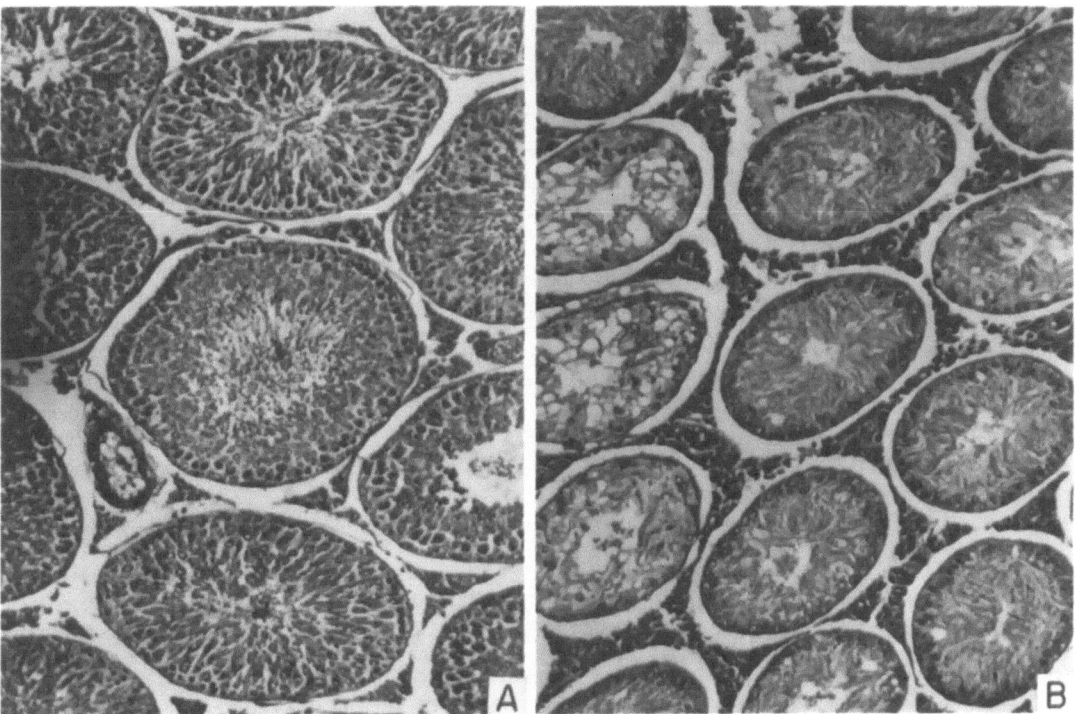

Figure 5. Pregnant dams were irradiated at 20 days of gestation with 125 rads. The pups were grown to 110 days of age. The testes were removed for histologic preparation: A) testis of control animals, B) testis of animals irradiated at 20 days of gestational life (200×). There is no evidence of spermatogenesis in the smaller tubules of the irradiated animals.

makes the Leydig cell an unlikely candidate as a putative MIS producer. Josso irradiated human testicular cells in vitro to destroy germ cells. In the present experiment fetal testes were irradiated in vivo to eliminate the germ cells. In both experiments, the irradiated testes demonstrated continued MIS activity, indicating that the functioning Sertoli cell is the cell most likely to produce MIS.

The smaller body weight of irradiated animals suggest a generalized decrease in DNA and RNA synthesis but no specific effect on the hormonal secretion of the Sertoli and Leydig cells. The smaller size of the testis of the 6-day animals treated with irradiation suggests an effect on the testis but neither Sertoli cell nor Leydig cells demonstrated morphological differences. In addition, MIS testicular levels and serum testosterone and dihydro-testosterone levels were the same in treatment and control animals.

5. SUMMARY

LH-RH-AS, which inhibited gonadotropin secretion in these studies, increased MIS production. Replacement with FSH returned MIS values to normal suggesting indirectly that FSH inhibits the production of MIS. Therefore, MIS appears to be under the control of the hypothalamic–pituitary axis. MIS secretion is not affected by irradiation during late gestation when germ cells are destroyed but Sertoli cells are spared. This study offers more indirect evidence to support the mounting evidence that Sertoli cells produce MIS.

REFERENCES

Arimura A (1976a) In vivo methods for studying the action of hypothalamic hormones with special reference to their antisera as tools for investigation. In Labrie F, Meites J, Pelletier G, eds. Hypothalamus and endocrine functions, p. 387. New York: Plenum Press.

Arimura A, Shino M, De la Cruz KG, Rennels EG, Schally AV (19786) Effect of active and passive immunization with luteinizing hormone releasing hormone and follicle-stimulating hormone levels and the ultrastructure of the pituitary gonadotropins in castrated male rats. Endocrinology 99: 291.

Bercu BB, Jackson IMD, Safaii H, Reichlin S (1976a) Testicular development requires luteinizing hormone releasing hormone (LH-RH) from birth. Evidence from studies of immunological blockade of endogenous LH-RH in the rat. Hamburg: 5th International Congress of Endocrinology.

Bercu BB, Jackson IMD, Safaii H, Sawin CT, Reichlin (1976b) The development of the pituitary gonadal axis in the male rat requires the luteinizing hormone releasing hormone (LH RII) decapeptide from birth. San Francisco: Endocrine Society Meeting, Abstract No. 365, p. 239.

Bercu BB, Jackson IMD, Safaii H, Reichlin S (1977) Permanent impairment of testicular development after transient immunological blockade of endogenous LH-RH in the neonatal rat. Endocrinology 101: 1871.

Bercu BB, Hayashi A, Poth M, Alexandrova M, Soloff MS, Donahoe PK (1980) LH-RH induced delay of parturition. Melbourne: 6th International Congress of Endocrinology.

Blanchard MG, Josso N (1974) Source of the anti-Müllerian hormone synthesized by the fetal testis: Müllerian inhibiting activity of fetal bovine Sertoli cells in tissue culture. Pediat Res 8: 968.

Donahoe PK, Ito Y, Marfatia S, Hendren WH (1976) The production of Müllerian Inhibiting Substance by the fetal, neonatal, and adult rat. Biol Reprod 15: 329.

Donahoe PK, Ito Y, Hendren WH (1977a) A graded organ culture assay for the detection of Müllerian Inhibiting Substance. J Surg Res 23: 141.

Donahoe PK, Ito Y, Price J, Hendren WH (1977b) Müllerian Inhibiting Substance activity in bovine fetal, newborn, and prepubertal testes. Biol Reprod 16: 238.

Goldman BD, Grazia YR, Kamberi IA, Porter JC (1975) Serum gonadotropin concentrations in intact and castrated neonatal rats. Endocrinology 97: 898.

Groenendijk-Huijbers M, Burggraaff J (1974) Experimental studies on capability of embryonic and young chicken testes to regress embryonic chick oviducts. Anat Anz Bd 135: 43.

Hansson V, Ritzen EM, French FS, Mayfeh SH (1975) Androgen transport and receptor mechanisms in testis and epididymis. In Hamilton DW, Greep R, eds. Handbook of physiology, Section 7: Endocrinology, Vol V: Male reproductive system, p. 173. American Physiological Society.

Jackson IMD, Reichlin S (1974) Thyrotropin releasing hormone (TRH): distribution in hypothalamic and extrahypothalamic brain tissue of mammalian and submammalian chordates. Endocrinology 95: 854.

Josso N (1973) In vivo synthesis of Müllerian inhibiting hormone by seminiferous tubules isolated from the calf fetal testis. Endocrinology 93: 829.

Josso N (1974) Müllerian inhibiting activity in human fetal testicular tissue deprived of germ cells by in vitro irradiation. Pediat Res 8: 755.

Koch Y, Chobsieng P, Zor U, Fridkin M, Lindner H (1973) Production and characterization of an antiserum to synthetic gonadotropin releasing hormone. Biochem Biophys Res Commun 55: 623.

Maraud R, Couland H, Stoll R (1969) Role inhibiteur de-l'hypophyse sur l'elaboration de l'inducteur testiculair responsable de la regression des canaux de muller chex l'embryon de poulet. CR Soc Biol 160: 964.

Maraud R, Stoll R, Couland H (1970) Donnés nouvelles sur les role du testicule et de l'hypophyse dans la differenciation sexuelle du poulet. CR Soc Biol 55: 442.

Means AR, Huckins C (1974) Coupled events in the early biochemical acticus of FSH on the Sertoli cells of the testis. In Dufau MD, Means AR, eds. Current topics in molecular endocrinology: hormone binding and target cell activation in the testis, p. 145. New York: Plenum Press, 1974.

6. ONTOGENY OF 5α-REDUCTASE AND THE ANDROGEN RECEPTOR IN THE PENIS

JACOB RAJFER, PEARL C. NAMKUNG and PHILIP H. PETRA

One of the variable factors affecting the ability of certain androgen target tissues to respond to androgens appears to be the age of the tissues. There is sufficient clinical data from the human to'suggest that the penis is quite responsive to exogenous androgenic stimulation during the prepubertal and pubertal years, whereas it is relatively inert to the same androgenic stimulation later on during adulthood (Vest and Howard, 1938; Turner, 1950; Feldman and Smith, 1975; Smith, 1977). Since the androgen induced response in most androgen target tissues requires (1) the ability of the target tissue to convert testosterone (T) to dihydrotestosterone (DHT) by the 5α-reductase enzyme (Anderson and Liao, 1968; Bruchovsky and Wilson, 1968) and (2) the binding of DHT to a cytoplasmic androgen receptor (cAR) (Fang et al., 1969; Mainwaring, 1969), it may be theorized that the lack of a response to androgens by the adult penis or, for that matter, by any androgen target tissue may be caused by a relative deficiency or complete absence of either the 5α-reductase enzyme or the cytoplasmic androgen receptor or both. This paper will describe some of the experimental observations from our laboratory regarding the age-related changes in these two parameters of androgen function in the penis.

1. ANIMAL MODEL

In our laboratory, the rat has been utilized as an animal model to investigate the age-related changes in the male reproductive system mainly because the time period between the beginning of the differentiation of the male reproductive system and the onset of puberty, which in man lasts for approximately 12 years, is displaced in relative time to about 8 weeks in the rat (Fig. 1). In fact, the same endocrine events

that occur in the human during the entire first trimester of gestation, i.e., the differentiation of the testes, internal ducts, and external genitalia, begins in the rat around the 13th day of gestation and is completed by the 21st and final day of gestation. In effect, what takes 13 to 15 weeks in the human the rat quickly accomplishes in approximately eight days. Penile growth, which occurs in the human during the second and third trimester of gestation (Smith, 1977; Walsh et al., 1978), occurs sometime during the early postnatal period in the rat (Goldman et al., 1972; Walsh et al., 1978). Consequently, in the rat, part of the time period between the birth of the animal and the onset of puberty should correspond to the latter two trimesters of gestation in the human.

These observations concerning the timing of some of the major endocrine events that occur during the life cycle of the rat allowed us to utilize this animal species in our investigations into the age-related changes in the level of both the 5α-reductase enzyme and the cAR in the developing penis.

2. ANDROGENIC RESPONSIVENESS OF PENIS AND ONTOGENY OF PENILE 5α-REDUCTASE ENZYME

In reviewing the literature, it is evident that an experimental investigation concerning the ability of the penis to respond to androgens has never been properly conducted. Since the rat penis undergoes its maximum growth sometime between the neonatal and pubertal periods (Fig. 1) and since penile growth is considered to be an androgen dependent event, it may be assumed that the rat penis, like the human's is maximally responsive to androgens during the immature time period. However, the ability of the penis to respond to androgenic stimulation at adulthood,

RELATIVE CHRONOLOGICAL EVENTS IN THE
MALE REPRODUCTIVE TRACT OF THE RAT AND MAN

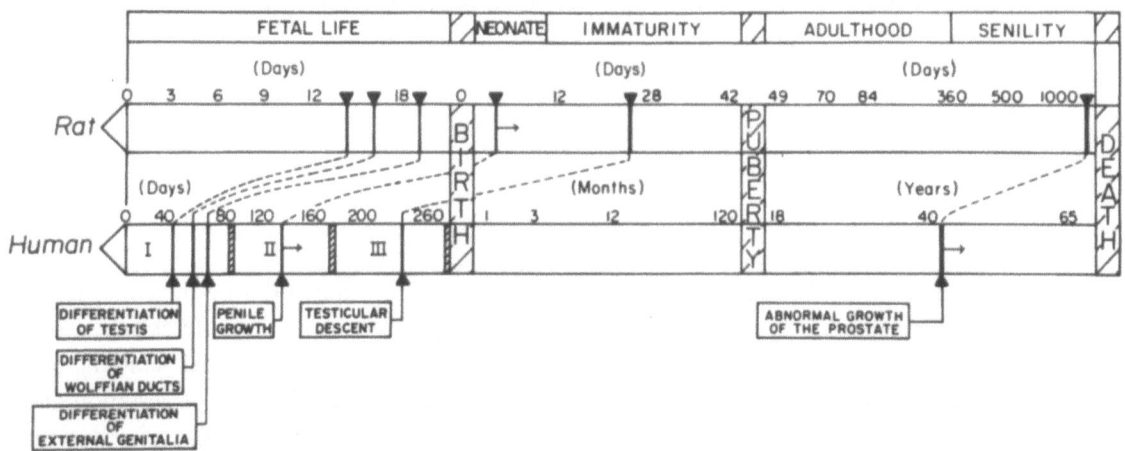

Figure 1. Comparison of the timing of the endocrine events in the male reproductive tract of the rat and human. Abbreviations: I, II, and III; first, second, and third trimesters of gestation.

after the period of maximal penile growth, has never been fully elucidated. In an attempt to determine whether the penis is capable of continued penile growth during adulthood and, if so, whether this is similarly an androgen dependent event, we conducted a series of experiments that are graphically represented by Fig. 2. Some of these data have been previously published (Rajfer et al., 1977). We found that androgen deprivation at adulthood due to castration (Group D) leads to a marked reduction in the penile weight when compared to untreated age-matched non-castrate animals (Group A), and this decrease in penile weight can be overcome by the administration of exogenous testosterone (Group E). This finding strongly suggests that the continued penile growth observed during adulthood (Group A compared to the 70-day-old controls), although very minimal, appears to be an androgen dependent event. Although there was some statistical significance between Groups A and B, we nevertheless concluded that 14 days of daily pharmacological doses of either TP (Groups B and E) or DHTP (Group C) at adulthood appeared to be no more effective than 14 days of physiological doses of androgens (Group A) in augmenting penile size. As a result, it appeared as if the adult penis, after attaining a certain size, will not respond further to either endogenous or exogenous androgenic stimulation regardless of the dosage or type of androgen

used. This is in marked contrast to what is seen in the prostate gland of the adult rat where the same androgenic stimulation results in a greater than 100% increment in prostate size (Rajfer and Coffey, 1979). Furthermore, the fact that DHTP was no more effective than TP in stimulating the adult penis suggests that this relative lack of androgenic responsiveness of the adult penis (in comparison to the prostate) is not solely due to a deficiency in the penile 5α-reductase activity.

To confirm the fact that this relative inertness of the adult penis to exogenous androgenic stimulation could not be due to a deficiency in the 5α-reductase enzyme, we simply measured the ability of the penis to convert testosterone to dihydrotestosterone in rats ranging from 16 to 84 days of age. For comparison, we also measured the total 5α-reductase activity of the ventral prostate gland in these animals. As can be seen in Fig. 3, the penis of the male rat contains measurable quantities of 5α-reductase activity, although the level gradually decreases with aging. In the ventral prostate gland, the level of total 5α-reductase activity is considerably greater on a per mg basis than in the penis, yet there appears to be a similar downward trend in the level of the enzyme in the prostate as the animal approaches adulthood.

Besides looking at the total 5α-reductase activity in the penis and prostate gland, we specifically measured in the penis the three major 5α-reduced products of testosterone: DHT, 3α-androstanediol (3α-diol), and 3β-androstanediol (3β-diol). We determined that in the immature penis, DHT appears to be the predominant product formed from the 5α-reduction of testosterone (Fig. 4). The fact that DHT is the major metabolite found in the penis during the time period the organ undergoes its maximum androgen-induced growth suggests that DHT, and not one of the diols, is the active androgen involved in the growth of the penis.

3. ONTOGENY OF THE ANDROGEN RECEPTOR

Since it was apparent that the relative lack of androgenic responsiveness of the adult penis was probably not due to a deficiency in the 5α-reductase en-

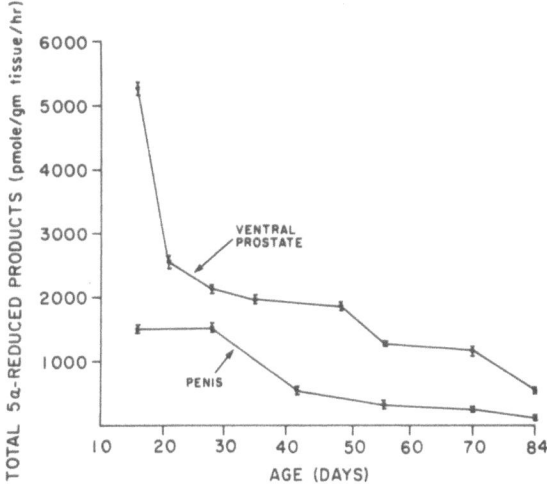

Figure 3. Age-related changes in the total 5α-reductase activity of the penis and ventral prostate gland of the male rat. An aliquot (100 μl) of tissue homogenate (diluted in 9 vols buffer, pH 6.6) was incubated for 15 min (ventral prostate) or 30 min (penis) with 37°C in a water bath with an equal volume of 5×10^{-8}m [³H] testosterone in the presence of 1×40^{-4}M NADPH. The reaction was stopped with 1 ml chloroform:methanol (2:1) solution. The layer containing the radioactive steroids was evaporated to dryness and the residue was suspended with carrier reference steroids. Thirty milliliters of this redissolved solution was applied to TLC plates and allowed to ascend twice in a chloroform:methanol (98.0:2.5) solvent at room temperature. The plates were sprayed with p-anisaldehyde reagent and each lane counted for radioactivity. Each homogenate was derived from the pooled prostates and penises of between 3 and 6 rats. Each point represents the mean ± SE of four separate assays performed on each homogenate.

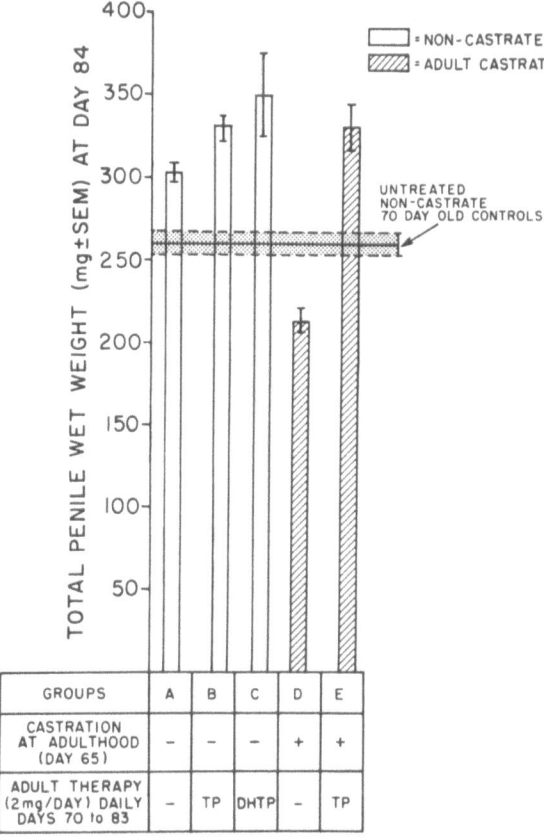

Figure 2. Effects of exogenous androgen therapy at adulthood on penile weight in both non-castrate and adult castrate rats. Penile weight was recorded at 84 days of age following 14 days of daily TP or DHTP treatment. For comparison, the penile weight of 70 day old non-castrate untreated male rats prior to the institution of androgen therapy is superimposed (Group A vs Group B, p = 0.01; Group A vs Group C, p = 0.10; Group A vs Group E, p >0.07).

zyme, an attempt was made to determine whether the relative androgenic unresponsiveness of the adult penis could be due to a deficiency in the cAR. For comparison, the cAR in the ventral prostate gland was also measured. Utilizing a dextran coated charcoal assay, it was determined that there is a relative absence of the cAR in the penis of the adult rat, whereas in the immature organ, the receptor is present in very high concentrations (Fig. 5). In fact, the penile cAR gradually decreases from a very high level at day 16 of age to almost undetectable levels at adulthood. It is entirely possible that this absence of the receptor at adulthood may explain the relative androgenic unresponsiveness of the adult penis. Similarly, the elevated levels of the receptor found in the penis during the sexually immature period are consistent with the clinical and experimental observation in humans that the maximum androgen-induced growth of the penis occurs during the sexually immature period (Vest and Howard, 1938;

56

Turner, 1950; Feldman and Smith, 1975; Smith, 1979).

For the ventral prostate gland, the receptor gradually increases from a level of about 25 femtomoles/mg cytosol protein at day 16 of age to reach a maximum of 87 ± 2 femtomoles/mg cytosol protein at day 49 of age. This level precipitously drops to approximately $19 \pm$ femtomoles/mg cytosol protein at day 70 of age (Fig. 5). The reason why the concentration of the cAR in the ventral prostate gland of the male rat is maximum at the time of puberty (day 49 of age) appears to remain somewhat of a mystery. It is entirely possible that the rapid growth of the ventral prostate gland during the prepubertal and pubertal periods may depend on the level of this receptor protein. On the other hand, it is known that the androgen imprinting of the ventral prostate gland occurs sometime between day 35 and day 65 of age (Rajfer and Coffey, 1978), and therefore it is also possible that the marked elevation in the cytosolic receptor of the ventral prostate gland at day 49 of age may be due to this imprinting phenomenon.

Nevertheless, the question of what actually regulates the level of the androgen receptor remains unanswered. It is known that some hormones regulate the level of its own receptor in some target tissues. One common mechanism involves a negative or down-regulation of the receptor in which the observed pattern is that the hormone will decrease the level of its own receptor. One example of this is the

effect of LH on its receptor in the Leydig cell (Hsueh et al., 1977; Catt and Dufau, 1977). Alternatively, the hormone may increase the level of its receptor as with prolactin and angiotensin (Aguilera et al. 1978). Another mechanism involves the regulation of certain receptors by other classes of hormones. For example, the regulation of the progesterone receptor by estrogen (Lippman and Allegra, 1978). In the penis, the observed decrease in the level of the cAr with aging at the same time the serum testosterone is gradually rising (Miyachi et al., 1973; Resko et al., 1968; Lee et all., 1975) suggests that down-regulation of the receptor by testosterone may be involved here. For the prostate gland, the regulation of the receptor appears more intriguing. It is entirely possible that testosterone may increase the level of the

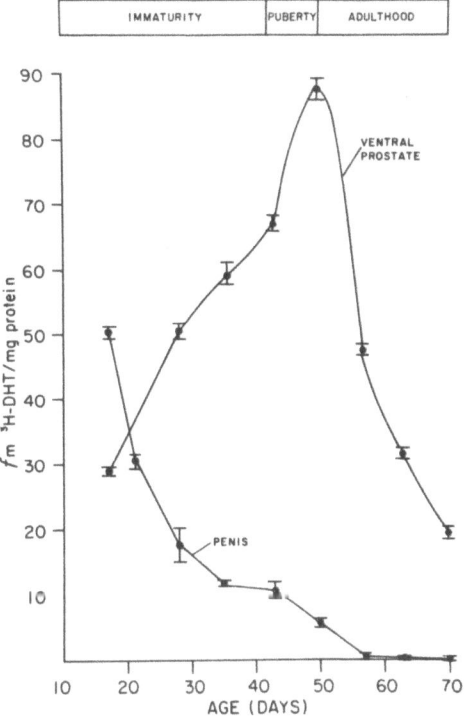

Figure 5. Age-related changes in the cytoplasmic androgen receptor of the penis and ventral prostate gland of the male rat. For each group, the prostates and penises of between six and nine animals were homogenized in 3 vols TED buffer, pH 7.4, at 4°C, and spun at 105,000 g × 90 min at 4°C. The resultant cytosol was incubated with 5 nM [³H] DHT for 2 h at 0°C with and without a 200-fold molar exces radioinert DHT. Free steroid was removed with dextran coated charcoal. An aliquot (50 μl) of the charcoal extracted solution was counted for radioactivity. Nonspecific binding was subtracted in all instances. Protein was measured by the Folin phenol reagent (Lowry et al., 1951). Each point represents the mean expressed as femtomoles [³H] DHT binding per mg cytosol protein $\pm$ SE of four single point assays performed on each cytosol preparation.

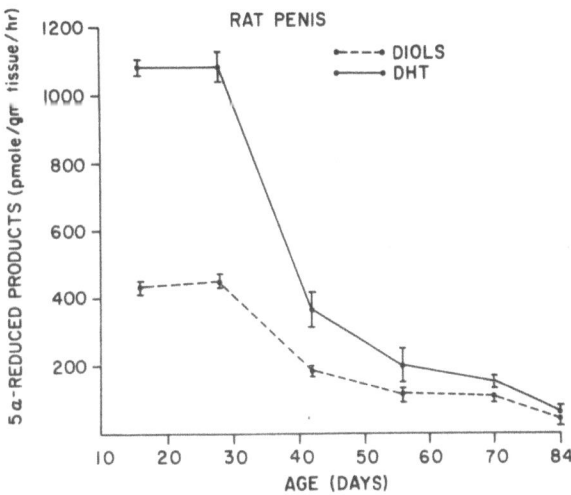

Figure 4. Ratio of diols (3α-androstanediol and 3β-androstanediol) to DHT in the maturing rat penis. Each point represents the mean $\pm$ SE of four assays performed for each age group. For methods, see Fig. 3.

prostatic receptor as in the prepubertal and pubertal animals. However, the abrupt decline in the receptor concentration in the prostate after puberty at the same time the serum testosterone is still continuing to rise (Miyachi et al., 1973; Lee et al., 1975) suggests the regulation of the prostatic cAR may change with age. In fact, there are some data to suggest that the regulation of the androgen receptor in the adult prostate is androgen independent (Sullivan and Strott, 1973; Blondeau et al., 1973). Whether testosterone initially increases the level of the receptor in the immature prostate and then causes down-regulation of the receptor in the adult gland or whether some as yet unknown mechanism is responsible for the regulation of the androgen receptor remains to be determined.

4. SUMMARY

The levels of 5α-reductase and the cAR were measured in the penis and ventral prostate gland of sexually maturing male rats. In the penis, the level of both 5α-reductase and the cAR decreased with aging, whereas in the prostate, the level of 5α-reductase actively also decreased with aging but the prostatic cAR gradually increased with aging until puberty at which time the receptor concentration began to precipitously drop to about 25% of the pubertal values. From these data, we concluded that the relative lack of androgenic responsiveness of the adult penis was probably due to the almost complete absence of the receptor at adulthood.

REFERENCES

Aguilera G, Hauger RL, Catt KL (1978) Control of aldosterone secretion during sodium restriction: adrenal receptor regulation and increased adrenal sensitivity to angiotensin II. Proc Natl Acad Sci USA 75: 975.

Anderson KM, Liao S (1968) Selective retention of dihydrotestosterone by prostatic nuclei. Nature 219: 277.

Blondeau JP, Corpechot C, LeGoascogne C, Baulieu EE, Robel P (1973) Androgen receptors in the rat ventral prostate and their hormonal controls. Vitam Horm 33: 319.

Bruchovsky N, Wilson JD (1968) The conversion of testosterone to 5α-androstan-17β-ol-3-one by rat prostate in vivo and in vitro. J Biol Chem 243: 2012.

Catt KJ, Dufau ML (1977) Peptide hormone receptors. Annu Rev Physiol 39: 529.

Fang S, Anderson KM, Liao S (1969) Receptor proteins for androgens. On the role of specific proteins in selective retention of 17β-hydroxy-5α-androstan-3-one by rat ventral prostate in vivo and in vitro. J Biol Chem 244: 6584.

Feldman KW, Smith DW (1975) Fetal phallic growth and penile standards for newborn male infants. J Pediatr 86: 395.

Goldman BD, Quadragno DM, Shyrne J, Gorski RA (1972) Modification of phallus development and sexual behavior in rats treated with gonadotropin antiserum neonatally. Endocrinology 90: 1025.

Hsueh AJW, Dufau ML, Catt KJ (1977) Gonadotropin-induced regulation of luteinizing hormone receptors and desensitization of testicular 3':5'-cyclic AMP and testosterone responses. Proc Natl Acad Sci USA 74: 592.

Lee VWK, deKretser DM, Hudson B, Wang C (1975) Variations in serum FSH, LH, and testosterone levels in male rats from birth to puberty. J Reprod Fertil 42: 121.

Lippman ME, Allegra JC (1978) Receptors in breast cancer. New Engl J Med 299: 930.

Lowry OY, Rosebrough NJ, Farr AL, Randall RJ (1951) Protein measurements with the Folin phenol reagent. J Biol Chem 193: 265.

Mainwaring WIP (1969) A soluble androgen receptor in the cytoplasm of rat prostate. J Endocrinol 45: 31.

Miyachi Y, Nieschlag E, Lipsett MB (1973) The secretion of gonadotropins and testosterone by the neonatal male rat. Endocrinology 92: 1.

Rajfer J, Coffey DS (1978) Sex-steroid imprinting of the immature prostate: long-term effects. Invest Urol 16: 186.

Rajfer J, Coffey DS (1979) Effects of neonatal steroids on male sex tissues. Invest Urol 17: 3.

Rajfer J, Coffey DS, Walsh PC (1977) Effects of hormones in the newborn period on the development of the penis. Surg Forum 28: 570.

Resko JA, Feder HH, Goy RW (1968) Androgen concentration in plasma and testis of developing rats. J Endocrinol 40: 485.

Smith DW (1977) Micropenis and its management. Birth Defects Orig Artic Ser XIII, No. 2, p 147.

Sullivan JN, Strott Ca (1973) Evidence for an androgen-independent mechanism regulating the levels of receptor in target tissue. J Biol Chem 248: 3202.

Turner HH (1950) The clinical use of testosterone. Springfield: Charles C. Thomas.

Vest SA, Howard JE (1938) Clinical experiments with the use of male sex hormones. J Urol 40: 154.

Walsh P-C, Wilson JD, Allen TD, Madden JD, Porter JC, Neaves WB, Griffen JE, Goodwin WE (1978) Clinical and endocrinological evaluation of patients with congenital microphallus. J Urol 120: 90.

7. STUDIES ON H-Y ANTIGEN: THE GENETIC BASIS OF ABNORMAL GONADAL DIFFERENTIATION

STEPHEN S. WACHTEL and MARIA I. NEW

According to Alfred Jost (1970), sex determination may be viewed as comprising sequential processes: (a) establishment of genetic sex (XX or XY) at fertilization, (b) translation of genetic sex into gonadal sex (ovary or testis), and (c) translation of gonadal sex into body sex (female or male). In the male, the last process is mediated by secretions of the newly-differentiated testis: *testosterone* from Leydig cells, and *antiMüllerian hormone*, from Sertoli cells. AntiMüllerian hormone suppresses development of the Müllerian ducts, whereas testosterone induces differentiation of the Wolffian ducts. Dihydrotestosterone, a metabolite of testosterone, induces orderly differentiation of the male external genitalia.

Thus testosterone plays a pivotal role in masculinization of the embryo. In the absence of testosterone (or its receptor) the embryo is feminized despite male "genetic" sex or gonadal sex. Accordingly testosterone may be said to impose the male phenotype against an inherent tendency to become female (Jost, 1970)

There is now a convincing body of evidence suggesting that the corresponding pivotal role in gonadal sex differentiation is played by H-Y antigen, a phylogenetically conservative cell surface component identified by serum from male-sensitized female mice. Based on occurrence of H-Y in a variety of species representing widely divergent pathways of vertebrate evolution, and on its association with the heterogametic-type gonad, we proposed that the molecule or group of molecules conferring H-Y antigenicity in mice directs differentiation of the initially indifferent embryonic gonad, causing it to become a testis in XX/XY species such as man (Wachtel et al., 1975). According to that view, the gonad should be feminized in the absence of H-Y (or its receptor?), despite karyotype or body sex. In the following paragraphs, we shall review a series of clinical and biological studies which clarify the role of H-Y antigen in sex determination and which provide new insights into the several abnormalities of gonadal differentiation, with implications for the differentiative process in general.

1. IN VITRO STUDIES

1.1. H-Y as the mammalian testis inducer

There are several direct indications that H-Y antigen is the inducer of the mammalian testis (reviewed in Wachtel and Koo, in press). When cells from a particular tissue are dispersed in culture, the cells have the tendency to reaggregate, thus forming structures characteristic of the tissue from which they were derived (Moscona, 1961). Dispersed Sertoli cells from the mechanically dissociated testes of newborn mice or rats organize tubular structures after 16 hours in slow rotary cultures for example. But when H-Y antigen is "lysostripped" from the surface membranes of these cells, by reaction with excess H-Y antibody, culturing and reaggregation result in the formation of spherical structures, many of which closely resemble the primordial follicles of the newborn ovary (Ohno, 1979).

It is possible to "sex-reverse" the reaggregation pattern of cultured ovarian cells as well. By exposure to soluble H-Y antigen (see below), dispersed cells of the newborn ovary are induced to form seminiferous tubule-like structures instead of follicles. One consequence of this exposure is the precocious appearance of LH/hCG receptors in the transformed XX cells (whereas LH/hCG receptors are present in the rat testis at birth, they do not normally appear in the rat ovary before six to eight days *after* birth) (Muller et al., 1978). Perhaps the most striking demonstration of a testis-organizing role of H-Y antigen was provided in the organ culture experiments of Ohno et al. (1979). When undifferentiated XX gonads of the fetal calf were exposed to concentrated sources of soluble H-Y antigen, "complete" testicular transformation was noted, beginning with the sudden appearance of seminiferous tubules after three days, and culminating in the appearance of a tunica albuginea after five days. The XX cells of the induced tubules resembled postpubertal Sertoli cells. Neither Leydig cells nor germ cells were observed.

1.2. Indications for the H-Y gonadal receptor

Evidently, H-Y antigen provides an *inductive signal* in transforming the XX presumptive ovary into a testis. This implies ability to identify such a signal in both XX and XY indifferent gonads. In fact, it is possible to obtain H-Y antigen in soluble form (as in the supernatant fluid of testicular cell preparations), and there is now compelling evidence for occurrence of a gonad specific H-Y antigen receptor. For example, H-Y antigen secreted by testicular Sertoli cells binds selectively to cells of the ovary, and to a lesser extent to cells of the testis, but not to cells of the extragonadal tissues (Table 1). And we have already noted that attachment of soluble H-Y signals a program of precocious testicular differentiation in cells of the XX presumptive ovary.

Table 1. Expression, binding and secretion of H-Y antigen *

Tissue	Expression	Secretion	Binding
Gonadal XX	−	−	+
Gonadal XY			
Leydig cells	+	−	+
Sertoli cells	+	+	+
Diploid germ cells	−	−	?
Haploid germ cells	+	−	−
Extra gonadal XX **	−	−	−
Extra gonadal XY	+	−	−

* After Muller (in press): H-Y+ and H-Y− phenotype were determined by exposing cells to soluble testis-secreted H-Y antigen and using these H-Y exposed cells to absorb H-Y antiserum in the cytotoxicity test.
** Brain, epidermis, kidney, liver, spleen.

1.3. Indications for a stable membrane anchorage site for H-Y antigen

In view of a number of reports indicating close association of H-Y antigen and plasma membrane components of the major histocompatibility complex (HLA in man), it has been suggested that H-Y is actually coupled with HLA on the cell surface (Ohno, 1977). The major histocompatibility complex is composed of a number of genetic loci including HLA-A and HLA-B in man (corresponding to H-2D and H-2K of the mouse), each of which determines formation of a serologically detectable polypeptide (MW, 45,000) associated with some 3000 sugar residues. The NH_2 terminal ends of the HLA molecules are exposed at the cell surface, linked to a smaller molecule called beta-2-microglobulin (β_2m) (MW, 12,000); the carboxy terminals of HLA are buried inside the plasma membrane. Thus HLA antigens may be said to constitute a "stable" portion of the human cell surface. According to Ohno (1977), β_2m-HLA dimers serve as the stable membrane anchorage sites not only for H-Y antigens, but for all "inducer" molecules, in all tissues, gonadal and somatic; i.e., H-Y antigen occurs on the surfaces of somatic cells (skin, brain, spleen, etc.) held in place as, it were, by molecules of β_2m-HLA.

There is evidence for and against this proposal (see for example Flaherty et al., 1979). Suffice it to say here that in β_2m($-$), HLA($-$) cells of the cultured male Burkitt lymphoma called "Daudi", H-Y is virtually undetected on the cell surface, and that it is released into the surrounding medium. Daudi culture medium is therefore an excellent source of "free" H-Y antigen; this H-Y has been used to transform XX gonads of the fetal calf (as described above).

Our model thus requires two membrane attachment sites for H-Y antigen: (a) the gonad specific receptor for (disseminated) H-Y and (b) the stable carrier (β_2m-HLA) for membrane-bound H-Y. It follows that H-Y may exist in at least three different states: (a) bound to its specific receptor, (b) as a part of the plasma membrane, and (c) free in solution. It may be inferred that testicular organization of the indifferent embryonic gonad is secondary to synthesis and secretion of H-Y, and to enagagement of H-Y and its specific receptor. Evidently these events signal a program of differentiation in Sertoli cells and their precursors (leading to formation of the seminiferous tubule) with consequent secretion of antiMüllerian hormone and H-Y, and to a corresponding program of differentiation in Leydig cells (leading to elaboration of the LH/hCG receptor) with consequent secretion of testosterone. In the following paragraphs, we shall review a series of clinical studies which support these inferences, and which clarify possible modalities of H-Y function and dysfunction in normal and abnormal differentiation of the mammalian testis.

2. GENETIC STUDIES

2.1. A gene on the Y-chromosome

H-Y transplantation antigen was discovered with the observation that within certain highly inbred strains of the laboratory mouse, male-to-female skin grafts were rejected, whereas skin grafts exchanged among the other sex combinations were not rejected (Eichwald and Silmser, 1955). Since the outstanding genetic difference between male and female members of the same highly inbred population is the Y-chromosome, it was assumed that the male grafts were rejected because they possessed a foreign antigen determined either directly or indirectly by Y-situated gene(s). For similar reasons it was assumed that expression of the serologically detectable H-Y moiety was determined either directly or indirectly by Y-situated genes.

The question was approached in humans by assaying for presence or absence of H-Y in patients exhibiting numerical or structural abnormalities of the Y-chromosome. In an early series of tests, excess H-Y antigen was detected serologically in the white blood cells of males with two Y chromosomes (47,XYY and 48,XXYY). Gene dosage effects are recognized for several systems of histocompatibility antigens; the amount of antigen on the plasma membrane often may be correlated roughly with the number of genetic determinants in the nucleus. Excessive H-Y in association with supernumerary Y chromosomes therefore seemed to imply occurrence of a Y-situated genetic determinant for H-Y.

Further study revealed that H-Y was present in subjects retaining at least a portion of the Y-short arm (Yp), and absent in subjects who lacked the Y-short arm (Yp−). The Y-situated H-Y gene was thus located on the short arm near the centromere (Table 2). In one patient a locus on the long arm (Yq) could not be excluded (Koo et al., 1977a).

Table 2. Mapping the H-Y gene on the human Y-chromosome

Phenotype	Gonads	Karyotype	H-Y antigen expression
Normal male	Testes	46,XY	+
Normal female	Ovaries	46,XX	−
Male	Testes	47,XYY	+ +*
Male	Testes	46,XYq⁻ **	+
Female	Streaks	46,X,i (Yq) ***	−

Evidence for H-Y gene locus on the short arm of the Y chromosome; see Koo et al. (1977a).

* (+ +) denotes excess H-Y antigen. It is not clear whether this represents "double dose".
** Yq⁻ denotes absence of the long arm of the Y.
*** i(Yq) denotes isochromosome (i) of the long arm (q) of the Y.

2.2. A gene on the X-chromosome

In the Scandinavian wood lemming there is a 4:1 female: male sex ratio. Roughly half of the females have a male karyotype (32,XY), yet they are H-Y⁻, fertile and anatomically indistinguishable from their normal 32,XX female littermates. The XY female wood lemming condition is inherited as an X-linked trait. This indicates that there is a mutant gene on the wood lemming X-chromosome that is able to suppress production of H-Y and thereby promote ovarian differentiation in the XY primordial gonad. In view of the extreme evolutionary conservation of the mammalian X-chromosome, similar X-linked mutants may occur in the other mammalian species including man. Consider the following case report (Bernstein et al., 1980):

A 46,Xp⁺Y karyotype (additional band on the short arm of the X) was discovered in the cells of a profoundly retarded girl with multiple congenital abnormalities. The abnormal Xp⁺ was inherited from the mother (46,XXp⁺), who was unaffected. The Y-chromosome was indistinguishable from that of the father. The child, a phenotypic female with unremarkable external genitalia, died when she was 5 years old. Post mortem examination revealed female internal genitalia and microscopic ovarian stroma with degenerating primordial follicles bilaterally. There was no testicular tissue. When the mother became pregnant again, 46,Xp⁺Y cells were discovered in the amniotic fluid, and the pregnancy was terminated at 20 weeks of gestation. The fetus was a female with multiple congenital abnormalities similar to those of the proband. The internal genitalia of the fetus were female. The gonads were normal ovaries containing numerous primordial follicles. As in the proband, there was no trace of testicular tissue. Cells from fetus and proband were typed H-Y⁻.

The data favor the view that testicular differentiation is secondary to normal function of a gene on the mammalian X-chromosome. Mutation of this gene should suppress production of H-Y antigen in man as in the wood lemming. In humans this should be associated with development of a degenerative ovary (see section 3.3 below).

2.3. Where is the H-Y structural gene?

Given two genetic loci involved in the synthesis of a particular antigenic molecule, the question arises which may be structural, coding for a particular amino acid sequence (whereby the antigenic molecules assumes its specificity) and which may be regulatory, governing the function of the other gene. One might conclude that the Y-situated H-Y gene is structural because two Y-chromosomes seem to "produce" excessive amounts of antigen. But the fact is that two Y-chromosomes could *induce* excessive production by other, structural, genes.

What if the H-Y structural gene were situated on the X-chromosome? Then, according to what we have said, the Y-chromosome should be required for activation. Aberrant differentiation of XX testis or ovotestis could be due to "constitutive" activation of the X-linked structural genes in the absence of the Y. On the other hand, differentiation of the XY ovary could be due to mutation of structural or regulatory genes located on *any* chromosome (see section 3.3).

So for the time being, it is not clear whether X-situated genes synthesize H-Y or govern its synthesis. Indeed it could be argued that X and Y situated genes are *both* structural, each coding for discrete polypeptide chains that associate to form the functional testis-inducer. Or one might suggest that the structural testis-determining H-Y gene is on an autosome, suppressed by the X, and activated by the Y (Wolf, 1979; Muller and Wolf, 1979). In that case, testicular differentiation in XX subjects could represent "escape" from X-mediated suppression, and again, ovarian differentiation in XY subjects could represent mutation of genes on X, Y or autosome.

3. CLINICAL STUDIES

3.1. H-Y antigen in male pseudohermaphroditism

Male pseudohermaphroditism is a condition in which an individual with testes develops female or intersexual somatic characteristics. There are two main categories of male pseudohermaphroditism: (a) failure of Müllerian duct regression, and (b) failure of virilization. The latter can also be subdivided into two categories: failure of androgen synthesis and failure of androgen function (Wilson and MacDonald, 1978). Here we shall review our study of H-Y in four kinds of pseudohermaphroditism: testicular feminization syndrome, representing defective androgen function; 17α-hydroxylase deficiency, representing defective androgen synthesis in the gonad; 5α-reductase deficiency, representing defective metabolism of testosterone and ineffective androgen at the target sites; and an unclassified form in a 45, X/46XYq- patient with abnormal synthesis (or function) of AMH and testosterone.

3.1.1. Testicular feminization syndrome (TFS). The TFS is a classical form of male pseudohermaphroditism first described by Morris in 1953. In this condition, embryos with a normal male karyotype (46,XY) develop testes, and the testes produce anti-Müllerian hormone and testosterone, presumably to the same degree as in any 46, XY embryo. In the TFS however there is a mutation of a critical gene on the X chromosome *(Tfm)*; this causes failure of the nuclear androgen receptor. As a result the embryo is androgen-insensitive, and all androgen-dependent traits are abnormal or fail to develop. Despite presence of testes, individuals with "complete" androgen insensitivity develop as phenotypic females with conventional appearance and standard psychosexual orientation. Because of antiMüllerian hormone secreted by the fetal testes, however, these individuals lack uterus and tubes and the cephalad portion of the vagina; the vagina now terminates as a blind pouch.

The testes in TFS are cryptorchid or intralabial. In four cases they secreted an average of 44 μg/day of estradiol compared with 6 μg/day in normal males (MacDonald et al., 1979). According to Wilson et al. (1979), the "florid" feminization of TFS results from increased secretion of testicular estradiol in the absence of normally antagonistic or competitive effects of androgen.

We have studied expression of H-Y antigen in several cases of TFS. All were H-Y+ (Table 3), suggesting that presence of H-Y on the cell membrane is not secondary to any interaction of androgen and its receptor. It follows that synthesis of H-Y antigen is not hormone dependent.

3.1.2. 17α-hydroxylase deficiency.

There are five enzymes known to mediate synthesis of testosterone, each of which catalyzes a step in the biochemical metabolism of cholesterol. One of these enzymes, 17α-hydroxylase catalyzes the reaction in which progesterone is converted to 17-hydroxyprogesterone (this in turn is converted to androstenedione; the latter, into testosterone). Mutational deficiency of 17α-hydroxylase in embryos with the 46, XY karyotype leads to a form of male pseudohermaphroditism in which affected individuals develop ambiguous genitalia. One of us (New, 1970) has described a case notable for small vagina, rudimentary penis and bifid scrotum. Testes were present intra-abdominally and uterus and Fallopian tubes were absent, evidently suppressed by antiMüllerian hormone as in the TFS. Despite female appearing genitalia, the patient was raised as a male. Our preliminary data indicate that H-Y antigen is present in this male pseudohermaphrodite with 17α-hydroxylase deficiency.

3.1.3. 5α-reductase deficiency.

In the urogenital sinus and urogenital tubercle, testosterone is a substrate, i.e. a pre-hormone. In the presence of the enzyme Δ^4-steroid 5α-reductase, testosterone is converted into another androgen, 5α-dihydrotestosterone (DHT). As we have already pointed out, DHT mediates orderly differentiation of the male external genitalia; 46,XY embryos with 5α-reductase deficiency develop testes and produce normal amounts of testosterone, but there is a decreased conversion of testosterone to DHT. As a result, affected individuals are born with marked ambiguity of the external genitalia. Patients with this disorder have inguinal or intralabial testes, labial-like scrotum, blind vaginal pouch and hypertrophic clitoris. Epididymides and vasa deferentia are present internally; the Müllerian derivatives are absent. At puberty there is a remarkable turn of events. Patients develop a characteristic male body type; the clitoris enlarges, the scrotum becomes rugated and in some cases the testes descend; there may even be an ejaculate containing spermatozoa. In the population reported by Imperato-McGinley et al. (1974) post-

Table 3. H-Y antigen expression in cases of abnormal differentiation

Sex phenotypes	Sex abnormalities	Gonads	H-Y phenotype*	Reference
Normal male	XY	Testes	+	
Normal female	XX	Ovaries	−	
Female TFS	XY	Testes	+	Koo et al. (1977b)**
5α-reductase deficiency	XY	Testes	+	
Ambiguous: male pseudohermaphrodite	XX/XYq⁻	Testes	+**	Kaye et al. (1976)
Ambiguous: true hermaphrodite	XX	Left ovary, right ovotestis	+**	Saenger et al. (1976)
Male	XX	Small testes	+	Proband 1 in de la Chapelle et al. (1978)
Female	XY	Left dysgerminoma, right streak	+	Case 4 in Wachtel et al. (1980)
Female	XYp⁻	Dysgenetic ovaries	−***	Rosenfeld et al. (1979)
Female	Xp⁺Y	Microscopic ovarian remnants	−	Bernstein et al., (1980)

* H-Y phenotype determined in skin fibroblasts (Bernstein et al., 1980) and in blood and skin fibroblasts (Rosenfeld et al., 1979); in all other cases, in blood.
** Possible reduced expression of H-Y in these cases.
*** The possibility of residual expression of H-Y could not be excluded in one of three tests in this case.

pubertal psycho-sexual orientation was male.

We have studied the white blood cells of a 5-year-old child with 5α-reductase deficiency. The child was castrated at two years of age, placed on estrogen therapy and raised as a female. Phenotype was unequivocally H-Y$^+$.

3.1.4. Unclassified male pseudohermaphroditism in a 45,X/46,XYq- phenotypic female with ambiguous genitalia.

Occasionally deficiencies of testosterone synthesis or function, and failure of Müllerian suppression occur in the same individual. In a 19-year-old female with enlarged clitoris, separate vaginal and urethral orifices and normal cervix, laparotomy revealed infantile uterus and tubes, and bilateral testes with closely packed immature seminiferous tubules. There was no spermatogenesis. Blood karyotype was 45,X/46,XYq− with 45,X in 50% of the cells studied; blood leukocytes were typed H-Y$^+$ (Kaye et al., 1976). Incomplete differentiation in this case could accordingly be attributed to paucity of XY cells and consequent paucity of H-Y antigen in the developing gonad (see discussion of threshold effects in section 3.2). This could account for insufficient production of both testosterone and AMH.

3.1.5. H-Y phenotype: androgen mediated effects.

Although the foregoing observations suggest that expression of H-Y is dependent on neither synthesis of androgen, nor on reaction of androgen and its nuclear receptor, the question whether androgens (or sex steroids in general) may influence expression of H-Y remains open. For instance: (a) there are indications that H-Y expression may be reduced in some patients with TFS compared with its expression in normal XY males; (b) in the non-mammalian vertebrates H-Y is induced by treatment of the homogametic (XX) sex with steroid hormones (see Muller et al., 1979); (c) exposure to physiologic concentrations of testosterone causes selective approximation of H-Y and H-2D^b in mouse thymocytes (Flaherty et al., 1979).

There is some controversy regarding steroids and their effects on H-Y transplantation antigen: (a) according to one report H-Y is induced in skin grafts from female mice (XX) by transient residence in a male environment; but this was not borne out in other reports from laboratories following essentially the same protocols (reviewed in Wachtel, 1977); (b) there are reports that castration reduces expression of H-Y in male mice; there are also reports that castration has no such effect (reviewed in Wachtel, 1977).

At present it seems reasonable to infer that occurrence of H-Y on the cell surface is at least qualitatively independent of sex steroid synthesis or action. Indeed it is not easy to envision the operation in utero of a testis-inducer that is hormone-sensitive. Yet sex steroids may modify the expression of cell surface antigens generally, and the precise relationship between H-Y antigenicity and steroid hormones remains to be clarified, as we have already noted. In that context it is worth pointing out that H-Y is first detected in the 8-cell pre-implantation embryo, presumably well before testosterone is synthesized (Krco and Goldberg, 1976).

3.2. H-Y antigen in XX sex reversal

3.2.1. XX true hermaphrodites.

Evidently the various forms of male pseudohermaphroditism are errors of secondary sex differentiation due to functional absence of hormone (androgen or AMH) at the target site. Yet the disorder may be intrinsically an error of gonadal differentiation (primary sex determination) as in the mosaic patient just described. True hermaphroditism, on the other hand, is *always* a question of aberrant gonadal differentiation. The true hermaphrodite is an individual possessing both testicular and ovarian tissue, in any combination (Table 4). Hormonal instabilities resulting from this aberrant combination often cause ambiguity of the secondary sex characteristics. For example, Saenger et al. (1976) reported 4 cm clitoris, fused labia majora and single perineal opening in a 2-year-old child with female karyotype (46,XX) and

Table 4. Some examples of gonadal development in true hermaphroditism *

Gonad	vs	Gonad
Testis		Ovary
Testis		Ovotestis
Ovary		Ovotestis
Ovotestis		Ovotestis
Ovotestis		Not present
Ovary and testis		Ovary and testis

* See van Niekerk (1974).

male levels of circulating testosterone. H-Y antigen was detected in white blood cells, and the child was explored surgically. A hypoplastic uterus was present, and bilateral Fallopian tubes. There was a left ovary with epididymis, and a right ovotestis with epididymis and vas deferens. The ovotestis contained numerous sterile testicular tubules as well as follicles with germ cells (Table 3).

The picture is representative of human true hermaphroditism: 46,XX is the most common karyotype; the ovotestis is the most common gonad (van Niekerk, 1974). Yet both these characteristics have raised difficult questions. First, how do synthesis of H-Y antigen and differentiation of testis occur in the absence of the "male-determining" Y-chromosome; and second, if H-Y is disseminated in "hormone-like" fashion, why is testicular differentiation limited to only *part* of the hermaphroditic gonad(s)?

We have already alluded to the possibility that H-Y structural testis-determinants are located on the X-chromosome. Testicular differentiation in the XX primordial gonad could accordingly follow mutational release from Y-chromosome mediated regulation. Indeed one might attribute hermaphroditic differentiation to lyonization with only a portion of cells of the presumptive gonad carrying the mutated X. It should be noted that our statistical evaluation of serological data from four XX true hermaphrodites revealed a clear-cut and highly significant difference between the amount of H-Y carried on their skin fibroblasts and white blood cells, and the amount carried on corresponding cells from normal 46,XY males. True hermaphrodites are H-Y$^+$ but they are evidently *less* positive than normal males, an observation favoring the view that only a portion of their cells are carrying "switched-on" H-Y genes.

The situation becomes rather more complicated when we consider the possibility that the structural testis-determinant is on the Y. In that case testicular differentiation in the XX primordium should indicate retention of the structural locus as in any of the following conditions: (a) Y-to-autosome translocation; (b) Y–X interchange; (c) early loss of the Y from an XXY cell line; (d) hidden mosaicism involving an XY or XXY cell line; (e) mutational acquisition of Y-chromosome function by an autosomal or X-linked gene. The alternatives have been reviewed elsewhere (Wachtel and Bard, in press). In brief, there is some evidence for X-Y interchange as

an etiologic factor in human true hermaphroditism, but little evidence for Y-autosomal translocation as a factor. Yet it is difficult to rule out any of the other conditions as possible causes of true hermaphroditism. For example, human true hermaphrodites with the 46,XX/46,XY mosaic or chimeric karyotype have been described in several instances, but the 46,XX/46,XY karyotype is not necessarily associated with hermaphroditism or even abnormal sex differentiation generally (Simpson, 1976).

Regarding the question of hermaphroditic development in the face of a disseminated testis-inducer, Winters et al. (1979) have evidence that the ovotestis arises from an H-Y$^-$/H-Y$^+$ mosaic primordium: cells cultured from the ovarian portion of a scrotal ovotestis were typed H-Y$^-$; cells from the testicular portion were typed H-Y$^+$. Blood cells from the same patient, a 46,XX phenotypic "male" with gynecomastia, were typed H-Y$^+$. Thus it may be asked how H-Y is selectively excluded from a portion of the developing gonad.

Given abnormal presence of a testis-inducer, and given the original organogenetic dictate of the XX gonadal primordium, the gonad might be expected to differentiate towards either of two extremes: unambiguous ovary or unambiguous testis. The outcome would be determined by competition between factors promoting testicular differentiation (H-Y) and those promoting ovarian differentiation (an ovary-inducing molecule?). According to that scheme, general dominance of the testis-inducer would lead to development of the XX testis, and incomplete dominance (inconclusive competition), to the XX ovotestis. Indeed low levels of H-Y antigen have been detected in the *mothers* of 46,XX males homozygous for recessive H-Y genes (de la Chapelle et al., 1978). So there must be a threshold of H-Y expression above which the testis is induced, and below which it is not.

Factors blocking attachment of disseminated H-Y to its receptor (or anchorage site) would therefore be expected to promote ovarian differentiation in the developing XX gonad. Examples of possible blocking factors are: (a) molecules which compete with H-Y for anchorage sites; (b) molecules which prevent reaction of H-Y and its receptor; (c) receptors with low affinity for H-Y; (d) paucity of H-Y secretin cells (due to lyonization); (e) low levels of H-Y synthesis by a particular "constitutive-type"

66

mutant. Conversely factors favoring attachment of H-Y and its receptor would promote testicular differentiation. Examples are receptors with high affinity for H-Y; plenitude of H-Y-secreting cells, and so forth.

3.2.2. XX males. No doubt XX true hermaphroditism and XX male syndrome represent alternative facets of the same disorder. There are examples of both conditions within the same human sibship, and in dogs, Selden et al. (1978) discovered an XX male that had been whelped by an XX true hermaphrodite. Clinically, human 46,XX males resemble males with 47,XXY Klinefelter's syndrome, but in the former, as in 46,XX true hermaphrodites, one is confronted with paradoxical differentiation of testis in the absence of the Y-chromosome. If 46,XX male syndrome represents a more "complete" reversal of sex than 46,XX true hermaphroditism, one might expect a more positive H-Y phenotype in XX males than in XX true hermaphrodites. Certainly this is true in the gonad, and there is a hint that it may also be true in the somatic tissues (not *all* XX males that we have studied seem to have H-Y "intermediate" phenotypes). However it is not at all clear that a somatic H-Y phenotype accurately reflects the phenotype of the developing gonad; and as we have pointed out, differential expression of H-Y in the developing XX gonad could account for a range of phenotypes: from ovary, to ovotestis, to testis.

3.2.3. A note on gonadal growth rates. It has been suggested that the Y-chromosome determines sex by regulating the growth rate of the developing gonadal rudiment. According to one view, the gonad must reach a certain critical size at a particular stage of development to become a testis. Gonads failing to reach that size become ovaries instead (Mittwoch, 1977). In that connection, two points are worth noting: first, that in human fetuses, the gonads on the right side tend to be larger, containing more cells, than the gonads on the left; and second, that in human true hermaphrodites having different kinds of gonads (e.g. testis versus ovary, ovotestis versus ovary etc.) the more masculinized gonad tends to develop on the right. If the human testis is induced by a particular molecule, this kind of lateralism would indicate unilateral presence or absence of the molecule or its receptor. Why a particular molecule

should tend to be expressed on the right side is not clear. Indeed Mittwoch (1977) suggests that asymmetrical gonadal differentiation, and gonadal differentiation in general, cannot be explained in genetic terms, and should be expressed in so-called "epigenetic" or "developmental" terms instead.

3.3. H-Y antigen in XY sex reversal

Among humans, two X-chromosomes are required to sustain the differentiated ovary. In embryos with the 45,X karyotype (Turner's syndrome), ovarian development proceeds along normal lines during the first trimester of gestation, but the germ cells eventually die, the surrounding follicles become atretic, and the ovary is characteristically represented at around the time of birth by an endocrinologically inert tissue containing ovarian stroma but devoid of germ cells and follicles ("gonadal dysgenesis").

With respect to the number of X-chromosomes, embryos with the XY karyotype are like those with the "XO" karyotype. It follows that in cases of loss or mutational inactivation of the H-Y testis-determining portion of the Y, the 46,XY gonad should develop initially as an ovary, but because the second X-chromosome is missing, the ovary should degenerate, leading to the condition called XY pure gonadal dysgenesis ("pure", in the absence of the somatic stigmata of Turner's syndrome). Accordingly XY gonadal dysgenesis in man can be attributed to *functional absence* of the testis-inducer in gonadal cells bearing a single X-chromosome. By "functional absence" we refer to any of the following specific conditions (Table 5):

3.3.1. Suppressed production of H-Y antigen. We have already described X-chromosome-associated suppression of H-Y antigen synthesis in a $46,Xp^+Y$ female and in her $46,Xp^+Y$ female fetal sibling. This could be due to mutation of a structural element (direct loss of ability to synthesize H-Y) or alternatively, to mutation of a regulatory gene, in which case the Y-chromosome (or autosome) would be indirectly prevented from synthesizing H-Y.

3.3.2. Deletion of H-Y genes. It is said that the mammalian X-chromosome has remained essentially invariant in evolution while the Y has undergone

Table 5. Functional absence of H-Y antigen in 46,XY gonadal dysgenesis

Condition	Somatic H-Y phenotype	H-Y bound to specific gonadal receptor
Suppressed production of H-Y antigen	−(±)	−
Deletion of H-Y genes	−(±)*	−
Mosaicism	?**	−
Loss of receptor binding activity	+***	−
Mutational deficiency of receptor	+	−

* Presence or absence of H-Y indicated by (+) or (−); H-Y intermediate phenotypes have also been reported (Wolf, 1979).
** Presumably somatic expression of H-Y determined by frequency of antigen-positive cells as in XO/XY mosaic.
*** See description in text.

continued degeneration, losing most of its genetic material to become a specialized testis-inducer ("Ohno's Law"). Accordingly deletion (unbalanced loss) of a portion of the X-chromosome should prove lethal in an individual carrying only a single copy of the X, whereas loss of a portion of the Y should have no such effect, and indeed should not be expected to prejudice significantly the viability of the affected individual.

A case of Y-chromosome deletion involving testis-determining genes was reported recently by Rosenfeld et al. (1979). The proband was a phenotypic female with the karyotype: 46,XYp⁻ [signifying loss of part or all of the short arm of the Y-chromosome (Yp)]. External genitalia were normal. Laparotomy, performed when the patient was three months old, disclosed normal uterus and tubes, and small gonads bilaterally, containing fibrous stroma with aggregation of "undifferentiated cells" arranged in cords or circumscribed clusters. Neither follicles nor tubules were present.

The patient was re-evaluated at 9 years of age. Several of the somatic features of Turner's syndrome were apparent: mild webbing of the neck, low posterior hairline, cubitus valgus, broad chest, pigmented nevi, high arched palate, clinodactyly of the fifth digit. Levels of FSH (68 mIU/ml) and LH (24 mIU/ml) were elevated; this is often encountered in cases of gonadal dysgenesis. In addition baseline levels of testosterone (5 mg/dl) and estradiol (<10 pg/ml) were neither influenced by administration of human chorionic gonadotropin.

In serological tests, skin fibroblasts from the patient did not absorb H-Y antibodies and were typed H-Y⁻; blood leukocytes were also typed H-Y⁻ although it was not possible to rule out the possibility of residual absorption in one test (see footnote to Table 3). The data signify either absence of H-Y, or expression well below the critical threshold required for testicular differentiation. The data are consistent with location of H-Y structural genes on the X or on the Y. (Residual expression of H-Y in cells carrying a partially deleted Y could reflect loss of a critical majority of genes from a *family* of structural elements; see discussion in Wachtel and Koo, in press.)

3.3.3. Mosaicism. Sex chromosome mosaicism is often encountered in individuals with aberrant sexual development. Thus the karyotype 45,X/46,XY (for example) may be expected in a proportion of phenotypic females with gonadal dysgenesis. The etiology seems straightforward: in the presence of a majority of XO cells, the gonad develops along ovarian lines with eventual degeneration, as indicated above. Yet the question arises what constitutes a "majority" in this case, as XY gonadal cells ostensibly secrete H-Y, thereby inducing neighboring cells to organize a testis, whatever their karyotype. Given XO/XY mosaicism as a factor in gonadal dysgenesis, the H-Y phenotype of blood cells could conceivably vary from negative to positive depending on the frequency of XY bearing cells in a particular sample or individual. Thus the H-Y phenotype of blood need not indicate a corresponding differentiative state of the gonad. In collaboration with O.J. Miller (unpublished) we studied a female patient with 46,XY blood leukocytes and H-Y⁺ phenotype. Examination of fibroblasts from one of the streak gonads of this patients revealed only 45,X cells.

3.3.4. Loss of receptor binding activity. A mutant H-Y has now been described in vitro (Iwata et al., 1979). The mutant protein is secreted by a variant line of cultured Daudi cells. It has retained its antigenic determinants, and is therefore identified by H-Y antibody, but it has lost receptor-binding activity, and is therefore inert functionally. These observations suggest that the active site and the antigenic site of the H-Y molecule are discrete, that there may be a single H-Y structural locus (in this

Daudi genome at least), and that a similar in vivo mutation could generate a form of XY gonadal dysgenesis in an H-Y$^+$ propositus. The last suggestion may be tested: mutant H-Y secreted in a dysgenetic gonad should react with H-Y antibody in an absorption assay, but it should fail to inhibit attachment of "normal" H-Y in a receptor binding assay.

3.3.5. Mutational deficiency of the H-Y receptor. Absence or mutation of the gonadal H-Y receptor is tantamount to absence of the testis inducer itself, H-Y$^+$ cellular phenotype notwithstanding. About two-thirds of all cases of 46,XY gonadal dysgenesis that have been reported have been typed H-Y$^+$ in blood cells or skin fibroblasts. It is tempting to attribute the H-Y$^+$ phenotype in these cases to presence of membrane-associated molecules of H-Y (bound to plasma membrane anchorage sites), and to attribute the failure of testicular development to mutation of the gonad-specific H-Y receptor.

Many dysgenetic XY gonads contain male elements: fitful tubules, clusters of "Leydig-like" cells, etc. Residual male differentiation in the 46,XY dysgenetic gonad could be induced by residual specific attachment of H-Y, or perhaps even by the mere presence of membrane-associated H-Y. There is a high incidence of gonadal malignancy (gonadoblastoma, dysgerminoma) among cases of 46,XY gonadal dysgenesis. Many of these tumors are notable for presence of testicular elements of the sort just described.

4. CLINICAL H-Y TESTING AND ITS SIGNIFICANCE

The sperm cytotoxicity test that was use in our laboratory is one of several techniques available for detection of human H-Y antigen. For reasons that are not clear, normal white blood cells cannot be used directly as targets for H-Y antibody-mediated cytotoxicity, and must be used instead in indirect absorption assays (Wachtel and Koo, in press). Direct assays are available, using fluorescence for example, but these have met with limited success. Thus for reasons of reliability and convenience, we continue to count heavily on the sperm cytotoxicity test, and other similar assays, the mixed hemadsorption-hybrid antibody test and the protein A-

sheep red blood cell test, with an eye to new radioimmunoassays, now evidently close at hand. It should be emphasized that tests in current use are technically formidable and require expert personnel that have been specially trained. Still the assays provide a measure of presence and function of testis-determining genes and evidence for presence or absence of the testis determining portion of the Y-chromosome.

4.1. Presence of testis-determining genes

Expression of H-Y antigen in a female is almost always a sign of abnormality. Although we have registered occasional "false-positive" results, these are amended with repeated testing, and H-Y$^+$ phenotypes in female blood or skin fibroblasts generally indicate aberrant differentiation of the gonad. A remarkable example is the XX female carrying autosomal "recessive" testis-determining genes. Despite the fact that they are obligatory H-Y$^+$ heterozygotes, such females can be fertile. But three that have been identified are the mothers of "recessively-determined" XX males (de la Chapelle et al., 1978).

More characteristically, study of H-Y antigen in a phenotypic female might now provide a fuller understanding of sexual abnormality than was possible before the advent of H-Y typing. Thus absence of H-Y in an XYp$^-$ female with gonadal dysgenesis signals loss of testis-determining genes, whereas presence of H-Y in an XY female with gonadal dysgenesis signals loss of binding ability; and it is now within our grasp to determine whether the latter might be due to a mutational defect of the testis-inducer or its specific receptor.

4.2. Presence of the Y-chromosome

To the extent that there may be structural genes for H-Y antigen on the X-chromosome or on an autosome, mere expression of H-Y does not guarantee presence in the genome of Y-chromosomal material. Yet when a Y is indicated by cytogenetic analysis, serology may provide a more finely resolved picture of just what part of the Y it is. Consider for example the 46,X,i(Yq) female referred to in Table 2. Absence of H-Y in that case would seem to confirm loss of Yp. Whether or not this bears on the increased risk of gonadal malignancy in phenotypic females carrying portions of the Y-chromosome remains to be ascertained. And it may now be asked whether the increased risk of malignancy is correlated with presence of the Y per se or with that part carrying H-Y genes.

ACKNOWLEDGEMENTS

Supported in part by grants from the NIH AI-11982, CA-08748, HD-00171, HD-10065, and from the National Foundation – March of Dimes Birth Defects Foundation (6-247).

REFERENCES

Bernstein R, Koo GC, Wachtel SS (1980) Abnormality of the X chromosome in human 46,XY female siblings with dysgenetic ovaries. Science 207: 768.

de la Chapelle A, Koo GC, Wachtel SS (1978) Recessive sex-determining genes in human XX male syndrome. Cell 15: 837.

Eichwald EJ, Silmser CR (1955) Untitled communication. Transplant Bull 2: 148.

Flaherty L, Zimmerman D, Wachtel SS (1979) H-Y antigen: cell surface mapping and testosterone-induced supramolecular repatterning. J Exp Med 150: 1020.

Imperato-McGinley J, Guerrero L, Gautier T, Peterson RE (1974) Steroid 5α-reductase deficiency in man: an inherited form of male pseudohermaphroditism. Science 186: 1213.

Iwata H, Nagai Y, Stapleton DD, Smith RC, Ohno S (1979) Identification of human H-Y antigen and its testis-organizing function. Arthritis and Rheumatism 22: 1211.

Jost A (1970) Hormonal factors in the sex differentiation of the mammalian foetus. Phil Trans Soc Lond B 259: 119.

Kaye CI, Wachtel S, Rosenthal IM (1976) H-Y antigen in 2 patients with XYq-karyotype with female and male phenotypes. Clin Res 24: 568A.

Koo GC, Wachtel SS, Krupen-Brown K, Mittl LR, Breg WR. Genel M, Rosenthal IM, Borgaonkar DS, Miller DA, Tantravahi R, Schreck RR, Erlanger BF, Miller OJ (1977a) Mapping the locus of the H-Y gene on the human Y chromosome. Science 198: 940.

Koo GC, Wachtel SS, Saenger PS, New MI, Dosik H, Amarose AP, Dorus E, Ventruto V (1977b) H-Y antigen: expression in human subjects with the testicular feminization syndrome. Science 196: 655.

Krco CJ, Goldberg EH (1976) Detection of H-Y (male) antigen on 8-cell mouse embryos. Science 193: 1134.

MacDonald PC, Madden JD, Brenner PF, Wilson JD, Siiteri PK (1979) Origin of estrogen in normal men and in women with testicular feminization. J Clin Endocrinol Metab 49: 905.

Mittwoch U (1977) H-Y antigen and the growth of the dominant gonad. J Med Genet 14: 335.

Morris JM (1953) The syndrome of testicular feminization in male pseudohermaphrodites. Am J Obstet Gynecol 65: 1192.

Moscona A (1961) Rotation-mediated histogenic aggregation of dissociated cells. Exp Cell Res 22: 455.

Muller U Testis-determining H-Y antigen and the induction of the HCG receptor. In Segal SJ, ed. Chorionic gonadotropin. New York: Plenum (in press).

Muller U, Wolf U (1979) Discussion note on the paper of S.S. Wachtel of "H-Y antigen in the functional female". Ann Biol Anim Biochim Biophys 19: 1239.

Muller U, Zenzes MT, Bauknecht T, Wolf U, Siebers JW, Engel W (1978) Appearance of hCG-receptor after conversion of newborn ovarian cells into testicular structures by H-Y antigen in vitro. Hum Genet 45: 203.

Muller U, Zenzes MT, Wolf U, Engel W, Weniger J-P (1979) Appearance of H-W (H-Y) antigen in the gonads of oestradiol sex-reversed male chicken embryos. Nature 280: 142.

New MI (1970) Male pseudohermaphroditism due to 17α-hydroxylase deficiency. J Clin Invest 49: 1930.

Ohno S (1977) The original function of MHC antigens as the general plasma membrane anchorage site of organogenesis-directing proteins. Immunol Rev 33: 59.

Ohno S (1979) Major sex-determining genes. New York: Springer-Verlag.

Ohno S, Nagai Y, Ciccarese S, Iwata H (1979) Testis-organizing H-Y antigen and the primary sex-determining mechanism of mammals. Rec Prog Horm Res 35: 449.

Rosenfeld RG, Luzzatti L, Hintz RL, Miller OJ, Koo GC, Wachtel SS (1979) Sexual and somatic determinants of the human Y chromosome: studies in a 46XYp⁻ phenotypic female. Am J Hum Genet 31: 458.

Saenger P, Levine LS, Wachtel SS, Korth-Schutz C, Doberne Y, Koo GC, Lavengood RW, German JL, New MI (1976) Presence of H-Y antigen and testis in 46XX true hermaphroditism. Evidence for Y-chromosomal function. J Clin Endocrinol Metab 43: 1234.

Selden JR, Wachtel SS, Koo GC, Haskins ME, Patterson DF (1978) Genetic basis of XX male syndrome and XX true hermaphroditism: evidence in the dog. Science 201: 644.

Simpson JL (1976) Disorders of sexual differentiation. Etiology and clinical delineation. New York: Academic Press.

van Niekerk WA (1974) True hermaphroditism. Clinical, morphologic and cytogenetic aspects, pp 6–16. Hagerstown, MD: Harper & Row.

Wachtel SS (1977) H-Y antigen: genetics and serology. Immunol Rev 33: 33.

Wachtel SS, Bard J. The XX testis. In Josso N, ed. The intersex child Basel: S. Karger (in press).

Wachtel SS, Koo GS. H-Y antigen in gonadal differentiation. In Austin CR, Edwards RG, eds. Mechanisms of sex differentiation in animals and man. London: Academic Press (in press).

Wachtel SS, Ohno S, Koo GC, Boyse EA (1975) Possible role for H-Y antigen in the primary determination of sex. Nature 257: 235.

Wachtel SS, Koo GC, de la Chapelle A, Kallio H, Heyman SM, Miller OJ (1980) H-Y antigen in the 46,XY gonadal dysgenesis. Hum Genet 54: 25.

Wilson JD, Griffin JE, George FW (1979) The mechanism of phenotypic sex differentiation. Arthritis and Rheumatism 22: 1275.

Wilson JD, MacDonald PC (1978) Male pseudohermaphroditism due to androgen resistance: testicular feminization and related syndromes. In Stanbury JB, Wyngaarden JB, Fredrickson DS, eds. The metabolic basis of inherited disease, 4 ed, pp 894–913. New York: McGraw-Hill.

Winters SJ, Wachtel SS, White BJ, Koo GC, Javadpour N, Loriaux L, Sherins RJ (1979) H-Y antigen mosaicism in the gonad of a 46,XX true hermaphrodite. New Engl J Med 300: 745.

Wolf U (1979) XY gonadal dysgenesis and the H-Y antigen. Hum Genet 47: 269.

8. ABNORMAL SEXUAL DEVELOPMENT: A CLASSIFICATION WITH EMPHASIS ON PATHOLOGY AND NEOPLASTIC CONDITIONS

WILLIAM R. WELCH and STANLEY J. ROBBOY

1. INTRODUCTION

Recent advances in chromosome analysis and increased understanding of the principles of sexual development have stimulated interest in problems of intersex and encouraged identification and treatment of the intersexual patient at an early age so as to permit a more normal life. The present classification of abnormal sexual development (Table 1) has been developed as an outgrowth of a lecture series given at the Massachusetts General Hospital and Harvard Medical School. It is based upon gonadal and genital anatomy, chromosomal composition and specific identifiable genetic or metabolic defects, and has the advantage that it presents the spectrum of intersexual conditions in a comprehensive manner, while grouping those classes of patients who are at high risk for development of neoplasia if their gonads are not removed prophylactically.

2. GENERAL PRINCIPLES OF SEXUAL DEVELOPMENT

The normal development of the male and female genital tracts is determined by several factors, all of which are time-specific during embryogenesis (Fig. 1). First, the differentiation of the indifferent gonad into a testis or ovary is determined by the sex chromosomes (Short, 1979). Approximately three weeks after fertilization, primitive germ cells migrate from the yolk sac to the urogenital ridge (indifferent gonad) via the hindgut. If the germ cell is male, H-Y antigen, which is located on the nuclear membrane and is a protein under control of the Y chromosome, interacts with the somatic cells in the primitive gonad and initiates the development of seminiferous tubules (Wachtel, 1979). A gene of the X chromosome may be required in addition. The testis is anatomically distinct with early tubular formation by the 44th day (which precedes by 5 weeks the beginning of ovarian differentiation, i.e. development of primordial follicles).

Second, the Sertoli cells of the testis produce Müllerian Inhibiting Substance (MIS), a polypeptide protein that causes regression of the Müllerian (paramesonephric) ducts. In the absence of this substance the Müllerian ducts develop passively to form the Fallopian tubes, uterus and upper vagina. Although MIS is first secreted in an effective

Table 1. Classification of abnormal sexual development*

I. Disorders with apparently normal sex chromosomes
    A. Female pseudohermaphroditism
        1. Adrenogenital syndrome
        2. Treatment of mother with progestins or androgens
        3. Maternal virilizing tumor
    B. Male pseudohermaphroditism
        1. Primary central nervous system (CNS) defect
            a. Abnormal gonadotropin secretion
            b. No gonadotropin secretion
        2. Primary gonadal defect
            a. Testicular regression syndrome (gonadal destruction)
            b. Leydig cell agenesis
            c. Defect in testosterone synthesis identifiable
            d. Defect in Müllerian Inhibiting System
        3. End-organ defect
            a. Androgen insensitivity syndrome (testicular feminization)
            b. 5α-reductase deficienty
II. Disorders associated with obviously abnormal sex chromosomes
    A. Sexual ambiguity unusual
        1. Klinefelter's syndrome
        2. Turner's syndrome
    B. Sexual ambiguity frequent
        1. Mixed gonadal dysgenesis
        2. True hermaphroditism

* "Idiopathic" or "unclassified" conditions exist within each major category.

72

amount 62 days after fertilization and the process of Müllerian regression is normally completed by day 77, the testis is capable of MIS production at progressively lower levels through the first two years of postnatal life. MIS has a local inhibiting action on the ipsilateral Fallopian tube. To prevent development of the uterus and vagina, both testes must secrete adequate amounts of MIS. Thus, a patient with a testis and a contralateral streak, ovary, or ovo-testis generally has a uterus, vagina and contralateral Fallopian tube.

Third, testosterone is required for differentiation of the Wolffian (mesonephric duct) into epididymis, vas deferens, and seminal vesicle. The Leydig cells appear in the testis at day 64 and begin to produce testosterone on about day 71. The activity of the Leydig cells is probably related to the increased production of chorionic gonadotropin from the placenta at that time. Testosterone acts locally on the ipsilateral Wolffian duct. In the absence of a testis, or inability of a testis to produce testosterone, or insensitivity of the Wolffian duct anlage to testosterone, differentiation of the epididymis, vas deferens and seminal vesicle does not occur. Only rarely are abnormally elevated levels (often maternal in origin) reached early enough in embryogenesis in a female fetus to cause differentiation of the duct into definitive male organs (androgen administration to the mother during pregnancy, or congenital adrenogenital syndrome).

Fourth, development of masculine external genitalia and differentiation of the prostate are dependent not directly on testosterone, but on its local conversion to dihydrotestosterone (DHT). DHT causes the genital tubercle to enlarge and form the glans penis, the genital folds to enlarge and fuse (to form the penile shaft with migration of the urethral orifice along the lower border of the shaft to the tip of the glans), and produces fusion of the genital swellings to form a scrotum. This hormone also causes differentiation of the prostate from the urogenital sinus. An absence of male development of the external genitalia in the presence of testes may be due to a lack of adequate testosterone secretion into the systemic circulation, deficient enzyme (5α-reductase) at the end-organ level to convert testosterone to DHT, or complete end-organ insensitivity (testicular feminization). Lesser degrees of deficiency or end-organ insensitivity may result in only partial male development characterized by a small penis, hypospadias, deficient formation of the scrotum, or a persistent urogenital sinus (vaginal opening into urethra). The effects of DHT begin about day 70 with fusion of the labioscrotal folds and closure of the median raphe, and at day 74 closure of the urethral groove. Development of the external genitalia is complete by day 120–140 (18th–20th week).

Fifth, female internal organs and external genitalia develop without a need for hormones secreted by the fetal ovary and differentiate even when gonads are absent. Unless interrupted by the re-

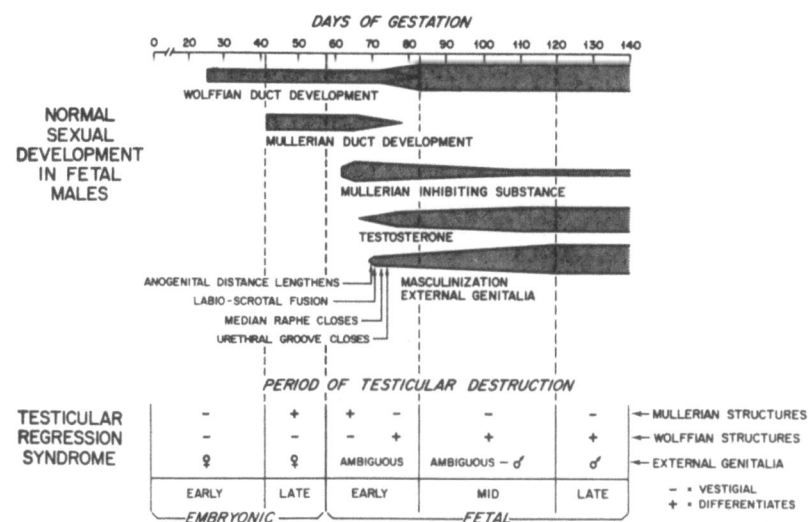

Figure 1. Normal sexual development in the male and application in testicular regression syndrome.

gressive influence of MIS, differentiation of the Müllerian ducts proceeds cephalocaudally to form Fallopian tubes, a uterus and a vagina. In the absence of the masculinizing effect of DHT, the external undifferentiated genitalia develop along feminine lines into a vulva. The genital tubercle develops into the clitoris, the genital folds into the labia minora and the genital swellings into the labia majora. Thus, the infant with ovaries or streak gonads has female internal and external genitalia at birth. Only in the female fetus with systemically elevated levels of androgens prior to the 10th to 12th week of gestation do varying degrees of masculine development occur; the external genitalia of an infant may appear to be ambiguous or that of a normal phenotypic male with a penis, but in which the vagina opens into the membranous portion of the urethra. If the androgens are not elevated until after the 20th week, by which time the external genitalia have fully formed, the only masculinizing defect is enlargement of the clitoris.

3. DISORDERS WITH APPARENTLY NORMAL SEX CHROMOSOMES

Specific genetic defects not detectable by usual chromosome analyis and intrauterine exposure of the fetus to virilizing hormones are responsible for the developmental defects of individuals in this category. Female pseudohermaphrodites must be 46,XX and male pseudohermaphrodites 46,XY to be included in this category. The gonads are usually recognizable grossly in the adult as ovary or testis, except in the case of testicular regression.

3.1. Female pseudohermaphroditism

Female pseudohermaphroditism is defined as a congenital state of relative androgen excess in an individual with two gross ovaries and female sex chomosomes (46,XX). The abnormal levels of androgen present during embryogenesis usually result in genital ambiguity but may result in the appearance of a phenotypic male.

3.1.1. Adrenogenital syndrome. Of all conditions responsible for the appearance of ambiguous genitalia in the newborn, congenital adrenal hyperplasia

is singular in that the lack of specific adrenal steroids may threaten the life of the patient and yet, with therapy, normal external genitalia and fertility can be achieved. Although the deficiency of any of seven specific adrenal enzymes involved in the synthesis of glucocorticoids and minerlo-corticoids can give rise to the condition, deficiencies of only two of these enzymes, 21-hydroxylase and 11β-hydroxylase, cause elevated levels of androgenic intermediates and in some cases ambiguity of genitalia in the newborn female. Deficiency of 3β-hydroxysteroid dehydrogenase is associated with clitoral hypertrophy but not with labial fusion or anterior displacement of the urethral orifice.

21-hydroxylase deficiency accounts for more than 95% of cases of congenital adrenal hyperplasia, occurs once in 50,000 births and is inherited as an autosomal recessive. In the female the clitoris may be enlarged; if androgen excess was present earlier than the 16th week of gestation, the vagina and urethra may open into a common urogenital sinus. More marked enlargement of the clitoris and an opening of the urogenital sinus at the base of the clitoris may mimic penile hypospadias and suggest an even earlier temporal effect. On occasion the changes have been of such severity that the female infants have been misdiagnosed as cryptorchid males with or without hypospadias.

Males who lack the enzyme have no evidence of genital ambiguity but may have an enlarged phallus and a hyperpigmented rugated scrotum. Bilateral testicular tumefactions may develop rarely and are composed of interstitial cells resembling Leydig cells or cells of adrenal rest origin (Fig. 2) (Kirkland et al., 1977).

3.1.2. Administration of progestins or androgens to the mother. Maternal ingestion of synthetic progestins was implicated as a cause of female pseudohermaphroditism in the late 1950s when such treatment was employed for threatened or habitual abortion; more recently, progestins have also been implicated in the development of hypospadias in male offspring (Aarskog, 1979).

Most cases of female pseudohermaphroditism in this category develop after the oral ingestion of Ethisterone (17α-ethinyl-testosterone) or Norlutin (17α-ethinyl-19-Nortestosterone), but occasionally after the ingestion of Enovid, diethylstilbestrol or

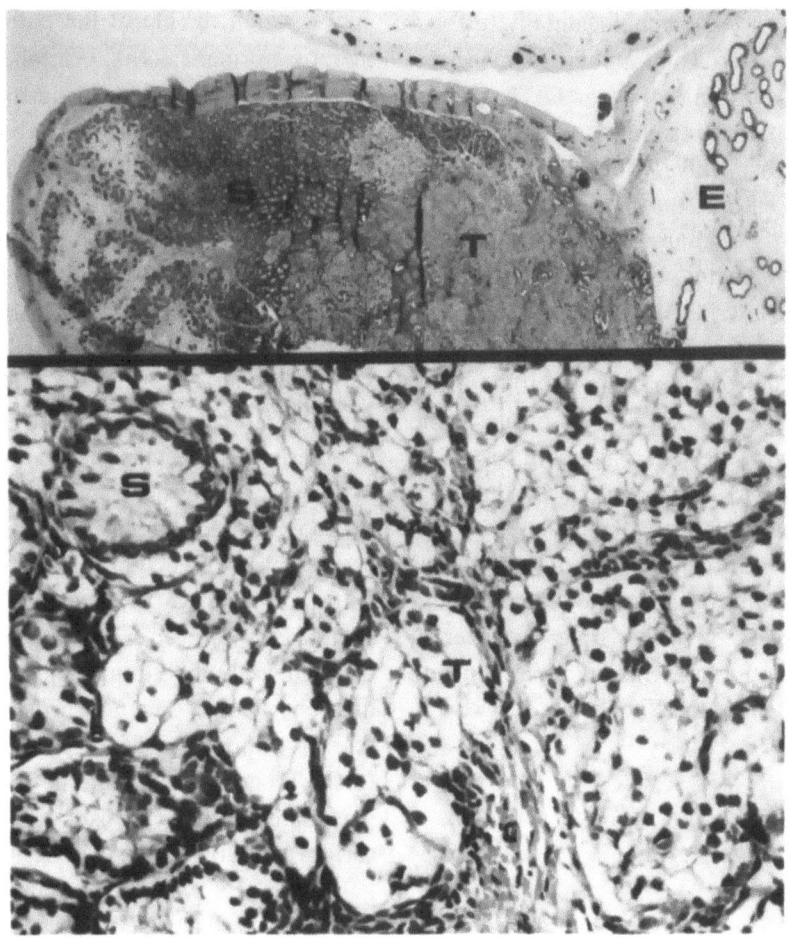

Figure 2. Interstitial cell tumor of the testis in a 4-year-old infant with adrenogenital syndrome. The tumor cells (T), which are illustrated at high magnification adjacent to immature seminiferous tubules (S) in the inset, resemble adrenocortical cells more closely than Leydig cells. The epididymis (E) is adjacent to the testis. (H&E, ×16, ×350.)

androgens or the intramuscular administration of progesterone (Wilkins, 1960). Masculinization usually consists of phallic enlargement and variable degrees of labio-scrotal fusion, depending on the time during gestation when the therapy was administered. Although the degree of masculinization is usually less than that associated with the adrenogenital syndrome, in some instances the sexual ambiguity in female infants has been of such severity to result in male sex assignment. The degree of virilization does not progress with age. The gonads and internal genital organs are unaffected, and ovulation, menstruation and normal secondary feminine characteristics appear at puberty.

3.1.3. Maternal virilizing tumor. A variety of tumors, both primary in, as well as metastatic to, the ovary have been associated with virilization of the mother and her female offspring (Haymond and Weldon, 1973). The luteoma of pregnancy, which is the most common tumor that causes maternal virilization during pregnancy, is a benign tumefaction of the ovary. It is most often encountered as an incidental finding at the time of cesarean section or postpartum sterilization, usually in women who are multiparous and black. Elevated levels of chorionic gonadotropin are thought to induce hyperplasia of theca-lutein or stroma-lutein cells. A small percentage of the female infants have become masculinized, with mild enlargement of the clitoris and occasionally minimal degrees of labio-scrotal fusion or rugate, hyperpigmented ("scrotal") labia. The nature of these changes indicates that the ovarian nodules do not function until the second half of gestation, which is in accord with the occasional onset of signs of masculinization in the mother during the third trimester.

At operation, one and often both maternal ovaries are enlarged by one or more soft, yellow-brown nodules that are well circumscribed but not encapsulated (Sternberg and Dhurandhar, 1977). Although most of them are less than 2 cm in diameter, they may be as large as 20 cm in greatest dimension. On microscopical examiniation, the nodules consist of large, polygonal cells with granular eosinophilic cytoplasm which are smaller and more eosinophilic than the luteinized granulosa cells of the corpus luteum but larger than the theca-lutein cells. Intracellular lipid is sparse, if at all present. Mitoses may be observed, but only rarely are they numerous.

Elevated levels of plasma (and tissue) testosterone, dihydrotestosterone, androstenedione and dihydroepiandrosterone have been detected in virilized patients; the plasma levels return to normal once the tumor is extirpated. Even without treatment, the nodules regress or disappear shortly after delivery (Malinak and Miller, 1963). A reappearance of the luteoma has been reported in only one patient during a subsequent pregnancy.

3.2. Male pseudohermaphroditism

Male pseudohermaphroditism is characterized by the combination of apparently normal chromosomes (46,XY), gross testes, or evidence that the testes were present during fetal development, and a state of relative or absolute androgen deficiency. The external genitalia are usually feminine or ambiguous, although in certain categories the genetic defect results in phenotypic male external genitalia.

3.2.1. Primary CNS defect. Park et al. (1975) have described this rare condition, in which there are relatively few pathological findings of the genitalia.

3.2.2. Primary gonadal defect. These conditions are associated with regression (destruction) of the gonads or their anlage during embryonic or fetal life, testes with Leydig cell agenesis, and testes with specific enzymatic defects in testosterone synthesis

or elaboration of Müllerian Inhibiting Substance (MIS).

Testicular regression syndrome. Recently Coulam (1979) introduced the concept of the testicular regression syndrome to bring together under one umbrella a variety of conditions where testes are thought to have regressed at some point during prenatal life. The various names given in the earlier literature to aspects of the syndrome ("pure gonadal dysgenesis"*, Swyer's syndrome, true agonadism, testicular dysgenesis, rudimentary testis, vanishing testis, complete bilateral anorchia) denote the constellation of findings that reflect the probable time of gonadal destruction during gestation. The key features of the testicular regression syndrome reflect the timing of gonadal regression in relation to the development of the urogenital ridge and Müllerian ducts, the appearance of Sertoli cells and subsequent synthesis and secretion of Müllerian Inhibiting Substance, and the development of Leydig cells capable of testosterone secretion. Regression of the testes during the critical periods for each of these events results in a slightly different phenotypic expression and a spectrum of differentiation or atrophy of internal genital structures (Fig. 1).

At one end of the spectrum, the external genitalia are feminine, the internal genital organs are absent, and the gonads are streaks. Presumably, the urogenital ridge was destroyed in its entirety during the early embryonic period before the anlage of the Müllerian or Wolffian ducts began to differentiate (i.e., prior to day 43).

At the other end of the spectrum, which is close to the end point of normal genital development, the patients are phenotypic males with infantile to nearly normal male external genitalia, normally differentiated Wolffian duct structures and inhibited Müllerian duct development. Testicular regression presumably occurred during the late fetal period (after 120 days) when Müllerian structures had already atrophied under the influence of Müllerian Inhibiting Substance and testosterone and dihydrotestosterone had exerted a major influence in the normal development of internal and external genitalia.

---

* Pure gonadal dysgenesis is a category which may represent several distinct disorders (Brøgger and Strand, 1965). Some but not all of the patients with pure gonadal dysgenesis should be included in the testicular regression syndrome.

Intermediate in the spectrum are patients with genital ambiguity and various combinations of Wolffian and/or Müllerian duct development. If the testes regress during the late embryonic period (day 43–59), testosterone will not have been synthesized and Wolffian structures will not have developed. The production of Müllerian Inhibiting Substance will have been variable resulting in poorly differentiated Müllerian structures or rudiments thereof. In the absence of systemic androgens, the external genitalia appear feminine.

Regression of the testes during the early fetal period (day 59–84) after Sertoli cell (Müllerian Inhibiting Substance) and Leydig cell (testosterone) function have begun or are about to begin results in an individual with ambiguous external genitalia and various combinations of Wolffian and Müllerian development depending upon the duration of androgen secretion and Müllerian inhibition.

Regression of the testes during the mid-fetal period (day 90–120) results in more advanced masculinization of the external genitalia, although degrees of ambiguity are usually present. Since Müllerian duct inhibition is normally completed by day 80, the Müllerian structures will have been suppressed; Wolffian structures are developed.

Leydig cell agenesis. These cases are very rare (Berthezene et al., 1976).

Defects in testosterone synthesis. Congenital deficiency of any enzyme involved in the production of testosterone in the testis or adrenal gland (20- and 22-hydroxylases, 22-desmolase, 3β-hydroxysteroid dehydrogenase and isomerase, 17α-hydroxylase, 17,20-desmolase and 17 ketosteroid reductase) results in a state of relative estrogen excess. The degree to which the external genitalia fail to develop normally depends upon the severity of the defect.

Defect in Müllerian inhibiting system. The persistent Müllerian duct syndrome, also known as "hernia uteri inguinalis," is a rare familial condition in which 46,XY phenotypic males with unilateral or bilateral cryptorchid testes and normal, or almost normal, masculine external genitalia have an inguinal hernia into which prolapse an infantile uterus and Fallopian tubes (Weiss et al., 1979). The pubertal development is normal; a rare patient has

been fertile. If at operation any patient has a streak gonad or a tumor rather than bilateral testes, the diagnosis of mixed gonadal dysgenesis should be considered. The underlying defect in the persistent Müllerian duct syndrome relates theoretically to deficient synthesis of Müllerian Inhibiting Substance, synthesis of a biologically inactive compound, abnormality in the timing of its secretion, or end-organ resistance.

3.2.3. End-organ defects. The normal development of the male derivatives of Wolffian duct origin (epididymis, vas deferens, seminal vesicle) and the external genitalia requires that both are responsive to androgen and the latter can bind and convert testosterone to dihydrotestosterone. If the androgen binding system is disordered, e.g. because of an unstable receptor or lack of a receptor (testicular feminization syndrome), neither internal nor external genital organs respond normally (Griffin and Wilson, 1980). If only 5α-reductase, the hormone which converts testosterone to dihydrotestosterone, is absent, the abnormalities in the reproductive tract are confined to the external genitalia and prostate.

Androgen insensitivity syndrome (testicular feminization). Testicular feminization is the most common form of male pseudohermaphroditism. In the complete form the external genitalia show unambiguous female differentiation for which reason the condition is rarely diagnosed before puberty unless an inguinal hernia or a labial mass is encountered or the disease is familial. The most common chief complaint is primary amenorrhea. The history usually reveals that breast development occurred normally at puberty. Pubic and axillary hair are scant, the vagina is short and the uterus and cervix are absent, as are the epididymides, vasa deferentia and seminal vesicles. The testes are cryptorchid and located in the inguinal canal, the pelvis or rarely the labia.

The gonad uninvolved by nodular growths is usually small and on section is tan to brown and traversed by thin white bands. A 1–2 cm firm, white nodule of hyalinized smooth muscle is present at one pole of the gonad and may represent abnormally hypertrophied gubernaculum. Microscopical examination of the testicular parenchyma discloses seminiferous tubules that are immature and usually sparsely distributed or clustered in small aggregates, sometimes on a background of stroma resembling ovarian stroma. Spermatogonia may be present but spermatogenesis is absent. Leydig cells may be abundant and resemble fetal Leydig cells.

The majority of testes contain multiple nodules that are discrete, yellow to brown, firm, and bulge above the sectioned surface of the testis (Fig. 3A). Most vary from about a millimeter to one centimeter, but some have been as large as 25 cm (Case Records, 1977). The nodules are almost always composed of solid tubules with Sertoli cells; spermatogonia may be present on occasion (Fig. 3B). Leydig cells are frequently present in the interstitium among the tubules and may form relatively pure stromal nodules which on a rare occasion may attain a size of over 1 cm and be considered as a Leydig cell tumor. In addition, the interstitium may contain stroma resembling ovarian stroma (Fig. 3C). Depending upon the components which are present, the nodules are classified as harmartoma, Sertoli cell adenoma, or rarely as Leydig cell tumor.

Atypical germ cells and even seminoma in situ may be observed within the tubules and are the source of the seminoma that is the second most frequent neoplasm, but most common cancer, in the gonad of patients with testicular feminization. Unlike mixed gonadal dysgenesis where tumors can develop in young individuals, the risk of malignancy in patients with testicular feminization is only 4% by the age of 25 years (Manuel et al., 1976). It reaches 33% by 50 years. Since tumors rarely develop until after puberty has been completed, castration can be delayed until after adolescence to permit the patients to undergo a normal pubertal spurt and develop feminine secondary sex characteristics at the expected time of puberty.

About 10% of patients have partial expression of the androgen insensitivity syndrome (incomplete testicular feminization), which to date has been associated only with thermo-unstable type of receptor (Griffin and Wilson, 1980). Individuals vary in the degree of masculinization of external or internal organs. Since virilization may accompany breast development in some individuals at puberty, gonadectomy should be performed before the expected time of puberty in prepubertal patients.

Although most patients who have disorders of androgen receptors have a female phenotype, some patients have the appearance of phenotypic males.

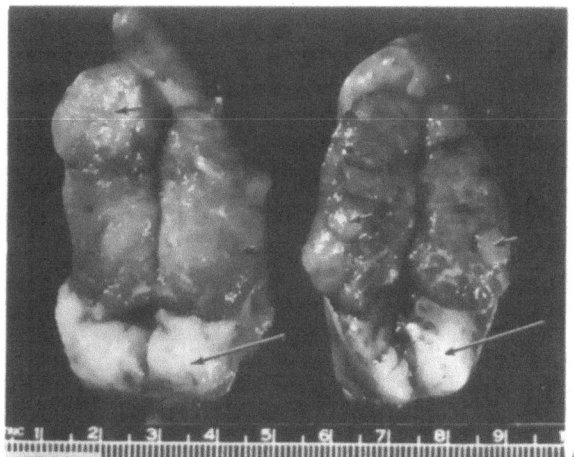

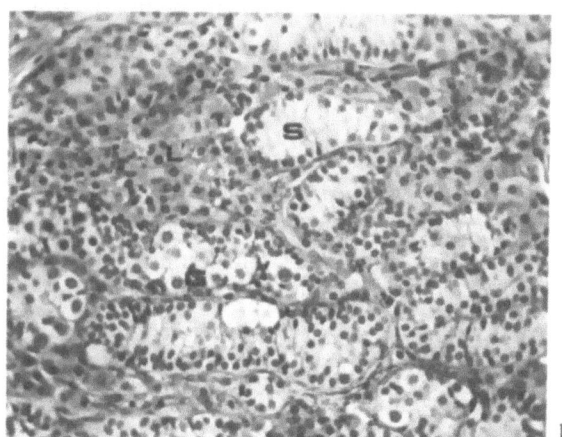

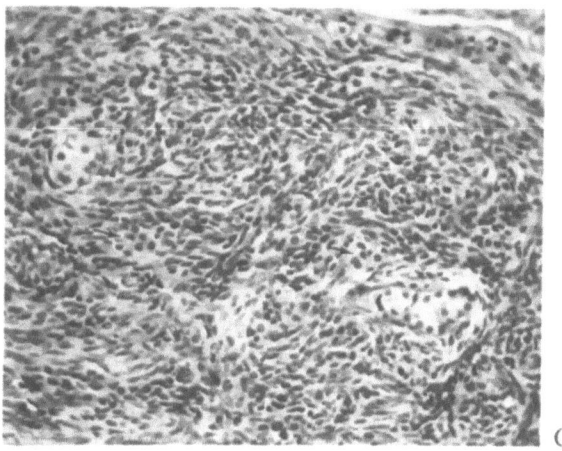

Figure 3. (*A*) Testis in a 17-year-old with testicular feminization syndrome. Numerous Sertoli cell adenomas (short arrows) are present in the parenchyma. The mass near one pole (long arrow) may represent an abnormally hypertrophied gubernaculum. (*B*) Hamartoma with immature seminiferous tubules (S), numerous germ cells (G), and numerous Leydig cells (L) in the interstitium. (H&E, × 175.) (*C*) Testis of testicular feminization syndrome with scattered immature seminiferous tubules embedded in a dense ovarian type cortical stroma. Occasional interstitial cells (arrows) are present, (H&E × 175.)

Various aspects of this syndrome, collectively called Reifenstein syndrome, have been described by Reifenstein, Lubs, Gilbert-Dreyfus, Rosewater and their associates. The range of features include hypospadias, breast development at puberty, feminine habitus, azoospermia and sometimes absence or hypoplasia of Wolffian duct structures. The mildest form of androgen insensitivity is represented by infertile males with gynecomastia who have no evidence of abnormal development of either internal or external genitalia.

The most likely mode of inheritance of testicular feminization is X-linked recessive. In the Reifenstein syndrome, additional, but as yet unidentified, factors that modify the androgen action in vivo are suspected, since various members within a family can display a spectrum of clinical abnormalities and yet have the same degree of receptor abnormality in in vitro assays.

5α-reducatse deficiency. This is a familial form of male pseudohermaphroditism in which the target organs cannot reduce testosterone, the prohormone, to dihydrotestosterone (DHT), the hormone that masculinizes the indifferent urogenital sinus (Imperato-McGinley et al., 1979). The disorder is transmitted as an autosomal recessive and is unique as an inherited disorder of steroid metabolism in that the carrier state is detectable.

Affected males have phenotypic female to ambiguous external genitalia at birth. The small clitoris-like phallus lacks a urethral orifice. In most affected individuals, the urogenital sinus opens on the perineum and within the sinus an anterior orifice leads to the urethra and a posterior orifice to a blind vaginal pouch. The testes are in the inguinal canal or labia. The Müllerian derived structures are absent whereas the vas deferens, epididymis and seminal vesicle, the anlage of which respond to testosterone, are developed normally.

At puberty, the penis lengthens, the bifid scrotum grows and becomes rugated and hyperpigmented, and the testes enlarge and descend. The prostate, however, remains impalpable. Erection, ejaculation and orgasm are possible. The appearance of virilization at puberty and the lack of breast development are in contrast to the complete form of testicular feminization and defects of testosterone synthesis.

4. DISORDERS ASSOCIATED WITH OBVIOUSLY ABNORMAL SEX CHROMOSOMES

Additions, deletions or mosaicism of the sex chromosomes characterize individuals in this category. The appearance of the gonads is variable and ranges from the presence of a streak to a nearly normal gonad on both gross and microscopic examination.

4.1. Sexual ambiguity unusual

4.1.1. Klinefelter's syndrome. Klinefelter's syndrome occurs in about one of every 600 newborn males (Gerald, 1976). The karyotype is usually 47,XXY or, occasionally, 47,XXY/mosaic. Although a rare infant may have hypospadias or a congenital anomaly such as hypoplasia of the middle phalanx of the fifth finger, the diagnosis is rarely suspected until adolescence when the patient presents with gynecomastia, obesity, or signs of eunuchoidism. Sparsity of beard and body hair is common. Laboratory tests reveal low testosterone levels and azoospermia. Clinically, the patients are often limited in their economic striving and sexual drive.

Adult 47,XXY individuals have small testes (Fig. 4A), which on microscopical examination disclose atrophy and hyalinization of the seminiferous tubules and a relative increase in the number of Leydig cells (Fig. 4B). The testis rarely exceeds 2 cm in maximal dimension in the adult. During the prepubertal period the primary spermatogonia are greatly reduced in number; the seminiferous tubules, however, are not atrophic. Shortly before the expected time of puberty, the seminiferous tubules begin to degenerate and the lamina propria becomes hyalinized. The absence of elastic fibers in the walls of the tubules indicates that the process of atrophy began prior to puberty. Although most of the seminiferous tubules in the chromatin-positive Klinefelter patient hyalinize completely, some may be preserved and lined only by Sertoli cells, while rare ones may contain germ cells in varying degrees of maturation. If sperm are detected, mosaicism, most likely of the 46,XY/47,XXY pattern, should be suspected.

The Leydig cells become pronounced in number some time after puberty. Although they appear hyperplastic relative to the atrophic appearance of the other elements, it is uncertain whether the absolute volume is greater than in normal testes. Functionally the Leydig cells are abnormal as evidenced by low levels of serum testosterone and a subnormal response to administration of chorionic gonadotropin.

Tumors of germ cell origin have been reported to develop rarely in patients with Klinefelter's syndrome. Most have occurred in extragonadal locations, especially in the mediastinum and in the form of choriocarcinoma (Sogge et al., 1979). The testicular tumors have been in the form of seminoma, teratoma, and embryonal cell carcinoma. Approximately 4% of males with breast cancer have Klinefelter's syndrome.

4.1.2. Turner's syndrome. In the classic form, Turner's syndrome is a disorder in which phenotypic females of short stature have various congenital anomalies, streak gonads and sexual immaturity; the cytogenetic hallmark is the 45,X karyotype.

In the newborn, the overt findings are related to lymph stasis, which is manifest usually as edema of the dorsum of the hands or feet or, less frequently, as swellings of the nape of the neck (cystic hygroma) (Gerald, 1976). Webbing of the neck or elevation of the distal portion of the nails are residua of more marked swellings present during fetal life and may still provide a clue to the correct diagnosis. The full range of somatic anomalies (more than 40) associated with this condition is presented elsewhere (Simpson, 1976; Engel and Forbes, 1965).

Patients who reach adolescence without a diagnosis may present because of primary amenorrhea. Examination reveals undeveloped secondary sex characteristics and a small uterus. Urinary excretion of gonadotropins is always elevated and the vaginal smear almost always reveals an absence of cornified cells. A buccal smear will usually disclose few if any Barr bodies, but about one-fifth of patients have a mosaic karyotype (usually 45,X/46,XX or 45,X/47,XXX) and in these instances the smear discloses some chromatin-positive cells. About 98% of fetuses with a 45,X karyotype abort; the frequency of Turner's syndrome is about 1:3000 in liveborn females.

At laparotomy, the internal genitalia are female

and although small, are in normal relation to each other. The gonads appear as white fibrous streaks, 2–3 cm long and 0.5 cm in diameter and are located in the position normally occupied by the ovary (Fig. 4C). On microscopical examination a streak consists of an attenuated cortex, a medulla and a hilus. The cortex is composed of characteristic ovarian stroma in which the cells are elongate, wavy and are composed largely of nuclei. Rete tubules (rete ovarii) and hilar cells are typically present in the hilus region. The fact that oocytes are present in normal numbers in 45,X embryos prior to the 12th week of gestation but reduced in older fetuses and almost always absent in adults has suggested that the second X chromosome controls granulosa cell development and primary follicular formation; in the absence of this X chromosome, granulosa cells fail to differentiate and it is believed that the oocytes not completely surrounded by granulosa cells degenerate.

Reports of gonadal tumors developing in patients who have a 45,X karyotype are exceedingly rare. Tumors of germ cell origin are undoubtedly rare due to the paucity of germ cells. Development of neoplasms of the so-called "common epithelial type" suggest that the coelomic epithelium encapsulating the gonad can undergo malignant change, even if the gonad is a streak (Murphy et al. 1979). Endometrial cancer may develop occasionally in those patients who have had long-term therapy with exogenous estrogens given to foster the appearance of the feminine secondary sex characteristics (Rosenwaks et al., 1979). Both natural estrogens and synthetic non-steroidal estrogens have been implicated. The duration of usage usually exceeds three years. In addition there is evidence that children and young adults may rarely develop other extragonadal tumors, most often of neurogenic origin (Wertelecki et al., 1970).

4.2. Sexual ambiguity frequent

Patients in this category exhibit a wide range of phenotypic appearances and internal genitalia. A "Y" chromosome is often present, usually as part of a mosaic complement. Sexual ambiguity is a common finding.

4.2.1. Mixed gonadal dysgenesis (MGD). MGD is a syndrome in which the most frequent features in-

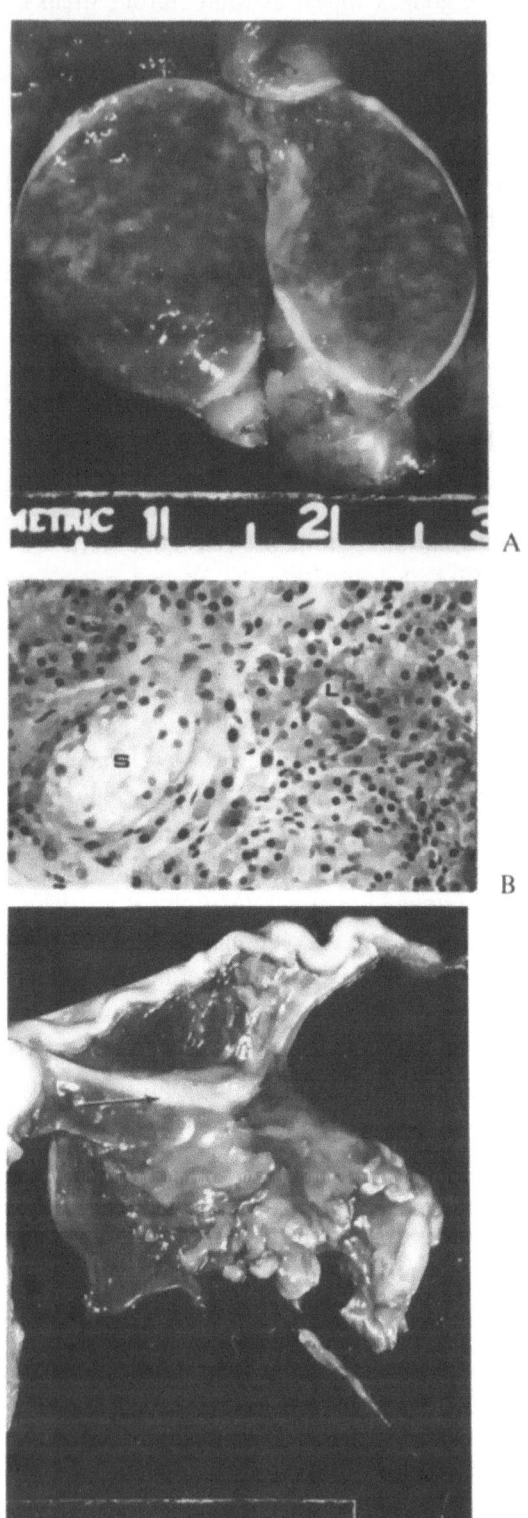

Figure 4 (A) Klinefelter's syndrome. The parenchyma of the 2 cm testis is golden-yellow to slightly brown. *(B)* Testis of Klinefelter's syndrome in which clusters of Leydig cells (L) surround a seminiferous tubule (S), (H&E, ×275.) *(C)* Streak ovary (arrow) in Turner's syndrome.

clude persistent Müllerian duct structures, chromosomal mosaicism with a Y chromosome component, and often asymmetry of the ambiguous external genitalia (Fig. 5A). In most patients one gonad usually resembles a differentiated testis, whereas the other is a streak (sometimes with slight differentiation towards ovary). Elsewhere the authors present data suggesting that the syndrome of MGD should be enlarged to include some patients with bilateral streak gonads (pure gonadal dysgenesis) or bilateral abnormal testes (dysgenetic male pseudohermaphroditism), since the clinical features of these syndromes so nearly resemble each other (Robboy et al. in preparation).

Most newborns with MGD exhibit some degree of fetal masculinization, even if the severity is insufficient to raise the suspicion of intersex. Most patients are assigned a female gender because of the presence of a single midline perineal orifice (actually an expression of hypospadias), a phallus that in size and position resembles a slightly hypertrophied clitoris rather than a penis, and absence of bilateral scrotal testes.

Organs deriving from the Müllerian duct are present in almost all cases (Fig. 5B). The uterus is usually infantile or rudimentary. The Fallopian tubes are frequently bilateral. If a testis is grossly near normal size and well differentiated, the fimbriated end of the ipsilateral tube may be absent, but in only one third of cases is the ipsilateral tube entirely absent. Organs of Wolffian duct derivation may be present also, but the frequency is variable. The epididymis is most commonly identified (two-thirds of cases) and is usually present on the side where there is a testis (Fig. 5B). The vas deferens is encountered less frequently. That the seminal vesicle is only rarely identified probably reflects the fact that the surgeon has not removed tissue near the bladder/prostate region.

The gonad may be a testis, streak, or the latter partially differentiated toward ovary or testis. Bilateral gross testes, frequently of an asynchronous degree of maturity, are found in about 15% of cases while a unilateral gross testis is found in 60%. In general, the state of architectural organization of the testis reflects the quantity and type of cellular components present. Some testes from infants have appeared normal for their age; the architecture was unremarkable, the seminiferous tubules contained a normal complement of spermatogonia, and occasional Leydig cells were present. More commonly, the gonads disclose varying degrees of immaturity and disorganization. The seminiferous tubules in these cases are irregular in diameter, shape and length and contain varying numbers of germ cells. Focal to extensive amounts of wavy, cortical-type ovarian stroma separate the tubules. Not uncommonly, the degree of organization varies among slides or even within fields in a single slide.

We have not observed a gonad that has been grossly identifiable as an ovary or a gonad with Graffian follicles, corpora lutea or corpora albicantia on microscopic examination. That a streak gonad has begun differentiation towards ovary is evident, though, by the presence of rare primordial follicles or, as in the fetal ovary, a myriad of germ cells partially surrounded by immature granulosa cells.

Gonads that are serially blocked frequently disclose substantial variation in tubular architecture in different areas. Typical testis may blend into a region of a streak gonad that more closely resembles a fetal ovary. In some gonads we have examined, the bulk has been typical testis, whereas the cortical region resembled fetal ovary and the hilar region contained bizarre tubules that appeared not yet fully committed as testis (Fig. 5C, D).

Morphological changes may occur over time in the gonads. Myriads of germ cells present in a

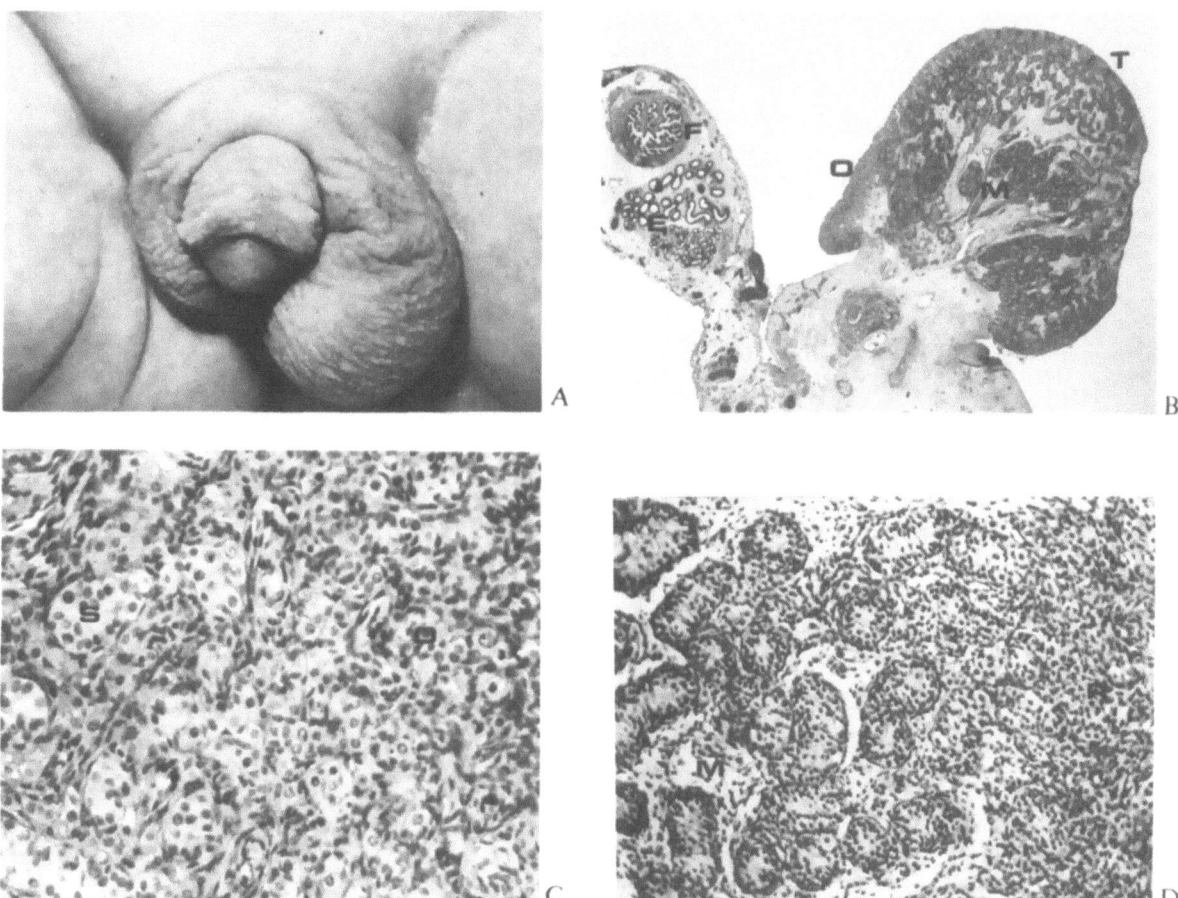

Figure 5 (A) Asymmetric scrotum in mixed gonadal dysgenesis. (*B*) Mixed gonadal dysgenesis with testis (T) and adjacent Fallopian tube (F) and epididymis (E). The medulla of the testis (M) contains immature seminiferous tubules with germ cells and interstitial cells while the region nearer the cortex resembles fetal ovary with immature sex cords (O) and rare primordial follicles. (H&E, ×9.) (*C*) Detail of Fig. 5B where testicular seminiferous tubules (S) merge into fetal type ovary (O). (H&E, ×190.) (*D*) Mixed gonadal dysgenesis. The parenchyma in the medulla of the testis (M) is composed of normal immature seminiferous tubules with germ cells and occasional interstitial cells, while the parenchyma in the region of the hilus near the rete testis (R) appears less committed as testis and is characterized by abnormal, pleomorphic seminiferous tubules. The photograph is taken at the junction of the two zones. (H&E, ×112.)

streak of an infant may degenerate and disappear by puberty, resulting in a gonad composed exclusively of fibrous tissue and a few rete ovarii (Fig. 6); similar changes occur in the streak gonads of Turner's syndrome (45,X karyotype) (Singh and Carr, 1966).

Patients with MGD are at high risk for the development of gonadoblastoma. Occasionally, it occurs also in patients with true hermaphroditism. Many of the isolated reports of gonadoblastoma associated with other forms of hermaphroditism describe clinical and pathological features more suggestive of MGD.

The gross appearance of the gonad with gonadoblastoma varies according to the size of the neoplasm, the presence of calcification, and whether the gonadoblastoma has been overgrown by a malignant form of germ cell tumor (usually germinoma) (Scully, 1970) (Fig. 7A). Approximately one-fifth of gonadoblastomas are discovered solely because a streak gonad was examined microscopically (Fig.

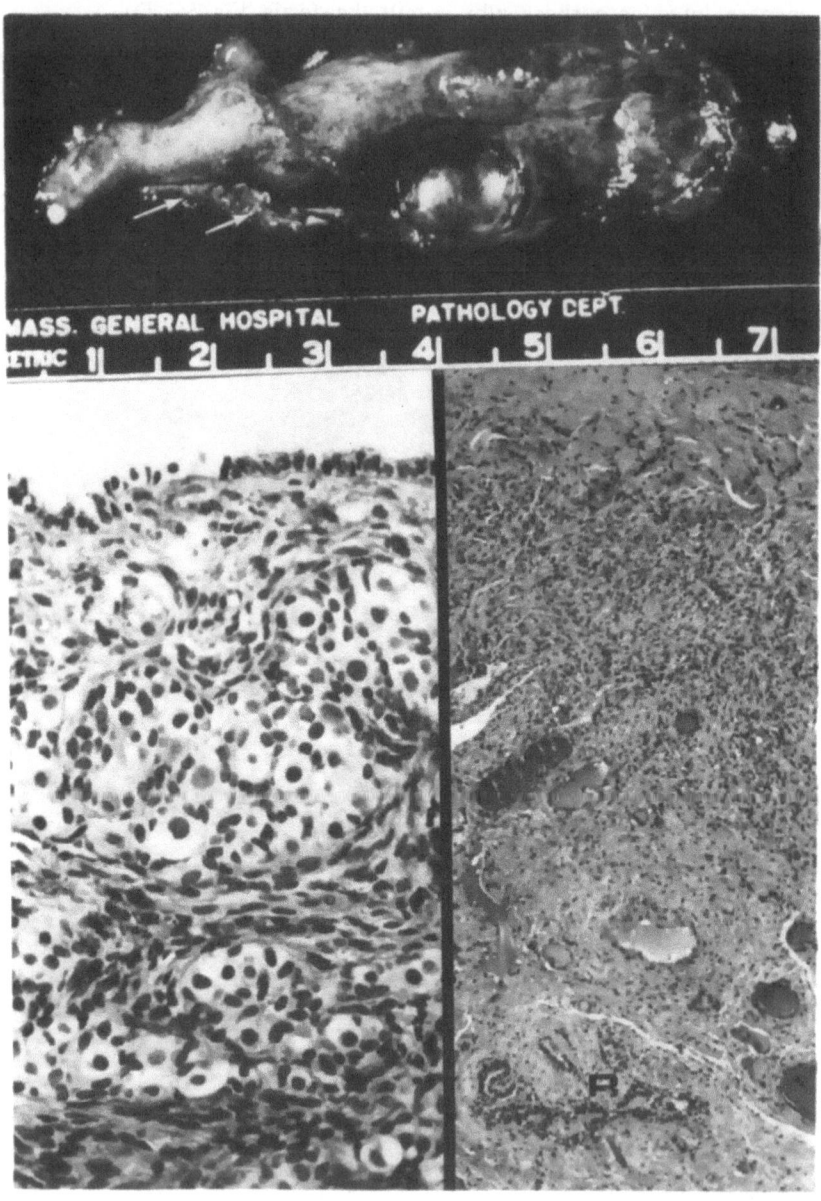

Figure 6. Mixed gonadal dysgenesis. When the patient was an infant the streak gonad resembled a fetal ovary with germ cells and immature sex cords (*left lower*, H&E, × 320). When the streak gonad was removed in entirety 13 years later (*top*–arrows), it existed only as several microscopical areas of whispy ovarian type stroma and rete ovarii (R) (*right lower*, H&E, × 100).

7B). The contralateral gonad also contains a gonadoblastoma in over one third of the patients.

On microscopical examination, the gonadoblastoma appears as circumscribed nests of neoplastic germ cells having the cytologic properties of germinoma (dysgerminoma and seminoma) and which are encompassed individually or in groups by sex cord derivatives with inconspicuous cytoplasm and small round to oval nuclei resembling immature Sertoli or granulosa cells. Hyaline, which is made up of basement membrane material, is found along the margin or as nodules within the nests of tumor. In four fifths of cases the hyaline material is calcified, initially appearing as small, laminated spheres, which eventually fuse and coalesce into large mulberry-like masses (Fig. 7C). Not infrequently, the only evidence that a dysgerminoma originated in a gonadoblastoma is the focal presence of the mulberry-like calcifications.

Hormonally active cells that resemble lutein and Leydig cells are found interspersed among the nests of tumor in about two thirds of cases. They are found least frequently in non-virilized phenotypic females, more often in virilized females, and most frequently in phenotypic males. To some degree, their appearance may be related to the postpubertal age of the patient when the gonad is examined.

Approximately one half of gonadoblastomas are overgrown by a malignant germ cell tumor, usually the germinoma; 8% are overgrown by endodermal sinus tumor, immature teratoma, embryonal carcinoma, or choriocarcinoma. Although the gonadoblastoma itself does not metastasize and therefore can be considered as an in-situ malignancy, the typical malignant behavior of the other tumors makes early prophylactic removal of the gonads in all patients advisable. Also, to avoid the consequences of onset of virilization if the patient is to be raised as a female, it is important that gonadectomy be performed before the patient reaches puberty (Donahoe et al., 1979). Patients who have been treated with long-term administration of estrogen may on occasion develop endometrial carcinoma.

4.2.2. True hermaphroditism.

True hermaphroditism is defined as the presence of both testicular and ovarian tissue in a patient. Because the wavy, cortical-type stroma typically seen in the female gonad can be found in both female and male gonads

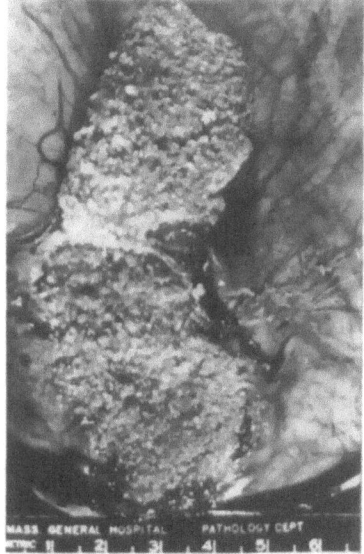

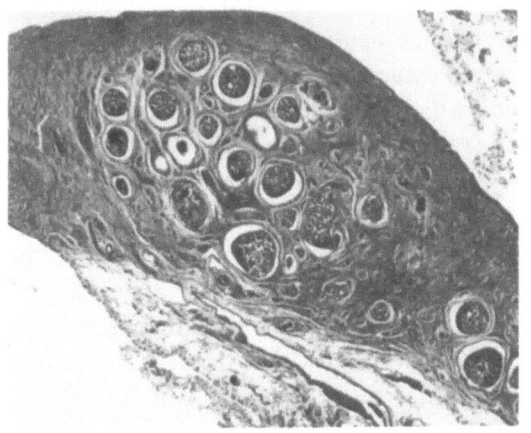

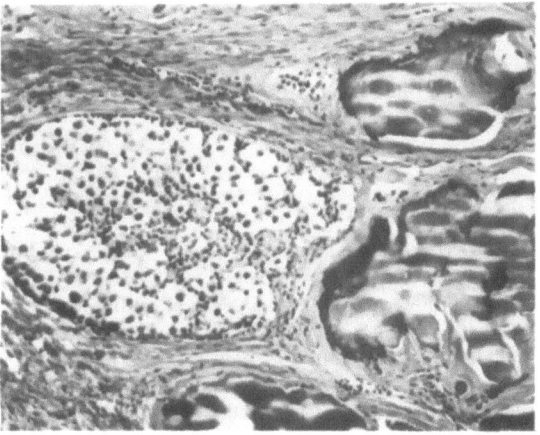

Figure 7 *(A)* 15 cm gonadal tumor composed largely of dysgerminoma. At one pole is a 5×2×0.5 cm calcified gonadoblastoma. *(B)* Gonadoblastoma occupying a gonadal steak, (H&E, ×16.) [Reproduced by permission of Scully (1970).] *(C)* Gonadoblastoma. Multiple mulberry-like calcific masses partially replace the tumor nests composed of germ cells surrounded by sex cord derivatives. (H&E, ×117.)

and therefore is nonspecific, follicular structures must be identified to classify the gonad as an ovary; seminiferous tubules must be identified to classify the gonad as a testicle. In true hermaphrodites, the gonads may be ovary and testis separately or combined in an ovo-testis.

The most common karyotypes in true hermaphroditism are 46,XX (60%), 46,XY (12%), and mosaic (28%), usually 46,XX/46,XY (van Niekerk, 1974). Of particular importance has been the recent discovery that even in some 46,XX individuals the ovarian portion of the gonad is H-Y antigen negative whereas the testicular portion is H-Y antigen positive (Wachtel, 1979). This finding implies that the hermaphroditic gonad may arise from a mosaic primordium regardless of the apparent karyotype.

The clinical presentations of true hermaphrodites vary, one factor being the patient's age at the time of diagnosis (Donahoe et al, 1978). Until recently, the condition often went undetected until adolescence when phenotypic male patients were evaluated for gynecomastia and phenotypic female patients were evaluated for amenorrhea or failure to develop secondary sex changes. Many patients have menstruated, however, and a few have become pregnant. With increasing awareness of intersex states, clinicians more often diagnose the condition in infants because of the ambiguous genitalia which are present in almost all patients. Like MGD, the degree of scrotal ambiguity may be asymmetric, with the larger, more normal appearing hemiscrotum containing a testis. The ovary is always in the abdomen whereas an ovo-testis may be abdominal, inguinal or scrotal in position. Fallopian tubes are frequently present bilaterally, but a vas deferens is usually adjacent only to a testis or an ovo-testis.

On microscopical examination, the gonadal tissue often appears normal if the patient is young. In two infants treated recently at the Massachusetts General Hospital the ovarian tissue contained numerous primordial follicles, while the testicular parenchyma disclosed normal appearing seminiferous tubules with spermatogonia (Donahoe et al., 1978). Patients in the reproductive years may have ovarian tissue even with corpora lutea but spermatogenesis is rare in the testicular portion.

At times, distinction between true hermaphroditism and MGD can be difficult. In the newborn, asymmetric ambiguous genitalia may be observed in both conditions. If a streak gonad from a patient with MGD is serially sectioned, a rare primordial follicle may be encountered in what otherwise appears to be a fetal type ovary admixed with testis with well developed seminiferous tubules. If the term true hermaphroditism is restricted to those patients in whom the ovarian and testicular tissue are both apparent grossly, it should be possible to segregate more clearly those individuals in whom the ovarian tissue may be functional.

The development of germ cell tumors, including gonadoblastoma, in the gonads of patients with true hermaphroditism has been reported to occur rarely (Radhakrishnan et al., 1978).

ACKNOWLEDGEMENT

Supported in part by a Junior Faculty Clinical Fellowship to Dr. Welch from the American Cancer Society.

REFERENCES

Aarskog D (1979) Maternal progestins as a possible cause of hypospadias. New Engl J Med 300: 75.

Berthezene F, Forest MG, Grimaud JA, Clastrat B, Mornex R, (1976) Leydig-cell agenesis. A cause of male pseudohermaphroditism. New Engl J Med 295: 969.

Brøgger A, Strand A (1965) Contribution to the study of the so-called pure gonadal dysgenesis. Acta Endocrinol 48: 490.

Case Records of the Massachusetts General Hospital (Case 8–1977) (1977) New Engl J Med 296: 439.

Coulam CB (1979) Testicular regression syndrome. Obstet Gynecol 53: 44.

Donahoe PK Crawford JD, Hendren WH (1978) True hermaphroditism: a clinical description and a proposed function for the long arm of the Y chromosome. J Pediat Surg 13: 293.

Donahoe PK, Crawford JD, Hendren WH (1979) Mixed gonadal dysgenesis, pathogenesis and management. J Pediat Surg 14: 287.

Engel E, Forbes AP (1965) Cytogenetic and clinical findings in 48 patients with congenitally defective or absent ovaries. Medicine 44: 135.

Gerald PS (1976) Current concepts in genetics. Sex chromosome disorders. New Engl J Med 294: 706.

Griffin JE, Wilson JD (1980) The syndromes of androgen resistance. New Engl J Med 302: 198.

Haymond MW, Weldon VV (1973) Female pseudohermaphroditism secondary to a maternal virilizing tumor. J Pediat 82: 682.

Imperato-McGinley J, Peterson RE, Gautier T, Sturla E (1979) Androgens and the evolution of male-gender identity among male pseudohermaphrodites with 5α-reductase deficiency. New Engl J Med 300: 1233.

Kirkland RT, Kirkland JL, Keenan BS et al. (1977). Bilateral testicular tumors in congenital adrenal hyperplasia. J Clin Endocrinol Metab 44: 369.

Malinak LR, Miller GV, (1963) Bilateral multicentric ovarian luteomas of pregnancy associated with masculinization of female infant. Am J Obstet Gynecol 91: 251.

Manuel M, Katayama KP, Jones HW jr. (1976) The age of occurrence of gonadal tumors in intersex patients with a Y chromosome. Am J Obstet Gynecol 124: 293.

Murphy GF, Welch WR, Urcuyo R (1979) Brenner tumor and mucinous cystadenoma of borderline malignancy in a patient with Turner's syndrome. Obstet Gynecol 54: 660.

Park IJ, Aimakhu VE, Jones HW Jr. (1975) An etiologic and pathogenetic classification of male hermaphroditism. Am J Obstet Gynecol 123: 505.

Radhakrishnan S, Sivaraman L, Natarajan PS (1978) True herm-aphrodite with multiple gonadal neoplasms. Report of a case with cytogenetic study. Cancer 42: 2726.

Robboy SJ, Miller T, Donahoe PK, Crawford JD, Welch WR (1980) Mixed gonadal dysgenesis; a clinicopathologic analysis. In preparation.

Rosenwaks Z, Wentz AC, Jones GS et al. (1979) Endometrial pathology and estrogens. Obstet Gynecol 53: 403.

Scully RE (1970) Gonadoblastoma. A review of 74 cases. Cancer 25: 1340.

Short RV (1979) Sex determination and differentiation. Br Med Bull 35: 121.

Simpson JL (1976) Disorders of sexual differentiation. New York: Academic Press.

Singh RP, Carr DH (1966) The anatomy and histology of XO human embryos and fetuses. Anat Rec 155: 369.

Sogge MR, McDonald SD, Cofold PB (1979) The malignant potential of the dysgenetic germ cell in Klinefelter's syndrome. Am J Med 66: 515.

Sternberg WH, Dhurandhar HN (1977) Functional ovarian tumors of stromal and sex cord origin. Hum Pathol 8: 565.

van Niekerk WA (1974) True hermaphroditism. Clinical, morphologic and cytogenetic aspects. Hagerstown, MD: Harper & Row.

Wachtel SS (1979) The genetics of intersexuality: clinical and theoretic perspectives. Obstet Gynecol 54: 671.

Weiss EB, Kiefer JH, Rowlatt UF, Rosenthal IM (1979) Persistent Müllerian duct syndrome in male identical twins. Pediatrics 63: 493.

Wertelecki W, Fraumeni JF, Mulvihill JJ (1970) Nongonadal neoplasia in Turner's syndrome. Cancer 26: 485.

Wilkins L (1960) Masculinization of female fetus due to use of orally given progestins. JAMA 172: 1028.

9. MALE PSEUDOHERMAPHRODITISM DUE TO ABNORMAL TESTOSTERONE BIOSYNTHESIS AND METABOLISM

PAUL SAENGER, LENORE S. LEVINE and MARIA I. NEW

The term male pseudohermaphroditism (MPH) describes an individual with ambiguity of the internal or external genitalia whose karyotype is 46,XY and who has testes. The purpose of this chapter is to describe enzymatic deficiencies of testosterone synthesis and metabolism resulting in male pseudohermaphroditism.

Complete differentiation of male external and internal genitalia requires the secretion of three hormones: antiMüllerian hormone, testosterone, and dihydrotestosterone. AntiMüllerian hormone and testosterone are secretory products of the fetal testis. AntiMüllerian hormone causes regression of the Müllerian ducts, the anlage of the uterus, Fallopian tubes and upper vagina. Testosterone stabilizes the Wolffian ducts and permits the development of the Wolffian ducts into vasa deferentia, epididymes, and seminal vesicles. For the development of the prostate from the urogenital sinus and in the development of the male external genitalia from the genital tubercle, genital folds and genital swelling, dihydrotestosterone is required. Therefore, testosterone acts only as a prehormone and it has to be metabolized peripherally by a steroid 5α-reductase to dihydrotestosterone (Wilson, 1975a) for the development of these structures.

1. ABNORMAL TESTOSTERONE SYNTHESIS AS A CAUSE OF MALE PSEUDOHERMAPHRODITISM

The biotransformations by which cholesterol is converted to steroid hormones are summarized in Fig. 1. Cholesterol can be synthesized, de novo, in the Leydig cells or can be derived from the plasma. There is now good evidence to suggest that the rate limiting step in testosterone synthesis is the conversion of cholesterol to pregnenolone (Dorfman, 1973).

Five enzymatic deficiencies involving the basic steps in testosterone biosynthesis from the substrate cholesterol have been described:

20–22	desmolase deficiency	adrenal
3β	hydroxysteroid dehydrogenase deficiency	insufficiency *and* male
17α	hydroxylase deficiency	pseudohermaphroditism
17–20	desmolase deficiency	male pseudohermaphroditism only
17β	hydroxysteroid dehydrogenase deficiency*	

The first three enzymatic deficiencies result in cortisol as well as testosterone deficiency and are forms of congenital adrenal hyperplasia.

The inheritance is autosomal recessive in 17-hydroxylase and 3β-hydroxysteroid dehydrogenase deficiency. In the other three defects, the inheritance is unclear. Heterozygous subjects are phenotypically normal.

Inhibition of the Müllerian ducts is usually complete in these patients and the uterus or Fallopian tubes are not present. Masculinization of the external genitalia is incomplete. Androgen action is normal in these patients in contrast to patients with androgen resistance (e.g. testicular feminization). Each enzyme deficiency shows considerable phenotypic heterogeneity. Different mutational events altering either structural or regulatory genes may explain the phenotypic variety these patients display (Imperato-McGinley and Peterson, 1976).

---

* Trivial name: 17-ketosteroid reductase deficiency.

S.J. Kogan and E.S.E. Hafez (eds.), Pediatric andrology, 87–97. All rights reserved.
Copyright © 1981, Martinus Nijhoff Publishers bv, The Hague/Boston/London.

1.1. Cholesterol desmolase deficiency

In 1955, Prader and Gurtner described a male pseudohermaphrodite with severe salt wasting and impaired synthesis of all three classes of adrenal corticosteroids: mineralocorticoids, glucocorticoids and sex steroids. Urinary 17-ketosteroid and 17-hydroxycorticosteroid excretion was low and was not stimulated by ACTH. In this genetic male, female external genitalia with male genital ducts were found at autopsy. The enlarged adrenals were remarkable in that the cortical cells were filled with lipoid material consisting of cholesterol and cholesterol esters, which prompted the name lipoid adrenal hyperplasia.

Several patients with this biosynthetic defect have been described since (Camacho et al., 1968; Kirkland et al., 1973). Most did not survive beyond infancy, and died in adrenal crisis because of deficient glucocorticoid and mineralocorticoid production. The biosynthetic defect involves the side chain cleavage converting cholesterol to pregnenolone. At least three enzymes are involved in this conversion: 20α-hydroxylase, 22R-hydroxylase and 20α-22R desmolase (Burstein et al., 1970; Luttrell et al., 1972; Hochberg et al., 1974). Degenhart et al., (1971) produced biochemical evidence that the deficient enzyme in their patient was the cholesterol 20α-hydroxylase. Any of these three enzymatic deficiencies leads to profound adrenal insufficiency. The severe ambiguity of the external genitalia in the male suggests that the defect is also present in the testes. Affected female infants have normal genital development. Since the defect impairs aldosterone and desoxycorticosterone secretion as well, salt wasting is attributable to the lack of mineralocorticoid secretion. Early recognition and proper treatment should permit survival of these infants as in Addison's disease of infancy.

1.2. 3β-Hydroxysteroid dehydrogenase (3βHSD) deficiency

An enzymatic deficiency of 3β-HSD, first described

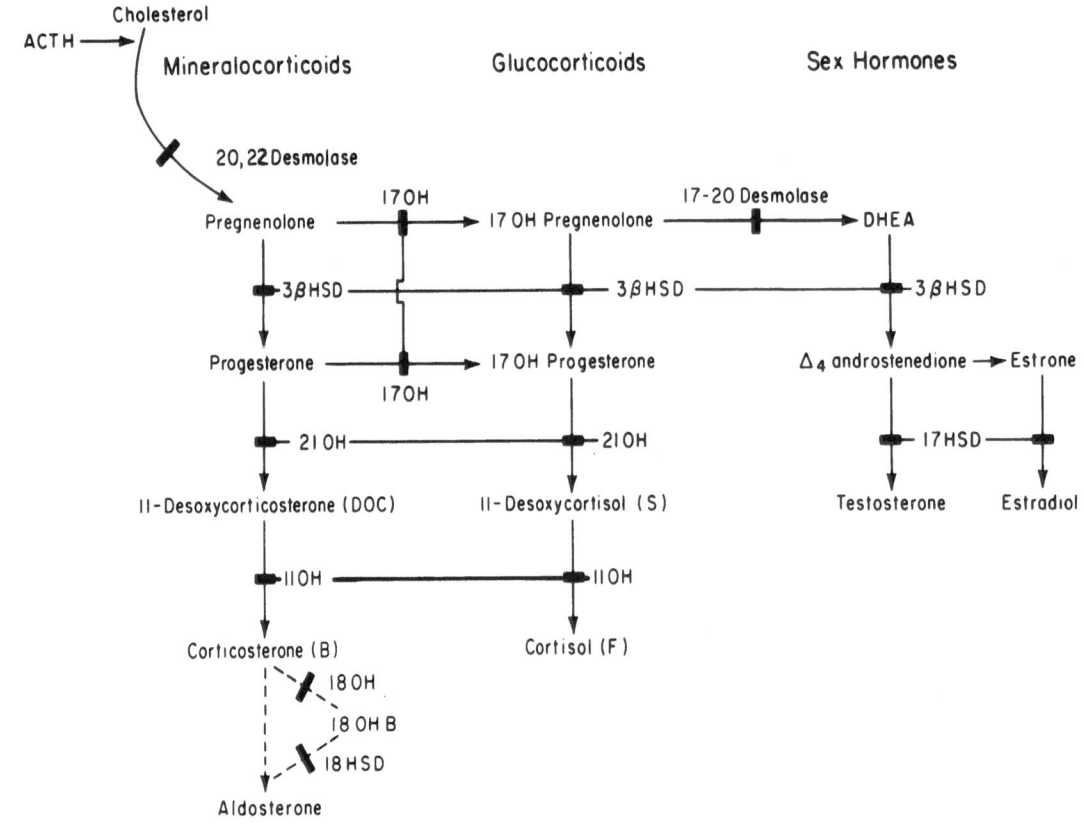

Figure 1. Biosynthesis of mineralocorticoids, glucocorticoids and sex steroids.

by Bongiovanni (1962), also results in decreased synthesis of all three classes of adrenal steroids. There is impaired secretion of aldosterone, cortisol, and testosterone, which leads to male pseudohermaphroditism and life threatening salt wasting in infancy. The female with 3β-HSD defect shows only minimal clitoral enlargement, probably due to the extremely high amounts of dehydroepiandrosterone (DHEA). Although it is secreted in very high amounts, DHEA is too weak an androgen to completely masculinize the external genitalia in the male. Congenital adrenal hyperplasia due to 3β-HSD deficiency must be suspected in a newborn with salt wasting symptoms who has ambiguous genitalia. The male with this disorder may resemble the virilized female with salt wasting due to 21-hydroxylase deficiency. The male with 21-hydroxylase deficiency shows no sexual ambiguity. Thus, in a genetic male with salt wasting and complete male differentiation, 3β-HSD is extremely unlikely. The female with 21-hydroxylase deficiency is more virilized than the female with 3β-HSD deficiency; labioscrotal fusion has not been reported in a female with 3β-HSD deficiency. The urine of patients with 3β-HSD deficiency predominantly contains steroids with a double bond at the C_5 position (Δ^5 steroids). Excessive urinary excretion of DHEA and its metabolite pregnenetriol, with markedly elevated DHEA and DHEA sulfate levels in plasma are diagnostic of 3β-HSD deficiency.

Since stress in the immediate postnatal period may elevate DHEA levels in infants with normal adrenal function, DHEA reference values for newborns should be consulted before the diagnosis of 3β-HSD is entertained (Levine et al., 1980).

The 3β-HSD enzyme in testes, adrenal, and liver may be under different genetic control. This, in turn, could result in varying degrees of enzymatic deficiency in different organs, the testes being less affected than the adrenal. Such a hypothesis may explain the advent of male puberty which has been described in some cases of 3β-HSD deficiency (Parks et al., 1971; Jänne et al., 1974; Schneider et al., 1975).

Florid pubertal breast development in this form of male pseudohermaphroditism may be the result of inadequate testosterone production in fetal life, leaving the breast anlage unsuppressed (Parks et al., 1971; Jänne et al., 1974; Schneider et al., 1975; Neuman and Elger, 1966).

1.3. 17α-Hydroxylase deficiency

A defect in 17α-hydroxylase will also result in diminished secretion of all glucocorticoids and sex steroids (Biglieri et al., 1966). Cases have been reported in both males and females (Goldsmith et al., 1967, Mallin, 1969; New, 1970; Mantero et al., 1971). The patients with a 46,XY karyotype are born with ambiguous genitalia, while females with this defect have hypogonadism presenting at puberty.

Prominent breast development was the only secondary sex characteristic which occurred at puberty in a male patient described by New (1970). The decrease in cortisol production results in increased ACTH secretion, which leads to an increase in the production of corticosterone (a weak glucocorticoid) and desoxycorticosterone (a mineralocorticoid) (New, 1970). Hypertension, hypokalemia and alkalosis are frequently present in this syndrome and are probably the result of the markedly increased desoxycorticosterone production (New, 1970; Tourniaire et al., 1976). The increased desoxycorticosterone levels result in sodium retention, decreased plasma renin activity and depressed plasma and aldosterone secretion. Urinary 17-ketosteroid excretion is low. Lifelong therapy with glucocorticoids is mandatory in males *and* females with this defect to maintain normal blood pressure and to correct the hypokalemic alkalosis (New, 1970).

The final two defects involve *only* testosterone biosynthesis.

1.4. 17–20 Desmolase deficiency

This defect was first described by Zachmann et al., (1972), in three patients – two first cousins and a "maternal aunt" – suggesting an autosomal recessive or X-linked mode of inheritance. All three patients had a 46,XY karyotype. These three patients shared a familial form of male pseudohermaphroditism, due to a partial defect in conversion of 17α-hydroxyprogesterone and 17-hydroxypregnenolone to C_{19} steroids by testes and adrenals. Only sex steroid biosynthesis is affected in this form of male pseudohermaphroditism. The patients presented with ambiguous external genitalia and inguinal or intraabdominal testes with no spermatogonia. All had third degree hypospadias but normal male ductal differentiation. One of the subjects had a rudimentary uterus and Fallopian tubes. Urinary pregnenetriolone, one of the metabolites of 17-hydroxypregnenolone, was increased and increased further after ACTH and HCG stimulation. However, testosterone or DHEA excretion did not rise appreciably. In vitro studies with testicular tissue also demonstrated the defect in testosterone biosynthesis. The results were, therefore, consistent with a deficiency of adrenal and testicular 17,20-desmolase activity. An unrelated 46,XY phenotypic female has recently been described with the same disorder except for the absence of Müllerian duct structures (Goebelsmann et al., 1976). Gynecomastia may occur at puberty (Goebelsmann et al., 1976) though it was not present in Zachmann's kindred.

1.5. 17-Hydroxysteroid dehydrogenase (17HSD) deficiency

Deficiency of the 17-HSD enzyme which also results in decreased testosterone synthesis is another known cause of male pseudohermaphroditism (Saez et al., 1971; Goebelsmann et al., 1973; Givens et al., 1974; Virdis et al., 1978). With one exception all previously reported genetic males were assigned to the female sex of rearing at birth because they were so incompletely masculinized. Only one patient who presented with sexual ambiguity noted in infancy (Knorr et al., 1973) was given a male sex assignment. In most patients, diagnosis was made at or after puberty when signs of virilization appeared, though recently Levine et al. (1980) demonstrated that this defect can be diagnosed in infancy by measuring testosterone and its precursors after an HCG stimulation test.

Common clinical features include: clitoral hypertrophy, testes in the inguinal canal or in the labia majora with absent spermatogenesis, a blind ending vaginal pouch, and absent Müllerian structures. Wolffian duct differentiation is normal. The hyperplastic Leydig cells in these patients secrete predominantly $\Delta 4$-androstenedione ($\Delta 4$), a testosterone precursor. In testicular effluent studies the $\Delta 4$/testosterone ratio was 96/5 (normal 3/75) (Virdis et al., 1978). Peripheral conversion of $\Delta 4$ to testosterone is apparently still intact; thus $\Delta 4$/testosterone ratio measured in peripheral blood is less elevated (5.8; normal 0.25–1.05) than that in the testicular venous effluent. This suggests that the enzymes controlling 17-hydroxysteroid dehydrogenase in testes and liver

are under different genetic control. Conversion of estrone to estradiol is also impaired, but usually to a lesser degree. The defect is probably only expressed in the gonad and can thus not be diagnosed after castration.

Follicle stimulating hormone (FSH) may be normal while luteinizing hormone (LH) is elevated. Serum testosterone levels are usually low in these patients. However, several patients with normal testosterone concentration have been reported. The relative lack of intrauterine virilization may be due to efficient aromatization of $\Delta 4$ to estrone in the placenta. Thus, very little $\Delta 4$ is available for extratesticular conversion to testosterone (Goebelsmann et al., 1973).

At puberty, these patients display remarkable heterogeneity in the phenotypes. Varying concentrations of circulating estrogens, particularly estradiol, may explain varying degrees of breast development noted in patients with 17-HSD. Increased gonadal $\Delta 4$ and estrone secreted at puberty are converted peripherally to testosterone and estradiol which may explain the simultaneous occurrence of gynecomastia and virilization in some of these patients (Goebelsmann et al., 1973). Data on the testosterone/dihydrotestosterone ratio suggest normal 5α-reductase activity, although as a consequence of low testosterone levels, the absolute DHT concentration is similarly decreased.

The defect in $\Delta 4$ and estrone metabolism is also demonstrable in vitro with testicular incubation studies (Virdis et al., 1978).

Demonstration that $\Delta 4$ is not converted normally to testosterone is necessary for diagnosis in 17-HSD deficiency. Thus, elevated $\Delta 4$/testosterone ratios in peripheral and spermatic blood are diagnostic. Since virilization develops at puberty, the patients given a female sex assignment require prepubertal castration and estrogen replacement therapy to make the puberty conform with the sex of assignment.

2. UNCLASSIFIED DEFECTS IN TESTOSTERONE SYNTHESIS

Berthezène et al. (1976) described a 35-year-old male pseudohermaphrodite who represents a specific defect in testicular Leydig cell differentiation. The patient had a female phenotype with a shallow vagina. No Müllerian structures were present. Testes were found intraabdominally, and vasa deferentia and an epididymis were present. At biopsy the testis contained no recognizable Leydig cells. Serum testosterone was low, luteinizing hormone was elevated, yet follicle stimulating hormone was normal. There was no response to HCG stimulation. The testes produced antiMüllerian hormone normally and testosterone at least sometime during fetal life since Wolffian differentiation was completed.

3. ABNORMAL TESTOSTERONE METABOLISM AS A CAUSE OF MALE PSEUDOHERMAPHRODITISM –5α-REDUCTASE DEFICIENCY

5α-reductase deficiency is a recently defined form of male pseudohermaphroditism (Walsh et al., 1974; Imperato-McGinley et al., 1974; Peterson et al., 1977; Saenger et al., 1978; Fisher et al., 1978), which greatly advanced our understanding of the hormonal control of male differentiation.*

This defect causes abnormally low conversion of testosterone to dihydrotestosterone, the androgen responsible for masculinizing the external genitalia of the male fetus. 5α-reductase deficiency is the first recognized inherited abnormality of steroid metabolism in which the basic defect resides in the hormone responsive target tissue.

While the female infants with this defect are normal, male infants with this deficiency of testosterone metabolism are born with ambiguous genitalia. The infant has a phallic clitoris. A urogenital sinus is present and depending upon the degree of masculinization, either a single orifice, or separate urethral and vaginal orifices may be present. Usually a blind ending vaginal pouch is present. The internal genitalia consist of testes and epididymis, which are found in the abdomen, the inguinal canal, or in the labioscrotal folds. Wolffian duct differentiation is normal in these patients and Müllerian structures are not detectable. At puberty, these patients virilize. The phallic clitoris enlarges, the testes also enlarge and descend into the labioscrotal folds. A male body habitus develops, the voice deepens and erections occur. The ejaculate may contain a normal number of sperm (Peterson et al., 1977). Testosterone rather than dihydrotestosterone appears to mediate these hormonal effects. In this form of male pseudohermaphroditism secretion of testosterone probably suppresses breast anlagen in utero; therefore, no gynecomastia develops. Acne is absent, beard growth is sparse, and the prostate remains small, suggesting that these events are dihydrotesterone dependent. The inheritance is autosomal recessive. Obligate heterozygous fathers of these patients are clinically normal.

The diagnosis of 5α-reductase deficiency can only be established biochemically. These patients have normal levels of testosterone before and after HCG stimulation and an abnormally low dihydrotestosterone response to HCG stimulation. In young infants in whom testosterone is normally transiently elevated, the testosterone/dihydrotestosterone ratio in the unstimulated state may be diagnostic (Pang et al., 1979).

In older infants, and in prepubertal males, when testosterone is normally very low, HCG stimulation is necessary to assess the testosterone/dihydrotestosterone ratio. In normal children a dihydrotestosterone rise paralleling the increase of testosterone is expected after a course of HCG injections. The normal ratio in children is 11 ± 4.4 S.D. The measurement of testosterone/dihydrotestosterone ratios after the administration of HCG is, therefore, a useful tool in diagnosing 5α-reductase deficiency in childhood (Peterson et al., 1977; Saenger et al., 1978), (Fig. 2). In adult, non-castrated patients with this form of male pseudohermaphroditism, unstimulated testosterone/dihydrotestosterone ratios will be diagnostic (Peterson et al., 1977) (Fig. 3).

In adult patients the circulating testosterone is often elevated, probably secondary to increased LH levels. The reason for the high LH levels is unclear. It is possible that low dihydrotestosterone results in higher LH, or that a relative insensitivity of the hypothalamus to testosterone exists (Peterson et al., 1977). The elevated FSH levels are probably due to the cryptorchidism present in these patients (Lee et al., 1974).

5α-reductase deficiency is also expressed in the urinary metabolites of testosterone. For a schematic presentation of the biotransformation of testosterone, see Fig. 4. The ratio of the urinary 5β-

---

* In the past, several groups described patients with "pseudovaginal perineoscrotal hypospadias" as a type of hereditary male pseudohermaphroditism; some of these patients had 5α-reductase deficiency. (Nowakowski and Lenz, 1967; Opitz et al., 1972.)

92

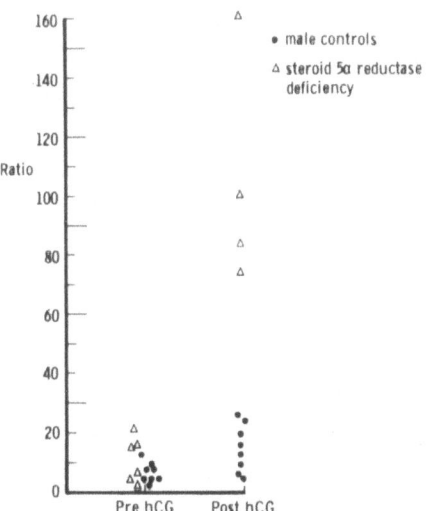

Figure 2. Ratio of plasma T/DHT in normal prepubertal male controls and prepubertal males with 5α-reductase deficiency before and after HCG stimulation. [Reprinted from Peterson RE, Imperato-McGinley J, Gautier T, Sturla E (1979) Hereditary steroid 5α-reductase deficiency: a newly recognized cause of male pseudohermaphroditism. In Vallet HL, Porter IH, eds. Genetic mechanisms of sexual development, p 155. New York: Academic Press].

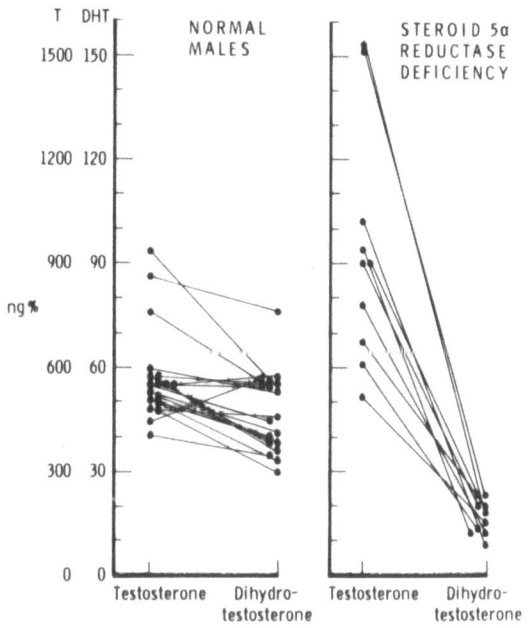

Figure 3. Plasma concentrations of T and DHT in normal adult males and males with 5α-reductase deficiency, 18 to 55 years old. [Reprinted from Peterson RE, Imperato-McGinley J, Gautier T, Sturla E (1979) Hereditary steroid 5α-reductase deficiency: a newly recognized cause of male pseudohermaphroditism. In Vallet HL, Porter IH, eds. Genetic mechanisms of sexual development, p 155. New York: Academic Press].

reduced 17-ketosteroid metabolite etiocholanolone (5β3α) to the 5α-reduced metabolite androsterone (5α3α) is less than 2 in normal children and adults (Peterson et al., 1977; Saenger et al., 1978). The urinary excretion of these 5β and 5α reduced androgen metabolites is another valuable and non-invasive test in the evaluation of patients with male pseudohermaphroditism. Measurement of urinary E/A ratios is also useful for the detection of obligate heterozygote carriers (Peterson et al., 1977).

This enzymatic deficiency can also be diagnosed by infusing ³H-testosterone at a constant rate as described by Horton and Tait (1966). This technique can be utilized to determine the plasma conversion of testosterone to dihydrotestosterone (Ito and Horton, 1971). In five controls the conversion ratio of testosterone to dihydrotestosterone was 5.3±3.0%; in two patients with 5α-reductase deficiency it was 0.4 and 0.3% (Saenger et al., 1978). Conversion of testosterone to dihydrotestosterone in seven patients with male pseudohermaphroditism of unknown etiology was normal (Saenger et al., 1978; Saenger and New, unpublished observations).

In addition to the above in vivo measurements, in vitro methods for the diagnosis of 5α-reductase deficiency have also been established: 5α-reductase activity in skin fibroblasts is decreased (Imperato-McGinley et al., 1974; Wilson, 1975b; Saenger et al., 1978; Pinsky et al., 1978). Measurement of 5α-reductase activity in genital skin fibroblasts is a sensitive means of detecting the enzyme deficiency (Griffin and Wilson, 1980). The enzymatic defect is not only expressed in the dihydrotestosterone dependent areas of the genitalia, but also in the non-genital skin (Peterson et al., 1977; Saenger et al., 1978).

Binding of ³H dihydrotestosterone to cytosol receptors of skin fibroblasts was normal in patients with 5α-reductase deficiency (Griffin et al., 1976; Saenger et al., 1978). This finding also provides additional proof that this form of male pseudohermaphroditism is a defect in testosterone metabolism and not in androgen binding. The clinical observation that dihydrotestosterone-proprionate treatment caused enlargement of the prostate, beard growth and acne, is in concordance with this biochemical finding (Peterson et al., 1977).

McGuire and Tomkins (1960) reported that several 5α-reductase enzymes with limited specificity

BIOTRANSFORMATION OF TESTOSTERONE

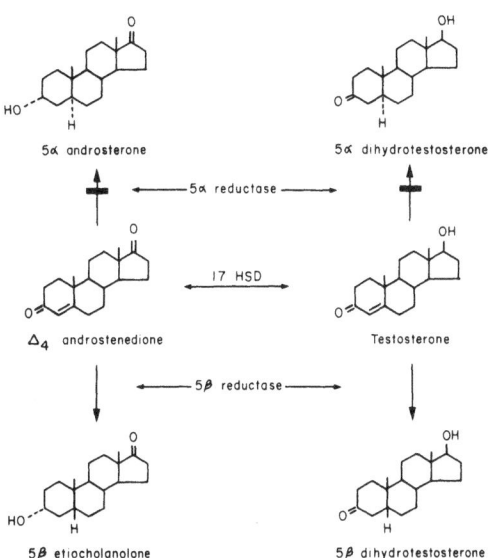

Figure 4. Biotransformation of testosterone. The black bars indicate the enzymatic block in conversion of testosterone and Δ4-androstenedion to their respective 5α-reduced metabolites (17HSD = 17-hydroxysteroid dehydrogenase).

are present in rat liver. These investigators assumed, therefore, that the enzymatic pathways for the 5α-reduction of androgens, particularly testosterone, and glucocorticoids are separate. If, indeed, there are several 5α-reductase enzymes present in the liver, then one would expect that patients with a 5α-reductase deficiency in testosterone metabolism should still excrete normal amounts of 5α-reduced metabolites of cortisol.

Detailed studies in two different pedigrees show, however, impaired 5α-reduction for both testosterone *and* glucocorticoids. Cortisol is metabolized almost exclusively to tetrahydrocortisol (5β) and only little allotetrahydrocortisol (5α) is formed (Peterson, R.E., personal communication). Elegant experiments using preparations of epididymal microsomes of a patient with 5α-reductase deficiency failed to show any 5α-reduction of either testosterone or cortisol (Fisher et al., 1978). Therefore, this form of male pseudohermaphroditism is characterized by impairment of 5α-reduction of androgens and glucocorticoids, although only the deficient 5α-reduction of testosterone is of physiologic importance.

A number of studies suggest heterogeneity of this enzyme deficiency

The patients studied by Walsh et al. (1974) had normal circulating testosterone and dihydrotesto-

sterone; 5α-reductase activity in slices of genital skin was deficient, however. Walsh et al. (1974) postulated, therefore, that the male pseudohermaphroditism in these patients was due to a deficient 5α-reductase in *target tissue only*. In contrast, the large kindred studied by Imperato-McGinley et al. (1974) shows deficient circulating dihydrotestosterone in all affected males. Therefore, a spectrum of deficiency of 5α-reductase may exist, with variable expression of the enzymatic defect. All patients, however, form some dihydrotestosterone after the time of expected puberty.

Wilson's group recently published evidence for several distinct mutations affecting in vitro 5α-reductase activity in the various pedigrees (Leshin et al., 1978). In one family, the mutation probably involves the interaction of enzyme and steroid substrate leading to a decreased conversion of testosterone to dihydrotestosterone. A study of another pedigree indicates the presence of an inherently unstable enzyme in certain in vitro conditions such as exposure to cycloheximide or elevated temperature (Leshin et al., 1978). Recently cells from a patient from a New York family were found to have intermediate levels of activity and stability of 5α-reductase (Imperato-McGinley et al., 1980). Griffin and Wilson (1980) point out that this genetic heterogeneity is akin to that noted in other enzymatic deficiencies, such as glucose-6-phosphate dehydrogenase deficiency (Yoshida et al., 1971; Beutler et al., 1973).

The largest pedigree with 5α-reductase deficiency has been found in an isolated village in the Dominican Republic (Peterson et al., 1977). It is unique to this remote community that when these individuals raised as girls, undergo a male puberty, the majority change their gender identity and their gender role in the village society (Imperato-McGinley et al., 1979). Sex reversal at the age of puberty has not been reported in the patients studied in the U.S. Change of assigned gender role after puberty has been reported sporadically in patients with MPH due to other causes.

The findings in the Dominican Republic raise the possibility that postnatal and pubertal androgen action contributes towards the development of male gender identity. (Imperato-McGinley et al., 1979). If this were true, this observation would certainly be at variance with the widely held concept that psychosexual orientation in man is irrevocably

Table 1. Clinical and laboratory features of various forms of male pseudohermaphroditism.

Clinical features							Urine					Blood						
Newborn with sexual ambiguity		Salt wasting	Hypertension	Postnatal virilization	Pubertal virilization	Enzyme deficiency	17KS	17OH	P'triol	Aldo	E/A	17OHP	DHEA	DS	Δ₄	T	DHT	T/DHT
Female	Male																	
O	+	+	O	O	O	cholesterol desmolase	↓	↓	↓	↓	?	↓	↓	↓	↓	↓	↓	?
+	+	+	O	O	+	3β HSD	↑*	↓	↓	↓	nl	↑	↑↑	↑↑	↓	↓	↓	?
O	+	O	+	O	O	17-hydroxylase	↓	↓	↓	↓	nl	↓	↓	↓	↓	↓	↓	?
O	+	O	O	O	O	17–20 desmolase	↓↓	nl	nl**	?	nl	↑	↓	↓	↓	↓	↓	
O	+	O	O	O	+	17 HSD	↑↑	nl	↑	nl	nl	↑	↑	↑	↑↑	↑	↑	nl
O	+	O	O	O	+ deficiency	5α-reductase deficiency	nl	nl	nl	nl	↑↑	nl	nl	nl	nl	nl	↓	↑***

* Mostly Δ5 17-ketosteroids (e.g. DHEA).
** Pregnanetriolone markedly elevated.
*** Abnormality in infancy; in prepubertal children only after HCG stimulation and adults.

Abbreviations: P'triol, Pregnanetriol; Aldo, Aldosterone; E, Etiocholanolone; A, Androsterone; 17OHP, 17OH Progesterone; DS, Dehydroepiandrosterone sulfate. For other abbreviations, see text.

Adapted from Saenger P, Levine LS, New MI (1980) Sexual ambiguity at birth. In Bain J, Hafez ESE, eds. Diagnosis in andrology, p. 46. The Hague: Martinus Nijhoff.

determined by the sex of rearing in the first 3 years of life (Money et al., 1955). Although it may not be applicable to children with 5α-reductase deficiency reared in rural Santo Domingo, the pressures to conform to the sex of rearing in a more modern society are very great.

When diagnosed in infancy, the choice of gender should be based on the infants' phenotype. If a female sex of rearing is assigned, castration should be performed well before puberty to avoid disturbing virilization.

For the salient clinical and laboratory findings in the enzyme deficiencies described, see Table 1.

4. MANAGEMENT OF PATIENT WITH MALE PSEUDOHERMAPHRODITISM

The birth of an infant with sexual ambiguity is a medical emergency presenting a challenge to the physicians caring for the infant to arrive expediently at a rational sex assignment.

The external genitalia will rarely be distinctive enough to allow diagnosis of a particular disorder. Different biochemical defects may lead to the same phenotype. Incomplete masculinization in a male individual, or virilization in a female may also result in identical phenotypes. Cytogenetic, endocrine, and radiological studies have to be initiated simultaneously. Particularly careful attention has to be given to potential electrolyte imbalance in patients with salt losing congenital adrenal hyperplasia. A panel of experts determines which sex to assign a patient with pseudohermaphroditism. It is important that the infant's capacity for future function as a male be considered. Androgen response to HCG stimulation and/or effects of systemic testosterone on penile size may be of help in arriving at a final decision (Burstein et al., 1979) although these diagnostic measures may lead to an undesirable delay in sex assignment.

The sex of assignment in infants with male pseudohermaphroditism should be guided by the anatomy of the external and internal genitalia, the possibility that puberty will conform to the assigned sex, and the capacity for sexual activity.

Recalling the complex time schedule of genital differentiation in man, it becomes clear that only transient disturbances in any of these processes may alter the male phenotype.

We would like to stress that even with the most sophisticated diagnostic techniques available to us, the pathogenesis of male pseudohermaphroditism remains obscure in many patients (Amrhein et al., 1977; Savage et al., 1978).

With present techniques testosterone synthesis *and* metabolism as well as androgen binding can be assessed; however, the steps required for androgen action following androgen binding (transcription and translation) cannot, at the present time, be tested in these patients.

ACKNOWLEDGEMENT

The preparation of this manuscript by Ms. Lorraine Miller is very much appreciated.

REFERENCES

Amrhein JA, Meyer WY, Danish RK, Migeon CY (1977) Studies of androgen production and binding in 13 male pseudohermaphrodites and 13 males with micropenis. J Clin Endocrinol Metab 45: 732.

Berthezène F, Forest MG, Grimand JA, Claustrat B, Mornes R (1976) Leydig cell agenesis: a cause of male pseudohermaphroditism. New Engl J Med 295: 969.

Beutler E, Yoshida A (1973) Human glucose-6-phosphate dehydrogenase variants: a supplementary tabulation. Ann Hum Genet 37: 151.

Biglieri EG, Herron MA, Brust N (1966) 17-hydroxylation deficiency in man. J Clin Invest 45: 1946.

Bongiovanni AM (1962) The adrenogenital syndrome with deficiency of 3β-hydroxysteroid dehydrogenase. J Clin Invest 41: 2086.

Burstein S, Kimball HL, Gut M (1970) Transformation of labelled cholesterol, 20α hydroxycholesterol, (22R)-22-hydroxycholesterol and (22R)-20α, 22 dihydroxycholesterol by adrenal acetone-dried preparation from guinea pigs, cattle and man. Steroids 15: 809.

Burstein S, Grumbach MM, Kaplan SL (1979) Androgen responsiveness is important in the management of microphallus. Lancet ii, 983.

Camacho AM, Kowarski A, Migeon CH, Brough AJ (1968) Congenital adrenal hyperplasia due to a deficiency of one of the enzymes involved in the biosynthesis of pregnenolone. J Clin Endocrinol Metab 28: 153.

Degenhart HJ (1971) A study of the cholesterol splitting enzyme system in normal adrenals and in adrenal lipoid hyperplasia. Acta Pediat Scand 60: 611.

Dorfman RI (1973) Biosynthesis of progestogens. In Greep RO, Astwood EP, eds. Handbook of Physiology, Section 7: Endocrinology, Vol II: Female reproductive system, Part 1, pp 537–546. Washington, D.C.; American Physiology Society.

Fisher LK, Kogut MD, Moore RJ, Goebelsmann U, Weitzman JJ, Isaccs H Jr, Griffin JE, Wilson JD (1978) Clinical, endocrinological and enzymatic characterization of two patients with 5α-reductase deficiency: evidence that a single enzyme is responsible for the 5α-reduction of cortisol and testosterone. J Clin Endocrinol Metab 47: 563.

Givens JR, Wiser WL, Summitt RL, Kerber IJ, Anderson RN, Pittaway DE, Fish SA (1974) Familial male pseudohermaphroditism without gynecomastia due to deficient testicular 17-ketosteroid reductase deficiency. New Engl J Med 291: 938.

Goebelsmann U, Horton R, Mestman JH, Arce JJ, Nagata Y, Nakamura RM, Thorneycroft IH, Mishell DR (1973) Male pseudohermaphroditism due to testicular 17β-hydroxysteroid dehydrogenase deficiency. J Clin Endocrinol Metab 36: 867.

Goebelsmann U, Zachmann M, Davajan V, Israel R, Mestman JH, Mishell DR (1976) Male pseudohermaphroditism consistent with 17–20 desmolase deficiency. Gynecol Invest 7: 138.

Goldsmith O, Solomon DH, Horton R (1967) Hypogonadism and mineralocorticoid excess: the 17-hydroxylase syndrome. New Engl J Med 277: 673.

Griffin JE, Punyashthiti KJ, Wilson JD (1976) Dihydrotestosterone binding by cultured human fibroblasts. J Clin Invest 57: 1342.

Griffin JE, Wilson JD (1980) The syndromes of androgen resistance. New Engl J Med 302: 198.

Hochberg RB, McDonald PD, Feldman M, Liebermann S (1974) Studies on the biosynthetic conversion of cholesterol into pregnenolone. J Biol Chem 249: 1277.

Horton R, Tait JF (1966) Androstenedione production and interconversion rates measured in peripheral blood and studies on the possible site of its conversion to testosterone. J Clin Invest 45: 301.

Imperato-McGinley J, Guerrero L, Gautier T, Peterson RE (1974) Steroid 5α-reductase deficiency in man. An inherited form of male pseudohermaphroditism. Science 186: 1213.

Imperato-McGinley J, Peterson RE (1976) Male pseudohermaphroditism: The complexities of male phenotypic development. Am J Med 61: 751.

Imperato-McGinley J, Peterson RE, Gautier T, Sturla E (1979) Androgens and the evolution of male gender identity among male pseudohermaphrodites with 5α-reductase deficiency. New Engl J Med 300: 1233.

Imperato-McGinley J, Peterson RE, Leshin M, Griffin JE, Cooper G, Draghi S, Berenyi M, Wilson JD (1980) Steroid 5α-reductase deficiency in a 65-year old male pseudohermaphrodite: The natural history, ultrastructure of the testes, and evidence for inherited enzyme heterogeneity. J Clin Endocrinol Metab 50: 15.

Ito T, Horton R (1971) The source of plasma dihydrotestosterone in man. J Clin Invest 50: 1621.

Janne O, Perheentupa J, Viinikka L, Vihko R (1974) Testicular endocrine function in a pubertal boy with 3β-hydroxysteroid dehydrogenase deficiency. J Clin Endocrinol Metab 39: 206.

Kirkland RT, Kirkland JL, Johnson C, Horning M, Librik L, Clayton GW (1973) Congenital lipoid adrenal hyperplasia in an eight-year old phenotypic female. J Clin Endocrinol Metab 36: 488.

Knorr D, Bidlingmaier F, Engelhardt D (1973) Reifenstein's syndrome: a 17β-hydroxysteroid-oxydoreductase deficiency? Acta Endocrinol (Copenhagen) Suppl 173: 37.

Lee PA, Hoffman WH, White JJ, Engel RME, Blizzard RM (1974) Serum gonadotropins in cryptorchidism. An indicator of functional testes. Am J Dis Child 127: 530.

Leshin M, Griffin JE, Wilson JD (1978) Hereditary male pseudohermaphroditism associated with an unstable form of 5α-reductase. J Clin Invest 62: 685.

Levine LS, Lieber E, Pang S, New MI (1980) Male pseudo-

hermaphroditism due to 17-ketosteroid reductase deficiency diagnosed in the newborn period. Pediat Res 14: 480.

Luttrell B, Hochberg RB, Dixon WR, McDonald PD, Lieberman S (1972) Studies on the biosynthetic conversion of cholesterol into pregnenolone. J Biol Chem 247: 1462.

Mallin SR (1969) Congenital adrenal hyperplasia secondary to 17-hydroxylase deficiency: two sister with amenorrhea, hypokalemia, hypertension and cystic ovaries. Ann Intern Med 70: 69.

Mantero F, Busnardo B, Riondel A, Veyrat R, Austoni M (1971) Hypertension arterielle alcalose hypokaliemique et pseudohermaphrodisme male par deficit en 17α-hydroxylase. Schweiz Med Wochenschr 101: 38.

McGuire JS Jr, Tomkins GM (1960) The heterogeneity of Δ4-3-ketosteroid reductases {5}. J Biol Chem 235: 1134.

Money J, Hampson JG, Hampson JL (1955) Hermaphroditism: recommendations concerning assignment of sex, change of sex and psychologic management. Bull Johns Hopkins Hosp 45: 284.

Neumann F, Elger W (1966) The effect of the anti-androgen 1,2α-methylene-6-chloro-Δ4,6-pregnadiene-17-α-ol-3,20-dione-17α-acetate (cyproterone acetate) on the development of the mammary glands of male foetal rats. J Endocrinol 36: 347.

New MI (1970) Male pseudohermaphroditism due to 17α-hydroxylase deficiency. J Clin Invest 49: 1930.

Nowakowski H, Lenz W (1961) Genetic aspects in male hypogonadism. Rec Prog Horm Res 17: 53.

Opitz JM, Simpson JL, Sarto GE, Summitt RL, New MI, German J (1972) Pseudovaginal perineoscrotal hypospadias. Clin Genet 3: 1.

Pang S, Levine L, Chow D, Sagiani F, Saenger P, New MI (1979) Dihydrotestosterone and its relationship to testosterone in infancy. J Clin Endocrinol Metab 48: 821.

Parks GA, Bermudez JA, Anast CS, Bongiovanni AM, New MI (1971) Pubertal boy with the 3β-hydroxysteroid dehydrogenase defect. J Clin Endocrinol Metab 33: 269.

Peterson RE, Imperato-McGinley J, Gautier T, Sturla E (1977) Male pseudohermaphroditism due to steroid 5α-reductase deficiency. Am J Med 62: 170.

Pinsky L, Kaufman M, Straisfeld C, Zilahi B, Hall C St-G (1978) 5α-reductase activity of genital and nongenital skin fibroblasts from patients with 5α-reductase deficiency, androgen insensitivity, or unknown forms of male pseudohermaphroditism. Am J Med Genet 1: 407.

Prader A, Gurtner HP (1955) Das Syndrom des Pseudohermaphroditismus masculinus bei Kongenitaler Nebennieren rinden Hyperplasie ohne Androgen-Überproduktion. Helv Pediatr Acta 10: 397.

Saenger P, Goldman AS, Levine LS, Korth-Schutz S, Muecke EC, Katsumata M, Doberne Y, New MI (1978) Prepubertal diagnosis of steroid 5α-reductase-deficiency. J Clin Endocrinol Metab 46: 627.

Saez JM, de Peretti E, Morera AM, David M, Bertrand J, (1971) Familial male pseudohermaphroditism with gynecomastia due to a testicular 17-ketosteroid reductase defect. I. Studies in vivo. J Clin Endocrinol Metab 32: 604.

Savage MO, Chaussain JL, Evain D, Roger M, Canlorbe P, Job JC (1978) Endocrine studies in male pseudohermaphroditism in childhood and adolescence. Clin Endocrinol 8: 219.

Schneider G, Genel M, Bongiovanni AM, Goldman AS, Rosenfeld RL (1975) Persistent testicular Δ5 isomerase-3β-hydroxysteroid dehydrogenase (Δ5-3β-HSD) deficiency in the Δ5-3β-HSD form of congenital adrenal hyperplasia. J Clin Invest 55: 681.

Tourniaire J, Audi-Parera L, Loran B, Blum J, Castelnovo P,

Forest MG (1976) Male pseudohermaphroditism with hypertension due to a 17α-hydroxylation deficiency. Clin Endocrinol 5: 53.

Virdis R, Saenger P, Senior B, New MI (1978) Endocrine studies in a pubertal male pseudohermaphrodite with 17-ketosteroid reductase deficiency. Acta Endocrinol 87: 212.

Walsh PC, Madden JD, Harrod MJ, Goldstein JL, McDonald PC, Wilson JD (1974) Familial incomplete male pseudohermaphroditism type 2: decreased DHT formation in pseudovaginal perineoscrotal hypospadias. New Engl J Med 291: 944.

Wilson JD (1975a) Metabolism of testicular androgens. In Greep RO and Astwood EP, eds. Handbook of physiology, Section 7: Endocrinology, Vol V: Male reproductive system pp 491–508. Washington, D.C.: American Physiology Society.

Wilson JD (1975b) Dihydrotestosterone formation in cultured human fibroblasts. J Biol Chem 250: 3498.

Yoshida E, Beutler E, Motulsky AG (1971) Human glucose-6-phosphate dehydrogenase variants. Bull WHO 45: 243.

Zachmann M, Völlmin JA, Hamilton W, Prader A (1972) Steroid 17,20-desmolase deficiency: a new cause of male pseudohermaphroditism. Clin Endocrinol 1: 369.

10. THE IMPACT OF ANDROGENS ON THE EVOLUTION OF MALE GENDER IDENTITY

JULIANNE IMPERATO-MCGINLEY, RALPH E. PETERSON, TEOFILO GAUTIER
and ERASMO STURLA

1. INTRODUCTION

Sex differences in behavior from infancy through adulthood have been documented in humans (Ounsted and Taylor 1972; Hutt, 1972) and animals (Reinisch, 1974; Goy and Goldfoot 1973). In animals, sexually dimorphic behavior is secondary to sex steroid induced differentiation and activation of the brain at critical periods. In humans, however, controversy exists as to whether gender identity formation is influenced by sex steroid "imprinting" of the brain at critical periods.

In man, pseudohermaphrodites were studied and conclusions were made concerning the supremacy of the sex of rearing as compared to biologic factors in the formation of gender identity (Chapman et al., 1951; Money et al., 1955a, b; Burns et al., 1960; Ghabrial and Girgis, 1962; Berg and Leeds, 1963; Brown and Fryer, 1964; Teter and Boczkowski, 1965; Dewhurst and Gordan, 1969; Money and Ogunro, 1974; Lev-Ran, 1974). However, most of the studies were conducted without adequate knowledge of the subjects' hormonal milieu (i.e. androgens) and therefore the conclusions which emphasized the dominant role of the sex of rearing were merely speculative.

Male pseudohermaphrodites with steroid 5α-reductase deficiency (Imperato-McGinley et al., 1974; Peterson et al., 1977; Walsh et al., 1974) are unique, since the biosynthesis and peripheral action of testosterone is normal and thus prenatal and neonatal testosterone exposure of the brain, proceeds as in the normal male. However, because of deficient 5α-reductase activity resulting in decreased dihydrotestosterone production in utero, there is such severe ambiguity of the external genitalia of the affected male fetus, that many affected male subjects are believed to be female at birth and consequently raised as girls. At puberty, however, masculinization occurs under the influence of normal plasma testosterone levels (Imperato-McGinley et al., 1974; Peterson et al., 1977). Thus, male pseudohermaphrodites with 5α-reductase deficiency raised as females, are extraordinary experiments of nature for evaluating the relative influences of testosterone and the sex of rearing in the determination of gender identity in man.

2. CLINICAL DESCRIPTION

At birth, the affected subjects have a scrotum that is markedly bifid, appearing more labial-like. The phallus is clitoral-like and they have a urogenital sinus with a blind vaginal pouch. The testes are in the abdomen, inguinal canal or scrotum (Imperato-McGinley et al., 1974; Peterson et al., 1977) (Fig. 1).

With puberty, a dramatic change occurs mediated by the normal to high plasma levels of testosterone. The voice deepens and the affected subjects develop a muscular habitus with substantial growth of the phallus (4–5 cm). The scrotum becomes rugated and hyperpigmented, and in the majority of cases the testes descend if they are not already in the scrotum. There is no gynecomastia. The subjects have erections and there is a ejaculate from the urethral orifice on the perineum. They are capable of intromission but because of the position of the urethra are not capable of insemination (Imperato-McGinley et al., 1974; Peterson et al., 1977) (Fig. 2). The post-pubertal affected males, have a scant to absent beard and decreased body hair. The prostate is small or absent (Imperato-McGinley et al., 1974; Peterson et al., 1977).

100

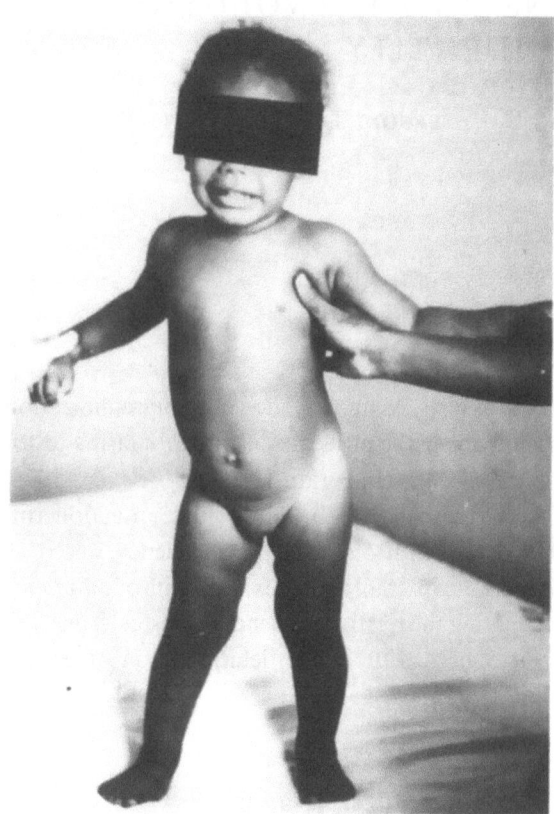

Figure 1. Subject #23 is a male pseudohermaphrodite at the age of 18 months with 5α-reductase deficiency.

3. METHODS AND RESULTS

There are 38 known male pseudohermaphrodites with 5α-reductase deficiency from 23 interrelated families spanning four generations in three rural villages, in the southwestern region of the Dominican Republic. The condition is inherited as an autosomal recessive trait (Imperato-McGinley et al., 1974; Peterson et al., 1977). Five of the affected subjects are deceased; two died in infancy and three in adulthood. Thirty-three males are living; 25 are postpubertal, three pubertal and five prepubertal.

Interviews concerning the psychosexual develop-

ment of the affected subjects were carried out in villages A and B. Historical data were obtained by interviewing the affected male subjects who were raised as females and those who were raised as males. Other males in the villages were interviewed as controls. Parents, siblings, wives, girl friends and neighbors of the affected subjects were interviewed when possible. The interviews were conducted in Spanish by members of our research group known to the community since 1972 and were independently translated into English by another member of the group.* The interviews were designed to determine any ambiguity in the female sex of rearing of the affected subjects and the validity of the change in those that appeared to adopt a male gender identity and gender role.** Data were obtained concerning the age the affected subjects who were raised as girls began to doubt their female gender. Information concerning their postpubertal male psychosexual orientation and behavior was also obtained. The social practices within the villages were investigated to discern the influence of cultural factors on the change in gender identity of the subjects.

From the interview data, 19 of 33 affected subjects from village A and B were found to have been unambiguously raised as females (Imperato-McGinley et al., 1979b). Adequate postpubertal psychosexual data were obtained from 18 of the 19 subjects. Sixteen of the 18 subjects successfully changed to a male gender identity and a male gender role. The two exceptions, are subject #4 and subject #25 (Fig. 3, Table 1). Subject #4 from village A adopted a male gender identity, but continues to dress as a female. Despite dressing as a female, this subject has the affect and mannerisms of a man and does man's work (see addendum) as a farmer and woodsmen. Subject #4 lives alone but engages in sexual activity with village women. Subject #25 (age 37) from village B (Fig. 3, Table 1), is the only postpubertal affected subject who has maintained a female gender

* Six of the affected subjects are now living and working in the hospital in Santo Domingo to which a member of the research team is affiliated. In addition, numerous trips to the community have been made since 1972 by various members of the team, and the villagers are now quite familiar with most of the team members. Also, six affected subjects and a father and sister of an affected subject have been hospitalized at The New York Hospital for a minimum of six to eight weeks. Presently four affected subjects are residing in New York. Thus, in addition to the formal interview sessions we have been able to observe these subjects over a protracted period of time and have become quite involved with both the subjects and their families.

** *Gender identity* — the sense of being male or female. The self awareness of knowing to which sex one belongs. The private experience of gender role. *Gender role* — the public expression of one's gender identity. This is manifested by what one does or says that indicates to others or to one's self the extent of being male or being female, or ambivalent.

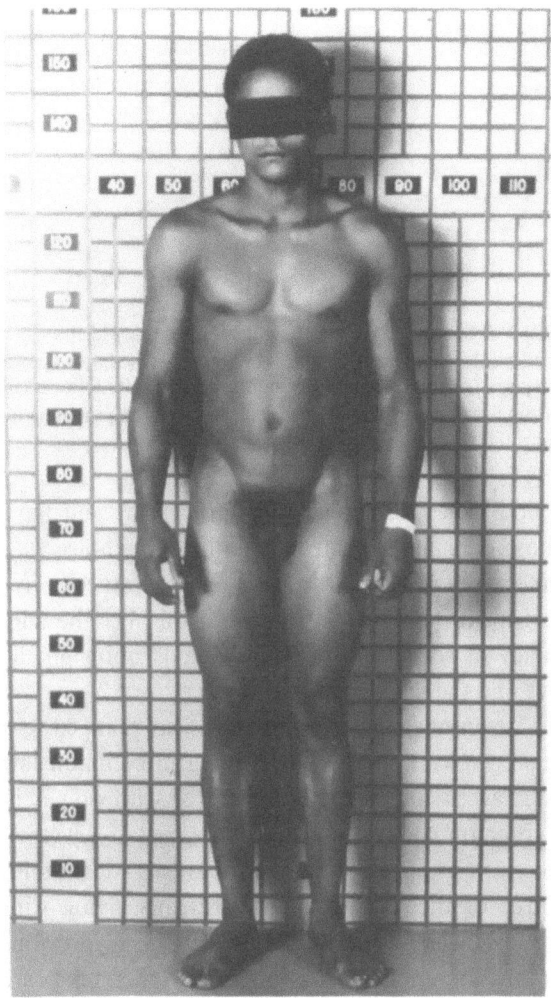

Figure 2. A 26-year-old male pseudohermaphrodite with 5α-re-ductase deficiency. Note the android build.

identity and female gender role. She was "married" at the age of 16 to a man in village B and they lived together for one year. He left her and she left the town shortly thereafter. Since moving to the Capitol she has been living alone and working as a domestic. She has not been sexually involved with other men and denies ever being attracted to women. Since puberty she has been wearing false breasts, yet despite this her build and mannerisms are quite masculine. She states that she wants surgical correction of the genitalia so that she can be a normal woman.

Between 7 to 12 years of age, those affected subjects raised as girls (with the exception of subject #25) began to realize that they were different from other girls in the village when they did not develop breasts. Serious self concern was raised over their

gender as they began to "feel like men," and as they noted their bodies begin to change in a masculine direction with masses noted in the inguinal canal or scrotum. A male gender identity evolved as they passed through stages of no longer feeling like girls, to "feeling like men" and finally to the self realization that they were indeed men. In all instances, there was a lag period from the time they began to realize differences from other girls their age, until the time they finally changed gender role from female to male (Fig. 4, Table 1). The change in gender role occurred either during puberty or in the postpubertal period after the affected subjects were convinced of their maleness, and were experiencing sexual interest in girls and were having morning erections and were masturbating. In a few instances, the change in gender role was delayed until they were confident of their ability to defend themselves if necessary. The average age of the gender role change was sixteen; although in three subjects, the change to a male gender role did not occur until they were in their twenties and in subject #4 the change did not occur at all (Table 1).

When the age of initiation of morning erections, nocturnal emissions, masturbation and first sexual intercourse were compared, there were no significant differences between those subjects raised as girls and those raised as boys. The time of first sexual intercourse was 15 to 18 years of age for those raised as girls, 15 to 17 years for those raised as boys and 14 to 16 years of age for 20 normal male controls in the village.

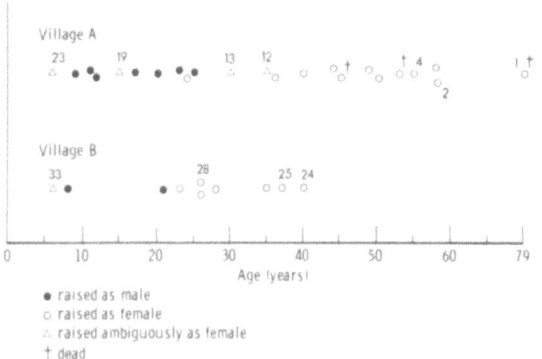

Figure 3. Thirty-three male pseudohermaphrodites with 5α-re-ductase deficiency from village A and B. Note that the condition is now recognized at birth or shortly thereafter in the younger affected subjects and they are being raised as boys; whereas in the older affected subjects, the condition was unrecognized throughout childhood and they were raised unambiguously as females.

Table 1. Male pseudohermaphrodites with 5α-reductase deficiency who were unambiguously raised as females

VILLAGE A

Subject	Age (years) 1978	Age of gender role change
1	59 (+ '58)	16
2	58	17
3	58	24
4	55	No change, male gender identity, female gender role
5	53 +	Puberty
6	50	15
7	49	16
8	45 (+ '74)	21
9	44	16
10	40	15
11	36	15
15	24	16

VILLAGE B

Subject	Age (years) 1978	Age of gender role change
24	40	20
25	37	No change, female gender identity and female gender role
26	35	Left town at 20 (no follow-up)
27	28	14
28	26	15
29	26	15
30	23	17

+ Deceased.

In the postpubertal subjects unambiguously raised as girls, the manifestations of male sexual behavior were evaluated according to the four patterns of sexual behavior differentiation (Diamond, 1965, 1977) 1 Sexual patterns (sex-related behavior) — for males it includes direct aggressiveness, assertiveness, large motor activity, occupation. 2. Sexual gender identity — the sex to which an individual ascribes. 3. Sexual object of choice — the sex of the individual chosen as an erotically interesting partner. 4. Sexual mechanisms — the features of sexual expression over which an individual has little control, i.e. for males it includes the ability to obtain and maintain an erection, and to achieve orgasm. With the exception of subject #25, all affected subjects perform male work in a society where there is a definite division of labor according to sex. All except subject #25 have a male gender identity and all except subject #4 and #25 have adopted a male

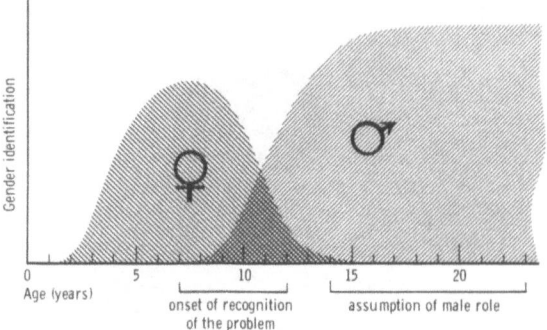

Figure 4. Schema depicting the change in gender identity and gender role from female to male. The cross hatched area depicts the period of confusion concerning their true gender followed by the final emergence of male gender identity in male pseudohermaphrodites with 5α-reductase deficiency.

gender role. All subjects have erections and have chosen females as their sexual object of choice with the exception of subject #25 who continues to live and identify as female (Fig. 3, Table 1). The adequacy of sexual intercourse depends upon phallic size and the severity of the chordee.

Fifteen of the sixteen subjects who changed to a male gender role are either living in common law marriages with women or have lived with women in a common law relationship in the past. They enjoy their role as head of the household (see addendum). Three of these subjects are presently living with women who have had children from previous unions. In a domestic setting, the women take care of the household activities while the affected male subjects work either as farmers, miners or woodsmen; as do the normal males in the town. The one exception is subject #24 from village B who lives alone in the hills where he works as a farmer since changing to a male gender role at age 20 (Fig. 3, Table 1).

Subject #28 in village B (Fig. 3) has been living with the same women for 9 years. During this time the woman has had three pregnancies and has four living children. Although this subject knows the children are not his, he now accepts them. His wife states that although she loves him she wants children and therefore becomes pregnant with other men. Subject #1 (Fig. 3) started living with his wife when he was 35 years old and she was 13 years of age. She stated that she loved him and was sexually satisfied by him. She remained faithful to him until he died at age 59 after 24 years of marriage. Only when she remarried did she realize that his genitalia were abnormal. Subject #2 (Fig. 3) a prominent man in village A, is both respected and feared. Everyone in town knows of his condition, but it is never discussed openly. He is married to a woman who has had three children from a previous union.

Although these subjects behave unequivocally as males, they experience certain insecurities because of the abnormal appearance of their genitalia. They view themselves as incomplete and this saddens them. They fear ridicule by members of the opposite sex and initially feel quite anxious about forming sexual relationships. They wonder why God made them this way, but feel that they cannot question what He has done.

Two postpubertal subjects #12 and #13 (Fig. 3) from village A were initially raised as girls, and later in childhood were changed to a male sex of rearing by their parents and have remained males. They are not considered to have been unambiguously raised as females. Subject #19 from village A (Fig. 3) was raised as a girl by her parents despite their knowledge that an older brother had changed gender identity and gender role at puberty, and despite the fact that they were raising two affected younger siblings as boys. Thus, subject #19 was not unambiguously raised as female. Likewise, subject #33 from village B (Fig. 3) is being raised as a girl despite family awareness of the situation. Subject #23 (Fig. 3) whose parents are descendants of the inhabitants of village A, was born in Santo Domingo and raised as a female. When she was hospitalized for a hernia repair at age 18 months, her parents were told of her condition (Fig. 1). They continued to raise her as a female however, until 5½ years of age when the father decided to raise the child as a boy.

Thus, the affected subjects in village A and B were raised as girls, until the townspeople became aware of the condition, i.e recognizing it at birth, and realizing that despite their female sex of rearing the affected subjects would change to a male gender identity and male gender role with the events of puberty. Subsequently, the villagers have either raised the affected subjects as males from birth, or have changed the sex of rearing to males as soon as the problem is recognized. As previously mentioned, two families have opted to raise two prepubertal affected subjects as females despite complete knowledge of what will transpire with puberty (Fig. 3).

Now that the villagers are familiar with the condi-

tion, the affected children and adults are sometimes objects of ridicule. The villagers refer to them as "guevedoce," "guevote" (penis at twelve) and or machihembra (first women, then man). The affected adult males are quite capable of defending themselves when necessary, since they are as tall and generally more muscular than the rest of the male community. Their comparative strength and ability to gain respect by physical force if necessary enables them to exist in the community.

4. DISCUSSION

Androgens administered prenatally and/or postnatally to either female animals or male castrate animals can induce both adult male sexual and nonsexual behavior and inhibit female sexual response. Although the amount of administered androgen and the critical period for treatment differ from species to species; comparable effects on the development of male sexual behavior have been obtained in the rat (Harris, 1964; Pfaff, 1971, guinea pig (Phoenix et al., 1959), mouse (Edwards and Burge, 1971), rabbit (Beyer et al., 1975), hamster (Paup et al., 1972) dog (Beach, 1975), sheep (Clarke, 1977), and rhesus monkey (Goy et al., 1977). The critical period for induction of male sexual response varies with the animal species, i.e. the dog requiring both pre- and postnatal exposure for optimal effect (Beach, 1975). Conversely, depriving the male animal of testosterone at a critical period will inhibit male sexual behavior and augment female sexual behavior in adulthood (Beach, 1975)

In addition to behavioral differences, androgen induced sex differences in brain morphology and function are well documented. In rats, perinatal androgen administration produces structural differences in brain areas associated with masculine sexual behavior (Pfaff, 1966; Dorner and Staudt, 1968, Raisman and Field, 1973; Gorski et al., 1978). In rats, under the neonatal influence of androgens, the preoptic suprachiasmatic area of the hypothalamus "differentiates" to regulate a tonic release of gonadotrophins from the pituitary; whereas in the absence of neonatal androgen exposure a cyclical release of gonadotrophins will occur (Barraclough, 1966). In canaries (*Werinus canarius*) and zebra finches (*Poephila gutata*), three vocal control areas in the brain are strikingly larger in males than in females (Notterbohm and Arnold, 1976) and a fourth area is absent in female zebra finches, and less well developed in female canaries. These differences correlate well with differences in singing behavior, as only males usually sing. In the squirrel monkey, sex differences have been found in the nuclear size of neurons in the medial amygdala which may be related to sex differences in the control of pituitary gonadotrophin secretion (Bubenik and Brown, 1973). The androgen effects on the brain causing sexual dimorphism in animals may be mediated either directly through androgens (i.e. testosterone) and/or via aromatization of androgens to estrogens in the brain (Reddy et al., 1974).

In man, the basic question of the relative influences of hormonal factors and environmental factors in the determination of gender identity remains unanswered. In 1955, the theory of sexual neutrality at birth was proposed (Money et al., 1955a, b). It stated that in man, sexuality was undifferentiated at birth, becoming differentiated as either masculine or feminine in the course of various experiences of growing. Later on the concept of sexual neutrality at birth was broadened to recognize that human male and female infants express sexually dimorphic behavior from birth. However, it was postulated that such sexually dimorphic behavior could be incorporated into either a male or female gender identity pattern and was not the exclusive property of either sex (Money and Ehrhardt, 1972). To test this hypothesis, pseudohermaphrodites were matched so that they were "chromosally, gonadally and otherwise diagnostically the same." "The matched pairs" were said to differ only in their sex of assignment and therefore their sex of rearing. The studies appeared to show that the gender identity of the individuals was concordant with the sex of rearing and not with the chromosomal or gonadal sex. Therefore, it was concluded that the sex of rearing predominated in establishing gender identity in man.

Although the subjects of those aforementioned studies may have been matched chromosomally and gonadally, they were not matched for a similar hormonal milieu; as the methodology for adequate plasma steroid evaluation was not available at that time. Thus, the amount of androgen exposure was assumed to be similar for the "matched pairs" of

pseudohermaphrodites but not known to be so. Therefore in these studies the issue of nature (i.e. androgen) versus nurture (ie.e sex of rearing) in the determination of a male gender identity cannot be adequately resolved due to lack of sufficient hormonal data. Furthermore, since the etiology of most cases of male pseudohermaphroditism is secondary to either inadequate testosterone production or action, many of the subjects described were probably testosterone deficient (Imperato-McGinley et al., 1976), and are inappropriate models (as are female pseudohermaphrodites) for determining the relative importance of the sex of rearing versus nature (i.e. androgen) in the determination of male gender identity in man. Also in most cases studied, where the gender identity was concordant to the sex of rearing and discordant to the chromosomal and gonadal sex, castration and sex hormone therapy were usually initiated to coincide with the sex of rearing thereby interrupting the natural sequence of events (Money et al., 1955a, b; Money and Ehrhardt, 1972).

In this study of human male pseudohermaphrodites with 5α-reductase deficiency, 18 subjects were unambiguously raised as girls. Despite the female sex of rearing, 17 subjects changed to a male gender identity and 16 subjects changed to a male gender role during or following puberty. These events occurred in a setting without physician intervention and/or other social factors which might have acted to interrupt the natural sequence of events. Intervention by a physician, i.e. reassurance, surgical correction of the external genitalia to coincide with the female sex assignment, or administration of hormone therapy concordant with the female sex of rearing, did not occur. Parental attitude when the change was occurring was one of amazement, confusion and finally acceptance, rather than hostility and prevention. Social pressure, i.e. embarrassment and possible harassment afterwards by the other villagers, were the major anxieties the affected males experienced, which may have caused them to hesitate for a time. However, with the exception of one subject (#4), the pressures were not strong enough to prevent the change to a male gender role from occurring in all 17 subjects who had adopted a male gender identity with puberty. The one affected subject (#25) who retained her female gender identity postpubertally, is a complete exception to this general phenomenon of pubertal gender identity change in these subjects. This highlights the fact that in humans because of higher cognitive processes and due to the multifactorial input in forming gender identity, there will always be exceptions to a general rule.

Normally the sex of rearing and testosterone imprinting of the brain act in unison to determine the complete expression of the male gender (Fig. 5).

NORMAL MALE

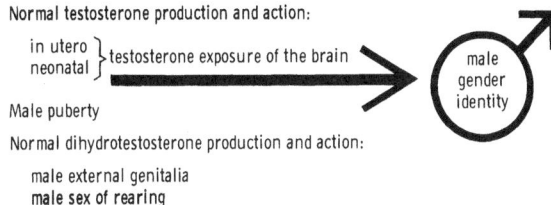

Figure 5. Schema depicting the hormonal factors and environmental factors, i.e. sex of rearing acting in unison to form male gender identity in the normal male.

However, the subjects of this study demonstrate that in a laissez-faire environment, when the sex of rearing (female) is discordant to the testosterone mediated biologic sex; the biologic sex prevails if normal testosterone activation of puberty is permitted to occur (Fig. 6).

From the data, it appears that the extent of testosterone exposure of the brain in utero, the early postnatal period, and at puberty, has greater impact in determining male gender identity than the female sex of rearing (Fig. 6). Theoretically, "masculinization" of the brain occurs under the influence of testosterone and together with the activation of a testosterone mediated puberty, male gender identity develops, overriding the female sex of earing.* This experiment of nature emphasizes the importance of androgens which act as inducers and activators in the evolution of male gender identity in man (Imperato-McGinley et al., 1979a, b).

In male pseudohermaphrodites with inadequate testosterone production or action, it is understandable that gender identity might coincide with the sex of rearing. Adequate androgen imprinting has not

MALE PSEUDOHERMAPHRODITES WITH 5α-REDUCTASE DEFICIENCY WHO WERE RAISED AS FEMALES

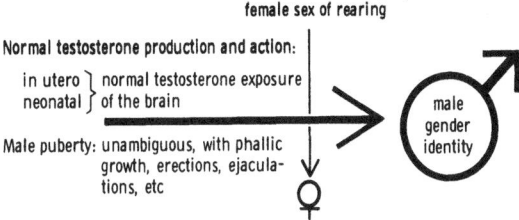

Figure 6. Schema depicting the dominance of testosterone imprinting and activation in the evolution of a male gender identity, completely overriding the unambiguous female sex of rearing in male pseudohermaphrodites with 5α-reductase deficiency.

occurred and therefore the sex of rearing becomes the predominant factor. Such individuals are a testimonial to the malleability of human beings in the acquisition of gender identity, but in no way approximate the normal sequence of events (Diamond, 1965) (Fig. 7 and 8.).

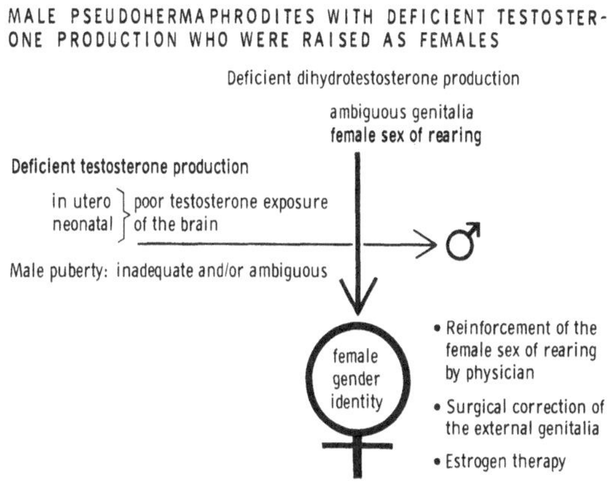

MALE PSEUDOHERMAPHRODITES WITH DEFICIENT TESTOSTERONE PRODUCTION WHO WERE RAISED AS FEMALES

Figure 7. Schema depicting the predominance of female sex of rearing in pseudohermaphrodites with deficient testosterone production.

It has been proposed that gender identity becomes fixed by 18 months to 4 years of age; around the time of language development (Money et al., 1955a, b; Money and Ehrhardt, 1972). At this time a child becomes aware of his or her gender. However, being aware of ones' gender and being unalterably fixed in that gender are two separate issues. From this

---

* We have recently investigated a 65-year-old male pseudohermaphrodite with 5α-reductase deficiency born in souther Italy and raised as a girl. The subject emigrated to the United States at age 16. Psychosexual evaluation shows that the subject gradually changed to a male gender identity with puberty and presently has a male gender identity but because of family pressure has retained a female gender role (Imperato-McGinley et al., 1980).

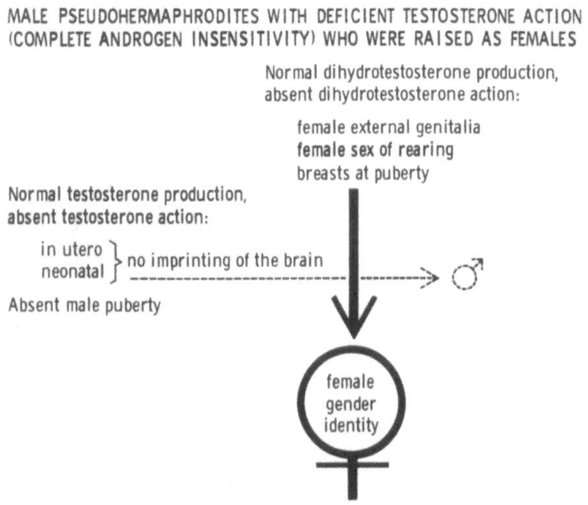

MALE PSEUDOHERMAPHRODITES WITH DEFICIENT TESTOSTERONE ACTION (COMPLETE ANDROGEN INSENSITIVITY) WHO WERE RAISED AS FEMALES

Normal dihydrotestosterone production, absent dihydrotestosterone action:

female external genitalia
female sex of rearing
breasts at puberty

Normal testosterone production, absent testosterone action:

in utero
neonatal } no imprinting of the brain

Absent male puberty

female gender identity

Figure 8. Schema depicting the predominance of the female sex of rearing in subjects with the complete androgen insensitivity syndrome (testicular feminization) who were raised as females.

study, it appears that the development of gender identity in man is continually evolving throughout childhood, becoming fixed with puberty.

Since the evolution of a male gender identity is initiated with early puberty in subjects with 5α-reductase deficiency, it is not surprising that either prepubertal or pubertal castration with the initiation of female hormone therapy might abort its development (Walsh et al., 1974; Saenger et al., 1978; Fisher et al., 1978). The time course for the development of a male gender identity with puberty appears to be unique to each individual (Fig. 4, Table 1). Thus, the age when successful interruption (i.e. castration, sociocultural factors, etc.) can be initiated to prevent the complete evolution of a male gender identity and/or the change to a male gender role will differ for each affected subject.

There are many reported cases of male pseudohermaphrodites with successful changes in gender from female to male occurring after the proposed "critical period" (Chapman et al., 1951; Burns et al., 1960; Ghabrial and Girgis, 1962; Berg and Leeds, 1963; Brown and Fryer, 1964; Teter and Boczkowski, 1965; Dewhurst and Gordan, 1969; Stoller, 1964; Zuger, 1970). In many of these cases, the change in gender role occurred during adolescence. Adequate hormonal evaluation would be important in these cases; as they also appear to challenge both the theory of the immutability of gender identity after the ages of 3 to 4 and the sex of rearing

as the major factor in determining male gender identity.

The data of this study show that in humans, environmental or sociocultural factors are not solely responsible for the formation of a male gender identity. Androgens make a strong and definite contribution. Analogous to the induction of the male phenotype from the inherent female phenotype, the formation of a male gender identity in man also appears to be at least partially induced by androgens from an undifferentiated and/or inherently female nervous system (Fig. 9).

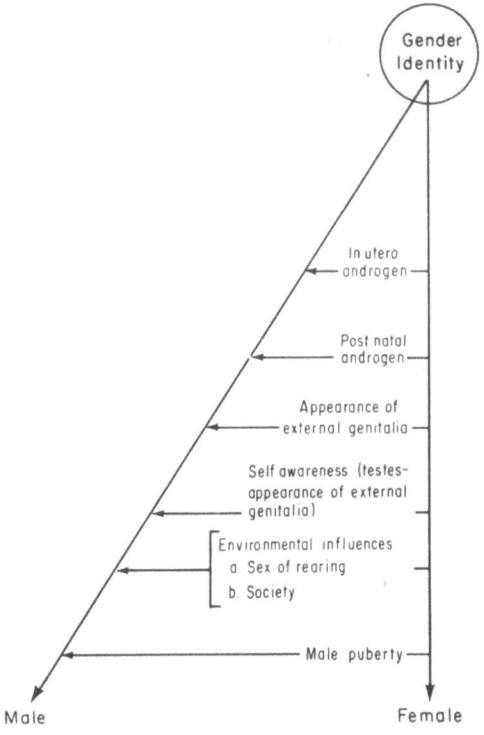

Figure 9. Schema depicting the critical factors involved in the evolution of a male gender identity in man.

ACKNOWLEDGEMENTS

This work was supported by Research Career Award (R.E.P.) K6-AM 14241-15, Clinical Investigator Award NIAMDD (J.I.-McG.) KO8-AM 00615-01, Clinical Research Center Grant RR-47, Research Grant HD0921, from the National Institutes of Health, National Foundation Research Grant 6-52, Shorr Fellowship Fund, and a grant from Gulf and Western (Dominican Republic).

REFERENCES

Barraclough CA (1966) Modification in the CNS regulation of reproduction after exposure of prepubertal rats to steroid hormones. Rec Prog Horm Res 22: 503.

Beach FA (1975) Hormonal modification of sexually dimorphic behavior. Psychoneuroendocrinology 1: 3.

Berg I, Leeds MB (1963) Change of assigned sex at puberty. Lancet ii; 1216.

Beyer C, de la Torre L, Larsson L, Perez-Palacio G (1975) Synergistic actions of estrogen and androgen on the sexual behavior of the castrated male rabbit. Horm Behav 6: 301.

Brown JB, Fryer MP (1964) Plastic surgical correction of hypospadias with mistaken sex identity and transvestism resulting in normal marriage and parenthood. Surg Gynecol Obstet 118: 45.

Bubenik GA, Brown GM (1973) Morphologic sex differences in primate brain areas involved in regulation of reproductive activity. Experientia 29: 619.

Burns E, Segaloff A, Carrera GM (1960) Reassignment of sex: report of 3 cases. J Urol 84: 126.

Chapman AH, Saslow G, Watson F (1951) Pseudohermaphroditism, a medical, social, and psychiatric case study. Psychosomat Med 13: 212.

Clarke IJ (1977) The sexual behavior of prenatally androgenized ewes observed in the field. J Reprod Fertil 49: 311.

Dewhurst CG, Gordan RR (1969) Case histories involving reregistration of sex. The intersexual disorder, pp 124–149. London: Balliere Tindall & Cassall.

Diamond M (1965) A critical evaluation of the ontogeny of human sexual behavior. Q Rev Biol 40: 147.

Diamond M (1977) Human sexual development: biological foundations for social development. In Beach FA, ed. Human sexuality in four perspectives, pp 22–61. Baltimore: Johns Hopkins University Press.

Dorner G, Staudt J (1968) Structural changes in the preoptic anterior hypothalamic area of the male rat, following neonatal castration and androgen substitution. Neuroendocrinology 3: 136.

Edwards DA, Burge KG (1971) Early androgen treatment and male and female sexual behavior in mice. Horm Behav 2: 49.

Fisher LK, Kogut MD, Moore RJ, Goebelsmann U, Weitzman JJ, Isaacs H Jr, Griffin JE, Wilson JD (1978) Clinical, endocrinological and enzymatic characterization of two patients with 5α-reductase deficiency. Evidence that a single enzyme is responsible for the 5α-reductase of cortisol and testosterone. J Clin Endocrinol Metab 47: 653.

Ghabrial F, Girgis S (1962) Reorientation of sex: report of two cases. Int J Fertil 7: 249.

Gorski RA, Gordon JH, Shryne JE, Southam Am (1978) Evidence for a morphological sex difference within the medial preoptic area of the rat brain. Brain Res 148: 333.

Goy RW, Goldfoot DA (1973) Hormonal influences on sexually dimorphic behavior. In Greep RO ed. Handbook of physiology, Section 7, Vol 2, Part 1, pp 169–186. Washington, D.C.: American Physiological Society.

Goy RW, Wolf JE, Eisele SG (1977) Experimental female hermaphroditism in rhesus monkeys: Anatomical and psychological characteristics. In Husaph H, Money J, eds. Handbook of sexology, Amsterdam: Excerpta Medica.

Harris GW (1964) Sex hormones, brain development and brain function. Endocrinology 75: 627.

Hutt C (1977) Male and females. Harmondsworth, M.ddx.: Penguin Education.

Imperato-McGinley J, Guerrero L, Gautier T, Peterson RE (1974) Steroid 5α-reductase deficiency in man: an inherited form of male pseudohermaphroditism. Science 186: 1213.

Imperato-McGinley J, Peterson RE (1976) Male pseudohermaphroditism: The complexities of male phenotypic development. Am J Med 61: 251.

Imperato-McGinley J, Peterson RE, Stoller R, Goodwin WE (1979a) Male pseudohermaphroditism secondary to 17β-hydroxysteroid dehydrogenase deficiency. Gender role change with puberty. J Clin Endocrinol Metab 49: 391.

Imperato-McGinley J, Peterson RE, Gautier T, Sturla E, (1979b) Androgens and the evolution of male gender identity among male pseudohermaphrodites with 5α-reductase deficiency. New Engl J Med 300: 1233.

Imperato-McGinley J, Peterson RE, Leshin M, Griffin JE, Cooper G, Draghi S, Berenyi M, Wilson JD (Steroid 5α-reductase deficiency in a 65 year old male pseudohermaphrodite: the natural history, ultrastructure of the testes and evidence of inherited enzyme heterogeneity. J Clin Endocrinol Metab (in press).

Lev-Ran A (1974) Gender role differentiation in hermaphrodites. Arch Sex Behav 3: 391.

Money J, Ehrhardt AA (1972) Man and woman/boy and girl — the differentiation and dimorphism of gender identity from conception to maturity. Baltimore Johns Hopkins University Press.

Money J, Hampson J, Hampson JL (1955a) Hermaphroditism: recommendations concerning assignment of sex, change of sex, and psychologic management. Bull Johns Hopkins Hosp 97: 284.

Money J, Hampson J, Hampson J JL (1955b) An examination of some basic sexual concepts: the evidence of human hermaphroditism. Bull Johns Hopkins Hosp 97: 301.

Money J, Ogunro C (1974) Behavioral sexology: ten cases of genetic male intersexuality with impaired prenatal and pubertal androgenization. Arch Sex Behav 3: 181.

Notterbohn F, Arnold AP (1976) Sexual dimorphism in vocal control areas of the songbird brain. Science 194: 211.

Ounsted C, Taylor DC (1972) Gender differences: their ontogeny and significance. Baltimore: Williams & Wilkins.

Paup DC, Goniglio LP, Clemens LG (1972) Masculinization of the female golden hamster by neonatal treatment with androgen or estrogen. Horm Behav 3: 123.

Peterson RE, Imperato-McGinley J, Gautier T, Sturla E (1977) Male pseudohermaphroditism due to steroid 5α-reductase deficiency. Am J Med 62: 170.

Pfaff DW (1966) Morphological changes in the brains of adult male rats after neonatal castration. J Endocrinol 36: 415.

Pfaff SW, Zigmond RE (1971) Neonatal androgen effects on sexual and non-sexual behavior of adult rats tested under various hormone regimens. Neuroendocrinology 7: 129.

Phoenix CH, Goy RW, Gerall AA, Young WC (1959) Organizing action of prenatally administered testosterone propionate on tissues mediating mating behavior in the female guinea pig. Endocrinology 65: 369.

Raisman G, Field PM (1973) Sexual dimorphism in the neuropil of the preoptic area of the rat and its dependence on neonatal androgen. Brain Res 54: 1.

Reddy VVR, Naftolin F, Ryan KJ (1974) Conversion of androstenedione to estrone by neural tissues from fetal and neonatal rats. Endocrinology 94: 117.

Reinish J (1974) Fetal hormones, the brain, and human sex differences: a heuristic, integrative review of the recent literature. Arch Sex Behav 3: 51.

Saenger P, Goldman AS, Levine LS, Korth-Schultz S, Muecke

EE, Katsumata M, Doberne Y, New MI (1978) Prepubertal diagnosis of steroid 5α-reductase deficiency. J Clin Endocrinol Metab 46: 627.

Stoller R (1964) A contribution to the study of gender identity. Int J Psychoanal 45: 220.

Teter J, Boczkowski K (1965) Errors in management and assignment of sex in patients with abnormal sexual differentiation. Am J Obstet Gynecol 93: 1084.

Walsh PC, Madden JD, Harrod MH, Goldstein JL, MacDonald PC, Wilson JD (1974) Familial incomplete male pseudohermaphroditism, type 2: Decreased dihydrotestosterone formation in pseudovaginal perineoscrotal hypospadias. New Engl J Med 291: 944.

Zuger B (1970) Gender role determination: a critical review of the evidence from hermaphroditism. Psychosom Med 32: 449.

ADDENDUM

The Towns and Social Practices

Villages A and B are in a remote and rural area in the southwestern section of the Dominican Republic. Both villages were virtually geographic isolates with access only via dirt roads. However, approximately 20 years ago, the government paved the road to village A in order to bring workers to the salt mine from a neighboring village. The access road to village B however is unchanged. The population of village A is approximately 5,000 and the population of village B is 2,500. The houses on the main street of the villages are constructed from woven palm leaves. The homes consist of two bedrooms and a living area. The other homes in the villages are huts with only two rooms; a community bedroom and a living area. They are constructed with sticks and have thatched roofs. In all the homes, the kitchen is separate and located behind the house. Very few homes have an outhouse and even fewer have shower facilities. The inhabitants of the towns, both adults and children bathe in the river.

The family unit consist of a mother and father who have not been married in either a legal or religious ceremony, and their offspring. The men earn a living either farming, mining or by chopping down trees to provide fuel (carbonero activity) for cooking. The farms are small agricultural plots and are worked individually by the head of the household (the father) or collectively by immediate male members of the family and other male skin. On the outskirts of village A, there is a salt and gypsum mine. Some of the men from the village are employed in the mine, but the majority of the miners are brought in by truck from a larger village nearby.

The women generally do not help in the carbonero activities or in cultivating the agricultural plots. They maintain the household, take care of the children, and cultivate small gardens in the back of the house. Female relatives of the mother usually come over during the day to participate in such household activities as cooking, cleaning, washing and babysitting. The children are taken care of by the mother or the grandmother, older sisters and other female relatives.

There is a definite socialization of the children according to sex. The boys are also allowed to go naked until the 7th or 8th year of life. However, the girls wear underpants from the time they are toilet trained. The boys and girls play together until the age of 6. Between the ages of 6 to 11, the children are encouraged to separate according to sex. From approximately the age of 7, the girls help their mothers with the household activities while the boys help their fathers during the planting and harvesting season or with the carbonero activities. In general, however, the boys have more freedom to romp and play. The girls are encouraged to stay with their mothers or play in close proximity to the house.

There is a primary school in the town and the children start their education at about 7 or 8 years of age. Boys and girls attend school together, with no segregation according to sex. Most of the children, however, do not go to school either because the parents don't have money to buy them books and pencils or because of lack of parental interest. Very few children in the town attend school beyond the 3rd grade.

From the age of 11 to 12, the boys seek entertainment at the bars and attend cockfights. The girls, on the other hand stay home and help with household chores and only occasionally go to the local bar to dance and socialize. In general, the girls marry earlier between the ages of 13 and 20, and the boys between the ages of 18 to 25. Fidelity is demanded from the women but not from the men.

There are no laws in the town against homosexuality, but there is strong social pressure against it and thus it is practiced furtively in both villages. Female prostitution also exist and is accepted as a fact of life. The boys in the town start going to prostitutes from the age of 14.

11. SEXUAL DIFFERENTIATION OF THE BRAIN

Roger A. Gorski and Carol D. Jacobson

1. INTRODUCTION

The brain is an integral component of the reproductive system since the secretory activity of the pituitary and thus gonadal function are under its control, as is reproductive behavior. Therefore, the fact that the brain undergoes sexual differentiation is of paramount importance to our understanding of the development of the reproductive system. As a working hypothesis which will be developed in this chapter, we may state that the brain, regardless of the genetic sex of the animal, has the potential to develop functional and morphological characteristics recognized as feminine in the adult. The establishment of masculine functional and morphological characteristics requires the exposure of the brain to effective levels of gonadal steroids particularly during a critical period of development. Although we cannot completely rule out neuronal genomic factors in the sexual differentiation of the brain, at the present time, such genomic factors if they exist, appear to be of lesser importance than the hormone environment.

In the present chapter we will focus on the process of sexual differentiation of the brain of laboratory animals, particularly the rat. This species is the subject of the authors' personal research but in addition, study of laboratory animals permits controlled invasive experiments which are not possible under clinical conditions. Given the apparent general applicability of the process of sexual differentiation of the brain to mammals and other vertebrates, we take the position that fundamental concepts, although possibly not accurate in terms of specific details, will be elucidated by the study of laboratory animals. Therefore, in this chapter, we will review data from the study of laboratory animals in order to establish fundamental concepts which can form the framework for speculative consideration of the possible sexual differentiation of the human brain.

2. SEXUAL DIFFERENTIATION OF THE NON-HUMAN MAMMALIAN BRAIN

Although the existence of sex differences in brain function and morphology in the adult obviously must be documented before we can consider the process of sexual differentiation, we must also establish that these sex differences are produced, or at least modified, by hormones during development and are not merely imposed on the brain by the hormonal environment of the adult. It is well recognized that gonadal steroids act on specific neurons of the adult brain. These neurons, the distribution of which has been thoroughly studied (Pfaff, 1976; Stumpf and Sar, 1978), contain cytoplasmic receptors specific for various steroids (Peck et al., 1979). Following translocation of the steroid–receptor complex into the nucleus and binding with chromatin, the steroid or steroid–receptor complex transiently modifies neuronal genomic activity. This transient action of steroids is called *activational* and can be contrasted, at least conceptually, with the permanent or *organizational* action of steroids which is responsible for sexual differentiation of the brain. Because of the different hormonal balance produced by the ovaries and testes, certain apparent differences in brain function of the adult could merely reflect the activational effects of a sexually dimorphic hormonal milieu. Therefore, it is necessary to characterize brain function under similar hormonal conditions in order to identify true sex differences in the brain. This has not been accomplished to the same degree for all potential sex dimorphisms.

2.1. Sex differences in brain function

In this section, experimental evidence for the existence of sex differences in brain function will be

S.J. Kogan and E.S.E. Hafez (eds.), Pediatric andrology, 109–134. All rights reserved.
Copyright © 1981, Martinus Nijhoff Publishers bv, The Hague/Boston/London.

110

reviewed briefly with emphasis on the ability of hormone exposure to organize the brain independent of the activational effects of these hormones in the adult. Citation of the extensive literature in each of the areas to be discussed below is beyond the scope of this discussion. When considering generally accepted concepts only recent reviews will be cited. It should be noted, however, that the proceedings of a workshop on the sexual differentiation of the brain, with a thorough bibliography, has recently been published (Goy and McEwen, 1980).

2.1.1. The pattern of gonadotropin (GTH) secretion.
In the laboratory rat, the pattern of GTH secretion is perhaps the most obviously sexually dimorphic characteristic and may be the most sensitive to the organizational action of steroids. The female reproductive system is characterized by cyclic activity in brain, pituitary and ovarian function, culminating every four or five days in ovulation (Fig. 1). In contrast, in the intact male the pattern of GTH and testicular secretion can best be described as tonic. Although there may be diurnal or seasonal fluctuations in hormonal activity, these do not compare with the dramatic cycle fluctuations characteristic

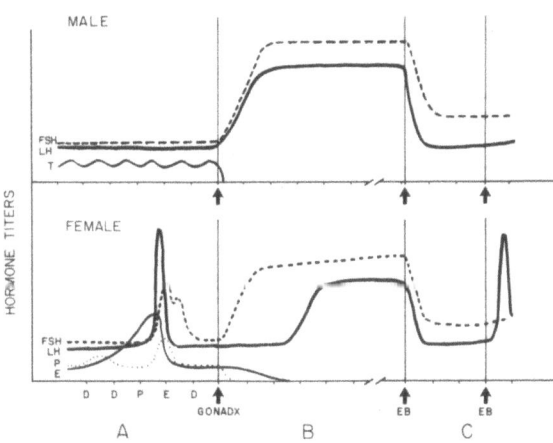

Figure 1. Highly schematic representation of the pattern of changes in plasma titers of gonadal (estrogens, E: progesterone, P; testosterone, T) and hypophyseal (luteinizing hormone, LH; follicle stimulating hormone, FSH) hormones in the intact male and female rat (A), following gonadectomy (B) and (C) subsequent administration of estradiol benzoate (EB). Although LH and FSH are secreted episodically following gonadectomy this is not indicated for simplicity. Abscissa in days with abbreviations: D, diestrus; E, estrus; P, proestrus. Data in Neill and Smith (1974) and Campbell and Schwartz (1977) were utilized in producing this figure ot highlight sex differences in the pattern of hormonal activity.

of the female. The importance of the activational action of gonadal steroids for the normal pattern of GTH secretion is demonstrated by the response to gonadectomy since in both sexes there is a marked increase in GTH secretion which is then episodic in nature. Although a sex difference in the rate of increase in LH secretion following gonadectomy has been reported (Fig. 1; Campbell and Schwartz, 1977.) the most significant sex dimorphism for the purposes of the present discussion has been demonstrated after equalizing the hormonal environment in both sexes. This was initially accomplished by grafting ovarian tissue in animals gonadectomized as adults. In the female, subcutaneous or intra-ocular ovarian grafts support vaginal cycles and ovarian follicles develop and luteinize at regular intervals. In contrast, in the castrated male rat, ovarian grafts become polyfollicular and fail to luteinize (Pfeiffer, 1936). This sex difference in the feedback action of gonadal steroids has also been demonstrated in the absence of ovarian tissue. When the ovariectomized female is appropriately treated with ovarian steroids (either a high dose of estradiol benzoate (EB), or EB followed by a second injection of EB or progesterone (P)), a time-dependent afternoon surge in LH is elicited. This positive feedback resonse does not occur in similarly treated male rats castrated as adults (Fig. 1; Harlan et al., 1979).

Since ovulation in the female rat is presently thought to be the product of an interaction between plasma steroid titers and an intracerebral cyclic stimulus with a potential 24 hour periodicity (Barraclough et al., 1979), the failure of the male to show this response could reflect a sex difference in cerebral function and/or pituitary sensitivity to hypothalamic or gonadal hormones. However, the results of pituitary grafting experiments have suggested that the sex difference resides principally in the brain (Harris, 1964).

It has also been clearly established that the neural substrate responsible for the cyclic patterns of GTH secretion typical of the normal female is sensitive to the organizational action of steroids postnatally. Thus, exposure of the female rat to a single injection of as little as 10 μg testosterone propionate (TP) within about the first week of life will lead to a permanent anovulatory condition. Although this response is dependent upon the dose of TP, the age at injection and at observation, it has been thoroughly documented that exposing the brain of the perinatal female to exogenous androgen prevents the development of the capacity of the hypothalamo-pituitary unit to release GTH cyclically in response to steroid priming (Gorski, 1971). Interestingly, the administration of estrogen is also capable of "masculinizing" GTH regulatory mechanisms (see Section 2.3.1 below). More importantly, castration within the first 1–3 days of postnatal life will result in a genetic male which, when adult, has the capacity to release GTH cyclically in response to ovarian hormones. In fact, ovarian transplants placed in the perinatally castrated male when adult will luteinize cyclically. Thus, the newborn rat, regardless of its genetic sex, has the potential to develop and express the cyclic regulation of GTH release (Fig. 2).

This developmental potential is not restricted to the rat as indicated by the fact that in the following species the ability of ovarian steroids to facilitate GTH secretion in the adult is sexually dimorphic and

the administration of testosterone during early development blocks this response in the female: mouse, hamster, guinea pig and sheep (Goy and McEwen, 1980). It is important to note that steroid treatment must be initiated prior to birth in the latter two species. More recently, androgen exposure, again prenatally, has been reported to block positive feedback in the pig (Elsaesser and Parvizi, 1979). The precise period during development in which the brain is sensitive to the organizational action of steroids apparently depends on the relative stage of neuroendocrine development at birth. However, treatment of the pregnant rhesus monkey with testosterone, although effective in masculinizing the external genitalia of her female offspring, does not inhibit their capacity for spontaneous ovulation (Goy and McEwen, 1980). However, in this species the adult male also exhibits a positive feedback response to estrogen treatment (Karsch et al., 1973). Although it may well be that the neuroendocrine response to positive feedback in this species is not sexually dimorphic, to our knowledge no one has demonstrated that ovarian grafts in the male rhesus monkey will luteinize.

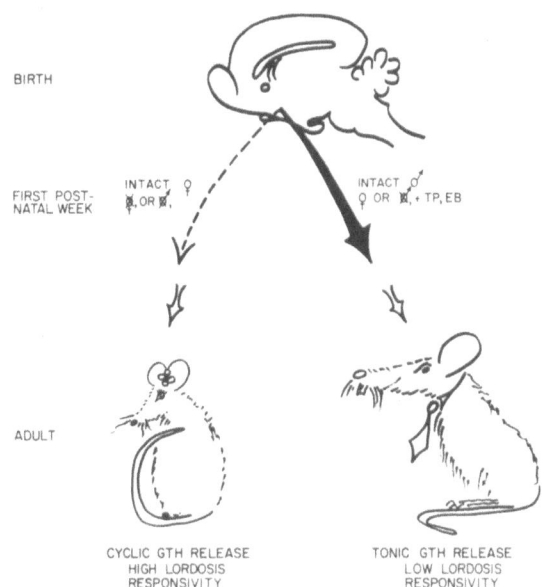

Figure 2. Schematic illustration of the concept of the sexual differentiation of the neural regulation of the pattern of gonadotropin (GTH) release and of feminine sexual behavior (lordosis responsivity) in the rat. At birth the brain is undifferentiated or inherently female. If development during the first week of life occurs without effective exposure to gonadal hormones (i.e., in the intact female, or the female (♀) or male (♂) gonadectomized on day one of postnatal life), the animal when adult displays the feminine neuroendocrine pattern. However, if the brain is exposed to endogenous androgen or exogenous testosterone proprionate (TP) or estradiol benzoate (EB) during approximately the first week of life subsequent brain differentiation produces the masculine pattern of neuroendocrine activity.

2.1.2. Feminine sexual behavior. The sexually receptive female rat, when mounted by a male, will characteristically assume the lordosis posture, thus permitting the male to achieve intromission. This behavior is clearly dependent on the activational effects of hormones since lordosis behavior is not exhibited by the gonadectomized female. In the ovariectomized adult, lordosis behavior can be restored to control levels by either prolonged (about one week of daily injections) treatment with EB, or by a shorter exposure to EB followed by P administration. Although both treatment paradigms have been used experimentally in the gonadectomized female, it is likely that lordosis behavior in the intact female is the result of the synergistic action of both estrogen and P (Gorski, 1974). Although there are other components of feminine sexual behavior, generally regarded as proceptive in nature, lordosis behavior per se is sufficient to illustrate another sexual dimorphism in brain function since the male rat, when castrated as an adult and primed with ovarian steroids, only rarely exhibits lordosis behavior in response to the mounting activity of a stud male. Although the display of lordosis per se may not be sexually dimorphic, the level of lordosis responding clearly is.

It is generally agreed that the genetic male, castrated as an adult, is relatively insensitive to the lordosis facilitating action of P. In the case of EB sensitivity, however, it has been reported both that the male is normally or hyporesponsive to this hormone (Gorski et al., 1979). The explanation of this apparent controversy may relate to the duration of exposure to exogenous hormones required to facilitate lordosis behavior compared to that of endogenous hormones which facilitate this behavior in the intact female. Suffice it to state that it is difficult to treat the male rat which has been castrated as an adult, with ovarian steroids and facilitate the high levels of lordosis responding typical of those of the female.

The experimental evidence for an organizational role of gonadal hormones in this behavioral system has documented the concept that the perinatal rat of either genetic sex has the potential to develop full lordosis responsiveness. Thus, perinatal castration produces an adult genetic male which can display female levels of lordosis responding, while a single injection of TP within the first week of postnatal life, although usually at a greater dose than that required to induce anovulatory sterility, suppresses the development of normal lordosis responsiveness in the female (Fig. 2).

Similar evidence for the sexual differentiation of the neural system which regulates feminine sexual behavior has been accumulated for the mouse, hamster, dog, guinea pig and sheep (Goy and McEwen, 1980), but again whether androgen exposure must occur pre- or postnatally varies with the species.

Because sexual differentiation of the neural mechanisms which regulate the pattern of GTH secretion and lordosis behavior, at least in the rat takes place postnatally, this species has been a convenient animal in which to define the period of greatest sensitivity to the organizing action of steroids, the so-called critical or competent period (Gorski, 1968). The male rat must be castrated prior to day three (although this age is strain specific) in order for him to develop the feminine functional patterns discussed above; in the intact male the critical period is apparently terminated by the action of endogenous hormones and completion of the masculinization process. In the female rat, which normally is not exposed effectively to gonadal steroids, it has been possible to define, on an empirical basis, the end of this critical period of hormone sensitivity. The single administration of a relatively physiological dose of TP is apparently ineffective when given beyond the first week or so of life, however, even when hormone exposure is maximal (e.g., when crystalline hormone is implanted into the brain) day 12 of postnatal life appears to mark the end of the critical period (Lobl and Gorski, 1974). The precise onset of the critical period is not well defined although injections of TP to the pregnant rat, or directly into the fetus, can induce anovulatory sterility (Gorski, 1968).

The fact that, even in the rat, the prenatal hormonal environment can influence sexual differentiation, has recently received an interesting confirmation. It has been shown that the intrauterine position of the female mouse (Gandelman et al., 1977) or rat (Clemens et al., 1978) fetus is a significant variable. The female fetus which is located between two males in utero is apparently affected by locally high testosterone titers (vom Saal and Bronson, 1980a). This is indexed by a significant increase in ano-genital distance when compared with that in female fetuses located between two other females, and in their behavior as adults (Clemens et al., 1978; vom Saal and Bronson, 1978). Vom Saal and Bronson (1980b) have also reported a greater incidence of irregular vaginal cycles in female mice interposed between two males in utero.

2.1.3. Masculine sexual behavior. In the rat and perhaps other mammalian species, masculine sexual behavior appears to be somewhat less sexually dimorphic than the two preceding characteristics. The normal behavioral sequence of the male rat includes mounting the female with or without penile intromission, and after approximately 8–12 intromissions, ejaculation. Although components of masculine sexual behavior may persist for a variable period of time, particularly if the animal is sexually experienced prior to castration, the activational effects of androgen clearly facilitate masculine sexual behavior (Larsson, 1979).

There is a definite sex difference in the level of intromission and ejaculatory behavior. (Note that experimentally these behaviors are recognized by specific dismount behaviors; therefore, it is possible for the female to exhibit intromission or ejaculatory behavior without actual penile insertion or seminal emission.) Mounting activity, however, is commonly exhibited by the female rat (and other mammalian species) and, in fact, it has been argued that mounting behavior in this species is not sexually dimorphic (Gorski et al., 1979). However, we have shown that the intrahypothalamic implantation of gonadal steroids in the perinatal female will significantly augment mounting behavior in the adult (Christensen and Gorski, 1978). We have, in fact, proposed that the prenatal hormone environment may facilitate the mounting activity displayed by the normal adult female. Although this could be attributed to intrauterine position (see above), it is also possible that endogenous estrogen may promote mounting behavior on an individual basis. It has been shown that estrogen levels are very high in the perinatal rat of both sexes (see Section 2.3.1) Although this hormone is currently thought to be functionally sequestered by a perinatal estrogen binding protein, it is possible that sufficient estrogen remains unbound to influence, perhaps on an individual basis, the neural substrate responsible for mounting behavior. The significance of individual differences in hormone secretion, "protective" binding mechanisms, or tissue sensitivity for the sexual differentiation of certain specific neural functions remains to be elucidated.

Masculine sexual behavior is facilitated, depending on the species, following pre- or postnatal exposure to androgen also in the mouse, hamster, ferret, dog, guinea pig, sheep and rhesus monkey (Goy and McEwen, 1980).

2.1.4. Other brain functions. Sexual differentiation is not limited to the regulation of GTH secretion or reproductive behavior; in fact, a large number of behaviors exhibit sexual differences which vary in their degree and in the role of the hormonal environment during development on their establishment. In fact, sexually dimorphic functions are not limited to behavior nor even to the central nervous system. In a detailed review Beatty (1979) has summarized the experimental evidence which suggests that aggressive behavior, running activity, social and play behavior, taste sensitivity, food intake and body weight regulation, territorial marking activity,

learning as indexed by the acquisition of avoidance behaviors and maze performance, and even the response to brain trauma, are all influenced by the organizational action of gonadal steroids. These observations appear to apply on an individual basis to the rat, mouse, hamster, gerbil and monkey. In addition, certain components of maternal behavior (Quadagno et al., 1977), and urination behavior in the beagle (Beach, 1974) also appear to undergo sexual differentiation.

Sex differences at the biochemical level have also been detected. Griffiths et al. (1976) have identified an influence of the perinatal hormone environment on the catabolism of the hypothalamic hormone luteinizing hormone releasing hormone. Peptidase activity in both the hypothalamus and cerebral cortex is increased by androgen treatment of the perinatal female rat.

In a followup of earlier studies in which she showed that perinatal hormone exposure alters the uptake of labeled amino acids in certain brain regions, Litteria (1977) has demonstrated that androgen treatment of the perinatal female rat induces a time dependent alteration in the uptake by the brain of the non-metabolizable amino acid, α-aminoisobutyric acid. Finally, the process of testosterone metabolism at the level of the liver also has been reported to undergo sexual differentiation (Denef, 1974). The list of sex differences in brain function is presumably incomplete and future research can be expected to uncover more examples.

2.2. Morphological differences in the non-human brain

2.2.1. Historical perspective. In the preceding section we have briefly reviewed the voluminous literature which supports the fundamental concept that many, if not all, sex differences in brain function are established under the influence of the perinatal hormone environment. Two fundamental questions remain: Are there morphological correlates of the functional differentiation of the brain? Where in the brain might such morphological correlates be found?

Early studies to identify possible sites of the organizational action of steroids involved an analysis of the neural substrates in the adult which regulate those functions which undergo sexual differentiation. This approach was based on the reasonable assumption that the identification of the neural substrate of the cyclic release of GTH, or of lordosis behavior, etc., would reveal probable loci of early hormone action. Another valid approach, perhaps with a similar rationale, was to focus on the regions of the brain in the adult known to be responsive to sex hormones. Such studies, for example, have suggested that the preoptic area (POA) is an hormone-sensitive integrative center important in the control of ovulation. Attempts to further define the neural substrate for the regulation of ovulation or for feminine and masculine sexual behavior, and other brain functions have continued; the progress in these areas is such that simplistic views have been gradually replaced by the concept that complex and multiple, even redundant, regulatory systems exist. With respect to the control of ovulation, for example, it is now clear that many extrahypothalamic brain regions contribute to the regulation of this event. Although the POA remains as a particularly important component of the ovulatory process, multiple inputs to this region are also of functional significance (Harlan et al., 1979). Because of this fact it is possible that the organizational action of gonadal steroids could take place at one, several or all of these levels. Just how pervasive is the organizational action of gonadal hormones on the brain remains unknown. The identification of specific anatomical markers of sexual differentiation could provide valuable insight into the nature of this phenomenon, first by identifying a specific focus of hormone action and second, as a potential model system to study possible mechanisms of this critical action of steroid hormones perhaps at the molecular level.

Before considering possible anatomical markers, it is important to point out that in functional terms, sexual differentiation of the brain is not necessarily an all or none process. The normal male rat will occasionally exhibit lordosis behavior. Therefore, the anatomical circuitry for this behavior must be present. Sexual differentiation may merely determine the ease by which this circuitry can be activated or perhaps disinhibited. Similarly, even with respect to the differentiation of the regulatory pattern of GTH secretion, sexual differentiation need not involve an all or none effect. Female rats exposed perinatally to a low dose of TP ovulate normally for a period of time following puberty and as a group gradually lose this ability over time (Gorski, 1968). At least for this postpubertal period, the neural circuitry which is required for ovulation must be present and active in the lightly androgenized female. If morphological changes in the brain accompany sexual differentiation, these could provide and anatomical explanation for this concept of the "accessibility" of a functional system.

Although we will focus on a relatively dramatic anatomical sex difference we have discovered in the rat hypothalamus, it is useful to put this discovery in proper perspective. Several studies had earlier revealed that nucleolar size of individual neurons varied with the endocrine status of an animal. Ifft (1964), and Pfaff (1966) reported that neuronal nucleoli in several brain regions (ventromedial hypothalamus, dentate gyrus and neocortex) were significantly larger in the male than in the female. Importantly, nucleolar size was reduced by perinatal castration of the male. Dörner and his colleagues have reported that the nuclear size of individual neurons in the POA (Dörner and Staudt, 1968), ventromedial hypothalamus (Dörner and Staudt, 1969), and amygdala (Staudt and Dörner, 1976) is significantly larger in the female rat. Once again, perinatal manipulation of the hormone environment had predictable effects on neuronal nuclear size. In contrast, Pfaff (1966) found that neurons of the ventromedial hypothalamus (as well as the dentate gyrus, parvicellular reticular formation and medial habenular nucleus) were significantly larger in the male.

A sex difference in the number of neurons in specific regions of the central nervous sytem has also been reported. In the male cat, there is a greater number of neurons within the thoraco-lumbar intermediolateral nucleus of the spinal cord than in this nucleus in the female (Henry and Calaresu, 1972). The medial amygdala of the male squirrel monkey has more neurons than the comparable area of the female (Bubenik and Brown, 1973). Similarly, in the cerebellum, male rats have a greater number of granular and Purkinje cells (Yanai, 1979), while the volume of pyramidal cells in the rat somatosensory cortex has also been reported to be greater in males (Gregory, 1975). From these studies, however, it is not clear whether or not these sex differences are influenced by the hormonal environment.

There also appear to be sex differences in neuronal connectivity at the morphological level. In an elegant study, Raisman and Field (1973) demonstrated the existence of a statistical sex difference in the number of synapses of neurons which do not travel via the stria terminalis on dendritic spines of neurons within the region of the bed nucleus of the stria terminalis. In these careful studies, perinatal hormone manipulations produced alterations in the pattern of synaptic input to this region consistent with the view that the hormone environment determined this sex difference. The concept that the arborization pattern of dendritic fields of preoptic neurons is sexually dimorphic was suggested by the work of Greenough et al. (1977) who demonstrated a sex difference in the dendritic branch patterns of Golgi impregnated POA neurons in the hamster. More recently, Matsumoto and Arai (1976) have reported that estrogen exposure during development stimulates synaptic formation in the arcuate nucleus in vivo, while Toran-Allerand (1980) has demonstrated that gonadal steroids, particularly estrogen, appear to be essential for neurite outgrowth from fetal mouse explants of hypothalamus grown in culture. It now appears that this neurite outgrowth clearly emanates from steroid responsive neurons (Toran-Allerand et al., 1980).

Although these elegant studies clearly suggest the existence of at least subtle morphological sex differences in the rodent brain, this concept received a new impetus from the report of a dramatic and relatively gross morphological difference in the neural components of the song system of the songbird (Nottebohm and Arnold, 1976). Although these studies initially only demonstrated the existence of this sex dimorphism in the adult, and characterized its response to the activational action of steroid in the adult (Arnold, 1980), recent results clearly implicate gonadal steroids in the development of this anatomical dimorphism (Gurney and Konishi, 1980).

Stimulated by the observation of Nottebohm and Arnold (1976), we compared brains of male and female rats at the light microscopic level and discovered a marked anatomical sex difference which turned out to be visible to the naked eye. Within the POA of the rat hypothalamus a limited component which stains more intensely is several fold larger in volume in the male than in the female (Gorski et al., 1978). A description of this region, which we have called the Sexually Dimorphic Nucleus of the POA (SDN-POA), and an evaluation of its potential significance as a marker of early hormone action is presented in the following section. Most recently, Breedlove and Arnold (1980) have discovered a nucleus within the rat spinal cord which is larger and distinct in the male and apparently absent in the female. This nucleus, for which the authors have proposed the name the spinal nucleus of the bulbocavernosus, was discovered by identifying neurons in the spinal cord which were labeled with horseradish peroxidase injected into the bulbocavernosus muscle of the rat penis. Once these neurons were identified anatomically in the spinal cord of the male, their absence in the female became apparent. Although it has not been established that this sexually dimorphic nucleus of the rat spinal cord is dependent upon, or influenced by, the hormonal environment during development, the concept that anatomical sex differences exist in the central nervous system seems well established. Only further research will determine the frequency of such differences in terms of neuroanatomical systems and species.

2.2.2. The sexually dimorphic nucleus of the preoptic area. The medial POA of the rat brain has been implicated in a number of neuroendocrine regulatory processes and on the basis of several observations, has been suggested as one probable site for the organizational effects of gonadal steroids. These observations include documentation of its role in neuroendocrine regulation as determined by the results of lesion, stimulation and deafferentation studies, the presence of a high concentration of steroid responsive neurons, and the effectiveness of local implants of steroids in this area in the perinatal rat in inducing functional masculinization (Harlan et al., 1979). Recently we have discovered that a more intensely stained component of this region is sexually dimorphic in terms of nuclear volume (Gorski et al., 1978) and in the estimated number of neurons (Table 1). On the basis of an increased cell and neuronal density within this component of the POA, we have named this area the SDN-POA (Gorski et al., 1980). Particularly in thick (60µm) sections of the brain, the size of the SDN-POA

Table 1. Sex differences in characteristics of the sexually dimorphic nucleus of the preoptic area (SDN-POA) of the rat

	Female	*Male*
Volume of SDN-POA (mm³ × 10⁻³)	3.7±0.9	28.1±1.6 *
Estimated number neurons/SDN-POA	640	1900 *
Neuronal density (number/1400 µm²)		
SDN-POA	3.2±0.2	3.6±0.3
Surround	2.7±0.1	2.3±0.3
Mean neuronal size (µm)		
SDN-POA	9.9±0.1	11.3±0.3 *
Surround	10.0±0.1	10.4±0.2

* Significantly greater than in female.
Data from Gorski et al. (1978); Gorski et al. (1980).

permits one to identify the sex of the animal with the unaided eye (Fig. 3).

The SDN-POA, at least on the basis of its overall volume, does not appear to be influenced by the hormonal environment in the adult since treatment with behaviorally effective doses of ovarian or testicular hormones fails to modify nuclear volume significantly (Fig. 4). However, the volume of the SDN-POA as seen in the adult rat is significantly influenced by its prior perinatal hormone environment. Castration of the 1-day-old male significantly reduces the volume of this nucleus, whereas the subcutaneous injection of 1 mg TP into the 4-day-old female, significantly increases nuclear volume measured in adulthood (Fig. 4). It is important to point out that these perinatal manipulations do not completely sex reverse the SDN-POA in terms of its

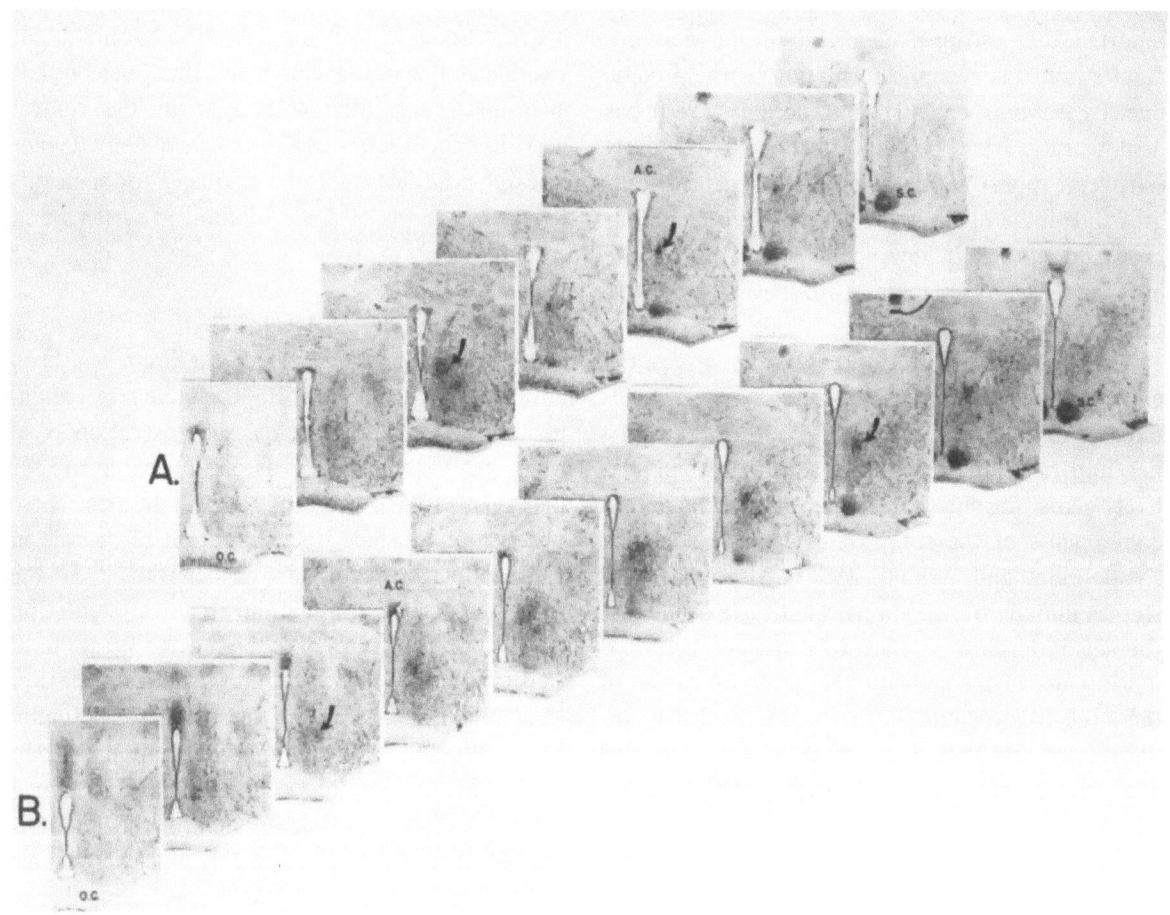

Figure 3. Thionin stained serial sections (60 µm) through the Sexually Dimorphic Nucleus of the Preoptic Area (SDN-POA) of the female (A) and male (B) rat sacrificed at 60 days of age. The arrows to the left indicate the SDN-POA on the second section after its beginning while those on the right indicate the nucleus two sections before its disappearance. Abbreviations: A.C., anterior commissure; O.C., optic chiasm; S.C., suprachiasmatic nucleus.

volume: the volume of the SDN-POA in the adult male following perinatal castration remains significantly greater than that of the genetic female, and although TP injection in the 4-day-old female increases adult SDN-POA volume, this does not reach that of the genetic male. Although the lack of complete sex reversal in terms of SDN-POA volume may relate to the dose of exogenous hormone, duration of exposure, or possible prenatal hormone action in the male, it may be that neuronal genomic factors may also contribute to this sex difference. In fact, it is likely that androgen exposure interacts with genomic factors to produce the SDN-POA of the male.

In this respect it is interesting to consider the results of a preliminary study. In collaboration with Dr. L. Krey (Rockefeller University), we evaluated the volume of the SDN-POA in normal and littermate male rats with testicular feminization mutation (Tfm). These animals are markedly deficient in brain androgen receptors (Naess et al., 1976) although estrogen receptors are apparently normal in the male mouse with the Tfm (Attardi et al., 1976). The animals have female appearing genitalia, small undescended testes, and lack seminal vesicles. They also exhibit feminine sexual behavior and reduced masculine performance (Beach and Buehler, 1977). In spite of these physiological anomalies, we did not find the volume of the SDN-POA to differ significantly from that of normal males. Since androgen levels in these animals are relatively high (Naess et al., 1976), this may indicate that the small number (15–20% of normal) of androgen receptors in the brain, are adequate to promote the development and differentiation of the SDN-POA. It is also possible that the volume of the SDN-POA is actually dependent upon estrogen titers during development. Although the adult male rat with the Tfm does not exhibit the cyclic pattern of GTH release following appropriate priming with ovarian steroids, perinatal castration does result in the retention of the positive-feedback response potential. Thus, the testes of the perinatal Tfm rat are functionally active in sexual differentiation of the brain at least to a degree (Olsen, 1979).

The data shown in Fig. 4 also emphasize our current ignorance as to the possible function(s) of the SDN-POA. Note that nuclear volume per se does not correlate either with cyclic GTH release or the level of lordosis responsiveness of the adult. Although the perinatally castrated male has the capa-

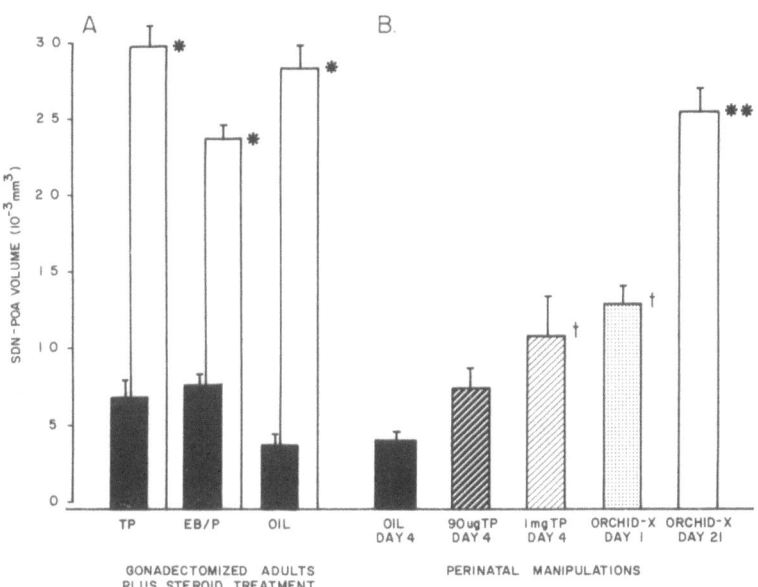

Figure 4. The influence of the steroid environment in the adult (A) and perinatal (B) rat on the volume of the Sexually Dimorphic Nucleus of the Preoptic Area (SDN-POA) as measured in the adult at least two weeks following gonadectomy. In A, ovarian steroids were administered according to an injection schedule known to facilitate sexual behavior in the rat: 2μg estradiol benzoate (EB) per day for three days followed by 500 μg progresterone (P) (feminine sexual behavior) or 150 μg testosterone propionate (TP) for 14 days (masculine sexual behavior). In B the influence of orchidectomy (orchid-x) or in the female, exogenous (TP) on the indicated days of postnatal life are shown. Data from males and females indicated by open and solid bars, respectively. * Significantly greater than that of any other perinatally treated group. + Significantly greater than that of oil treated control females. Data from Gorski et al. (1978).

city as an adult to release GTH cyclically and to exhibit high (female) levels of lordosis responsiveness, the volume of its SDN-POA is not different from that of the anovulatory androgenized female which does not exhibit lordosis behavior. Moreover, SDN-POA volume in the neonatally castrated male when adult is significantly greater than that in the normal adult female yet both exhibit high levels of lordosis responding and ovulatory potential. It is noteworthy, however, that the volume of the SDN-POA does appear to correlate reasonably well with masculine behavioral performance. Although it would be important to determine the specific (if any) function of the neurons of the SDN-POA, the significance of our discovery is limited to its heuristic value for our understanding of the processes of sexual differentiation and morphological development of the brain.

A recent report by Yamanouchi and Arai (1977) is potentially very important from a conceptual point of view. These investigators reported that transection of the dorsal connections of the POA in the adult male rat markedly facilitates his ability to display lordosis behavior. One interpretation of these results is that the knife cut has transected a neural input which inhibits lordosis responsiveness in the normal male. This suggests the concept that the perinatal hormone environment in the male promotes the development of neural systems which actively suppress neuroendocrine control mechanisms typical of the female. Although this concept would not necessarily explain the present lack of correlation between the volume of the SDN-POA and neuroendocrine potential in the adult rat, their observation strongly emphasizes that a particular functional system can be suppressed by decreasing activity within the neural substrate responsible for that function, and/or by promoting the development of inhibitory mechanisms which suppress its activity.

Comparison of the characteristics of neurons within the SDN-POA with those outside this nucleus for both males and females leads us to postulate that there are apparently no unique sexually dimorphic characteristics at the level of individual neurons with the possible exception of neuronal size (Gorski et al., 1980). Mean neuronal size in the SDN-POA of the male is slightly but significantly larger than that in the female (Table 1). Although more sophisti-

cated analyses of these neurons (e.g., immunocyto-chemical, ultrastructural) may reveal characteristics that are sexually dimorphic, current data suggest that the increase in the number of neurons in the SDN-POA of the male is due principally to an increased area of greater neuronal density.

Given this presumed morphological signature of the organizational action of gonadal steroids, we were able to ask and answer an important question: Is this action manifest immediately, or only after a delay? Note that in previous studies, with few exceptions, steroids were administered perinatally but the analysis of functional activity was performed in the adult animal. The data shown in Fig. 5 demonstrate that the sex difference in SDN-POA volume is established during the first ten days of postnatal life in the rat, the period during which sexual differentiation of the brain occurs.

Although the volume of the SDN-POA just prior to birth is not different in the intact male and female rat, on day one of postnatal life (day 23 postconception) and on day 3 (day 25 postconception) and thereafter, SDN-POA volume in the male is significantly greater than that in the female. Figure 5 suggests that this nucleus continues to grow in volume rather dramatically after birth but only in the male. In this study (Jacobson et al., 1980), we also evaluated the temporal change in other parameters of brain size including brain height and width, septal width, POA height, and the longest diameter of the caudate-putamen in a coronal section through the approximate center of the SDN-POA. Although each of these parameters significantly increased with increasing postnatal age, there were no sex differences. Thus, the sex difference in SDN-POA volume appears to be specific, at least in terms of these other measures of brain growth.

Although many sexually dimorphic aspects of brain function are not expressed until after puberty, this may be attributable to a dependence of these functions on the activational effects of gonadal steroids which attain effective levels only after puberty. At least in the case of this one example, morphological sex differences in the brain appear to be established early in postnatal life presumably under the influence of the hormonal milieu existing at that time (Weisz and Ward, 1980).

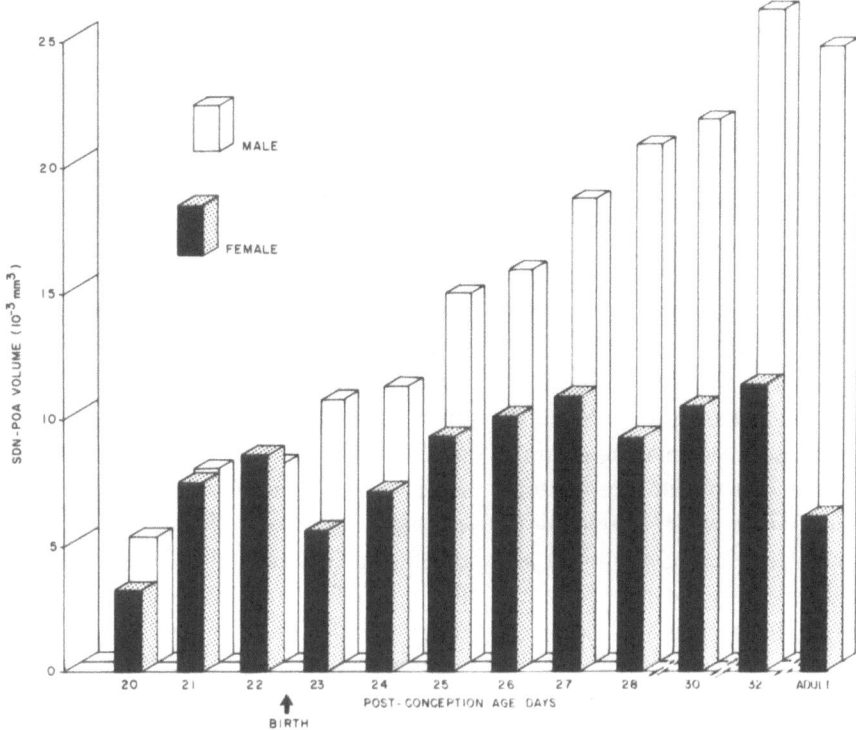

Figure 5. The influence of pre- and postnatal age on the mean volume of the Sexually Dimorphic Nucleus of the Preoptic Area (SDN-POA), in intact male and female rats. The volume of the SDN-POA in adult gonadectomized animals is also illustrated. Statistical analyses revealed a highly significant effect of age and sex and an interaction. Nuclear volume was significantly greater in the males on day 23 and on days 25 postconception and thereafter. Data from Jacobson et al. (1980).

2.3. Possible mechanisms of steroid induced masculine differentiation of the brain

Although the actual mechanism(s) by which sex steroids cause sexual differentiation of the brain is unknown, several hypotheses deserve further study. Before these are considered, however, we must emphasize an important fact. Although a number of functional systems undergo sexual differentiation (see above), each of these may be relatively independent. We have already pointed out that the neural mechanisms which regulate GTH secretion and feminine sexual behavior are differentially sensitive to exogenous TP in the female. The animal treated perinatally with a relatively low dose of TP, although anovulatory still can exhibit lordosis behavior when adult. In fact, such animals exhibit lordosis behavior daily rather than cyclically. This can best be explained on the basis that the normally (or perhaps hyper-) responsive neural substrate for lordosis behavior is continually exposed to estrogen because of its constant secretion by the polyfollicular ovaries.

A similar independence in terms of dose required to alter brain differentiation of specific functions has been observed in terms of the regulation of food intake (Tarttelin and Gorski, 1973). Moreover, there may be temporal differences in the differentiation of specific functions. Note for example, that the sexual differentiation of the external genitalia is essentially complete before birth even though that of the brain is not. Finally, in the rat it is generally held that the prenatal hormonal environment influences the neural substrates for masculine behavior (Clemens et al., 1978). Although one could postulate that a unique and single population of neurons, presumably those that are steroid responsive, differentiates at the same time and that this is translated into various functional effects at specific time periods because of subsequent neurochemical or morphological changes, it may be more reasonable to assume that the influence of hormones on the developing brain varies over time with specific functional systems. There may also be regional specificity as suggested by the finding that intrahypothalamic implants of crystalline hormones in the medial basal hypothalamus induced anovulatory sterility in females, while implants in the POA increased the potential to display mounting behavior (Christensen and Gorski, 1978).

This concept that specific functional (and perhaps morphological) systems undergo sexual differentiation independently is the basis for the division by some authorities of the process of sex differentiation into two processes: masculinization and defeminization (McEwen, 1978; Goy and McEwen, 1980). Inhibition of ovulatory capacity and lordosis behavior are the result of defeminization while the facilitation of masculine behavioral potential is masculinization. That these indeed may be separate processes is suggested by experimental procedures which produce a genetic male which exhibits both masculine and feminine behavior (Goldfoot et al., 1969). Although we do not deny the heuristic value of defining defeminization and masculinization as distinct processes, this could be interpreted as analogous to the inhibition of growth and development of the Müllerian duct by Müllerian Inhibitory Factor (Josso et al., 1977) and the stimulation of the Wolffian duct by androgen in the male. Although different hormones may be responsible for defeminization and masculinization, in the case of the genital duct system, there is essentially complete disappearance of either the Müllerian or Wolffian system. In the case of brain mechanisms it is possible that the response potential (and perhaps the neural circuitry) for the various sexually dimorphic brain functions are present in adults of both sexes and that the perinatal hormone environment in some way determines the accessibility of each system, albeit probably on an independent basis, to the normal environmental and hormonal stimuli required for its activation in the adult. Moreover, as discussed above, it is likely that sexual differentiation is not an all or none process and therefore, it also may be instructive to envision a continuum between "maleness and femaleness;" the exact degree of differentiation of a specific system being dependent on many factors.

Although the process of sexual differentiation of the brain has been clearly documented at the phenomenological level, our understanding of the mechanisms by which gonadal steroids permanently alter or determine brain development is minimal. At this stage in our understanding we can only suggest several speculative mechanisms, which for convenience, we will first consider as independent processes.

2.3.1. The identity of the active molecular species of steroid in differentiation. Although it is clear that the testes are the source of the hormone(s) which influences brain development, the precise identity of the steroid molecule(s) which is active at the cellular level remains controversial. As described above, it is clear that TP, when administered to the perinatal female, closely mimics testicular-dependent differentiation of the brain in the intact male. However, the administration of EB also produces similar effects whether this hormone is given to the perinatal female systemically or intracerebrally (Gorski, 1971). Moreover, EB is more potent than TP. In addition, estrogen administration masculinizes the brain of the male castrated on the second day of postnatal life (Gorski, 1966). On the other hand, the administration of dihydrotestosterone (DHT) to females is relatively ineffective, although DHT appears to be the metabolite which induces masculine differentiation of the external genitalia.

Although rapid peripheral metabolism of DHT could provide an explanation for its ineffectiveness, it is generally held that this is due to the fact that DHT is a non-aromatizable steroid. In fact, it has been assumed that testosterone is active because it is converted intraneuronally into estrogen (McEwen, 1978; Fig. 6). Consistent with this view is the fact that brain tissue, particularly from those regions implicated in neuroendocrine function, possesses aromatase activity (Naftolin et al., 1975). Moreover, treatment with anti-estrogens or aromatase-inhibitors blocks the action of endogenous or exogenous testosterone (McEwen, 1978; Harlan et al., 1979).

Although the ovaries of the perinatal rat had been considered hormonally quiescent as indicated by the lack of an effect of their removal, it is now apparent that estrogen levels are very high during the perinatal period in both male and female rats (Gorski et al., 1977). Although the precise source of this hormone (gonadal and/or adrenal) is not clear, the important question becomes: If estrogen is the "masculinizing" hormone, what protects the female from its influence? The answer to this fundamental question appears to be that the perinatal rat has a special estrogen binding protein (alphafetoprotein) which binds estrogen and apparently effectively sequesters it, thus preventing its biological action (McEwen, 1978). Since androgens are bound much less by alphafetoprotein, when secreted by the testes they are not sequestered and can enter neurons where they may be converted into estrogen (see Fig. 6). Although this hypothesis is currently popular, and as indicated above, affords the possibility that behavioral differences in individual females could be the result of the action of estrogen not effectively bound to alphafetoprotein, it may be too simplistic. Given the numerous components of brain function which undergo differentiation, it seems premature to rule out any effect of testosterone per se, DHT, or other metabolites.

In this respect, it should be mentioned that it has been postulated that estrogen-exposure of the brain may in fact be necessary for its normal development (Döhler, 1978; Dunlap et al., 1978). As will be reviewed below, estrogen has been shown to be required for the growth of neural processes in culture (Toran-Allerand, 1980), and to promote synapse formation (Matsumoto and Arai, 1976) as well as myelinization (Casper et al., 1967). Moreover, the presence of estrogen receptors in the cerebral cortex of the rat for the first 20 days or so of life (McEwen et al., 1975; Sheridan, 1979), also argues for a possible

role of this hormone in cortical development and/or functional organization. Undoubtably the action of the gonadal hormones on brain development is complex and not necessarily restricted to sexual differentiation. Any formal hypotheses about hormone action on the developing brain should recognize this possibility.

2.3.2. Relation to steroid receptors. Steroid receptor mechanisms could play an important role in sexual differentiation at two levels: as mediators of the action of these hormones in the perinatal period and/or during adult neuroendocrine function. However, because of the unique permanent nature of the organizing action of steroids on the perinatal brain, one could postulate that this effect is not mediated by the classical receptor system. Consistent with this speculative view were the results of biochemical studies, which suggested that estrogen receptors did not exist prior to about day five of postnatal life. In this context, the development of steroid receptors could be viewed as one factor which terminates the period of sexual differentiation since their presence only then could permit the regulation of chromatin exposure to steroids. Although such a hypothesis could well explain the permanency of steroid action in the younger animal, more recent data force a complete reversal of this hypothesis: the appearance

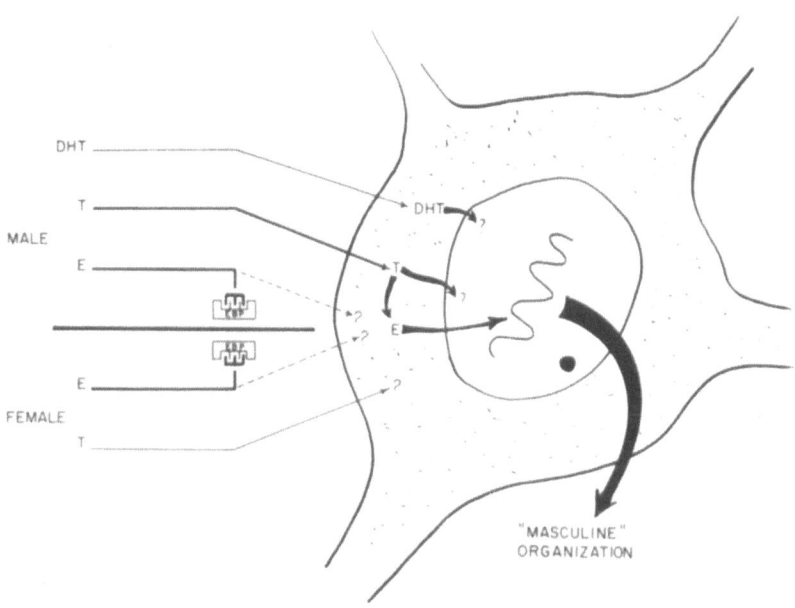

Figure 6. Schematic representation of the steroid hormone environment within plasma and neuronal compartments in the perinatal rat in relation to masculine organization of the latter. Abbreviations: DHT, dihydrotestosterone; E, estrogen; EBP, perinatal estrogen binding protein; T, testosterone.

of steroid receptors may signal the beginning of the period of sexual differentiation.

The existence of steroid receptors in the brain of the newborn rat was first inferred from autoradiographic evidence of steroid uptake (Sheridan et al., 1974). Subsequently, the existence of alphafetoprotein and the fact that the levels of estrogen are high became known, the biochemical approach was modified and it has now been established that steroid receptors appear in the brain several days before birth (MacLusky et al., 1979; Vito and Fox, 1979; Vito et al., 1979). Therefore, it may be assumed that the organizational actions of gonadal hormones is mediated via classical steroid–receptor–genomic interaction. Given the current view that steroid hormones alter RNA and protein synthesis in the adult, and the fact that their organizational effects appear to be permanent, it is likely that an alteration in these fundamental biochemical processes may underlie sexual differentiation. In this context, a number of antibiotics and other chemical agents when injected systemically or implanted directly into the POA of the neonatal rat attenuate androgenization (Gorski, 1979). Even if we assume that steroid action involves such biochemical steps, there is little definite information with respect to the mechanisms which translate these into altered function. Thus, it may be useful to consider possible alterations in steroid action in the adult animal, which might offer a clue to their effects during development.

The fact that many of the sexually dimorphic functions of the brain are dependent in the adult on the activational effects of gonadal steroids implies that a perinatally induced, permanent alteration in the general biochemical action of these hormones could explain functional sex differences in the adult. Alterations could occur at one or several levels: receptor-binding, translocation, chromatin binding, translation and/or in subsequent steps (see Fig. 7). There is experimental support for several of these possibilities.

In terms of receptor binding, the experimental data are somewhat controversial; some investigators report that steroid uptake in the adult androgenized female or the male is reduced relative to that in the normal female but others have not confirmed this observation (Harlan et al., 1979). Recently, Whalen and Olsen (1978) have reported a sex difference in chromatin-binding of estrogen in brain: males bind less estrogen than do females. Moreover, this sex

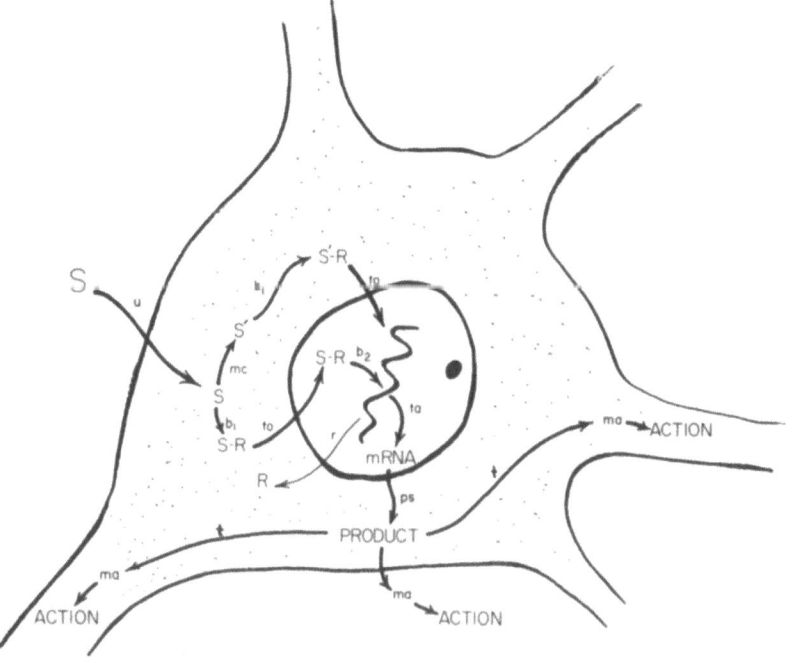

Figure 7. Schematic representation of the steps in steroid hormone action on the neuron of the adult which could be altered by perinatal exposure to gonadal hormones. Abbreviations: b_1, binding of steroid to cytoplasmic receptor; b_2, binding to chromatin; ma, metabolic activation; mc, metabolic conversion; ps, protein synthesis; r, receptor replenishment; R, cytoplasmic steroid receptor; S, steroid; S', steroid metabolite; S-R, steroid–receptor complex; t, transport to axonal or dendritic nerve terminals; ta, translation; to, translocation.

differences is modified by the perinatal hormone environment in parallel with alterations in feminine behavioral potential (Olsen and Whalen, 1980). Earlier, Vértes and King (1973) had reported that in the immature androgenized female translocation of the steroid–receptor complex into the nucleus is reduced while in the adult receptor replenishment is reduced.

At the present time, a permanent alteration in steroid action at the molecular level appears to be an attractive candidate for one mechanism of sexual differentiation. However, further evaluation of the process of hormone action in both the adult and neonate is necessary (see Fig. 7). When, and if specific proteins induced by hormone exposure of the brain can be identified, new avenues of research will be available. One difficulty with current research in this area is the fact that the sensitivity of the biochemical techniques demands tissue samples pooled from different regions of the brain and often from different animals. The former may be more significant because it precludes anatomical specificity. More sensitive techniques which would permit, for example, specific study of the SDN-POA might be more informative, but even in this case it is unlikely that the total neuronal population of this nucleus has the same function or the identical response to steroids.

2.3.3. Relation to the biogenic amines, neurotransmitters and neuromodulators. Neural function, whether of steroid responsive neurons or not, ultimately depends on the release and/or response to neurotransmitters and neuromodulators. Although the distinction between neurotransmitters and neuromodulators is currently a topic of wide discussion, resolution of this question is not necessary for the purposes of our discussion. Suffice it to say that neurochemicals released by presynaptic terminals which cross a synapse and briefly alter the postsynaptic membrane potential can be considered neurotransmitters. On the other hand, chemical substances, irrespective of their origin, which modulate this system either pre- or post-synaptically and perhaps on a different time scale can be called neuromodulators. Candidates for neuromodulators include various peptidergic substances and perhaps peripheral hormones. It is obvious that steroid hormone action perinatally could produce permanent

effects on adult brain function by altering chemical information processing in the brain.

The biogenic amines, in particular, appear to play a significant role in neuroendocrine function in the adult. Moreover, sex differences in aminergic activity have been detected in the adult and during development (Crowley et al., 1978; Harlan et al., 1979). Dyer et al. (1976) reported a sex difference in the electrophysiological response of POA neurons, which project to the median eminence, to electrical activation of the amygdala, although they have not as far as we know evaluated the influence of the perinatal hormone environment on this system. Obviously, a sex difference in electrophysiological connectivity such as this could have an anatomical or neurochemical basis, or both.

Although the biogenic amines are currently a popular focus of experimental study in neuroendocrinology, one reason for this effort is the fact that specific aminergic pathways have been demonstrated cytochemically and the amines and specific rate-limiting enzymes involved in their synthesis can be quantified relatively easily. In spite of the wealth of information linking the amines to neuroendocrine function, and thus possibly to sexual differentiation, other neurotransmitters or neuromodulators currently not studied may be equally important. It may be that a complex balance of chemical input may prove to be critical for specific neural functions. At this stage in our knowledge we can only point to chemical signaling as one system which could be a target for the organizational action of steroid hormones on the developing brain.

2.3.4. The induction of morphological differences in the brain. Given the recent observations of a number of morphological sex differences in the central nervous system as discussed above, it is now clear that one consequence of the organizational action of steroids can be permanent alterations in neuronal morphology and connectivity. Current concepts of neurobiology view the structure of the brain as surprisingly dynamic. Structural reorganization of the brain may be relatively common (Harlan et al., 1979; Lund, 1978), at least at the level of synaptic connections. Following a central lesion the brain probably exhibits a high degree of plasticity. Although the several anatomical sex dimorphisms reviewed above clearly indicate that the

124

hormonal environment during development alters the morphology of the brain, the important question, "How?", remains unresolved. Because the genomic and environmental factors which guide neural morphogenesis and the establishment of normal connectivity remain virtually unknown, it is difficult to put the probable action of steroid hormones in appropriate context. In this regard, however, we believe the discovery of the SDN-POA offers a valuable model system for further study since it provides a focus for histochemical and ultrastructural studies. Moreover, this nucleus has dimensions which would permit its sampling by the punch technique for neurochemical analyses and/or study of its growth in tissue culture and of the factors which may influence that growth.

Even without these additional studies the ontogenic history of the SDN-POA offers the opportunity to make and test several fundamental concepts of the action of steroid hormones during differentiation. Since the larger volume of the SDN-POA in the adult male rat correlates with an increase in the number of neurons within this nucleus relative to that in the SDN-POA of the female, it appears likely that exposure to steroids within the first few days of postnatal life in the rat determines, at least in part, final neuronal number in this nucleus. An interesting dilemma arises from this conclusion: it has been reported that neurons of the POA undergo their final mitotic division on or before day 16 postconception (Ifft, 1972; Altman and Bayer, 1978). Nevertheless, hormone action about 10 days after the neurons of the POA apparently become postmitotic alters volume and presumably final neuronal number in the SDN-POA.

In our opinion, there are four possible explanations for this effect (Fig. 8): 1) Mitotic activity in those cells which give rise to this nucleus may be prolonged by the hormone environment in the male; the hormonal environment may influence 2) the migration or 3) the aggregation of neurons into the region recognized as the SDN-POA; 4) the hormonal environment may prevent neuronal death, presumably by promoting the growth of neuronal processes and functional connectivity.

Experimental evidence to support or refute any of these hypotheses is minimal. Seress (1978) has reported that androgen treatment restores mitotic activity in the hypothalamus in the neonatal rat.

However, the animals were sacrificed one hour after the injection of labeled thymidine; thus, it is possible that this study was confounded by glial mitotic activity. Preliminary evidence of our own suggests that mitosis is still taking place perhaps specifically within the SDN-POA as late as day 18 postconception, and that there also may be a sex difference in this regard. In this respect it is interesting that Weisz and Ward (1980) have reported that there is a surge of testosterone in male fetuses on days 18 and 19 of gestation. With respect to the migration or aggregation of neurons into the SDN-POA, there appears to be little information regarding the factors which lead to the formation of specific nuclei. Therefore, there is no reason to dismiss the possibility that environmental factors, such as hormones, play a role in this basic aspect of developmental neurobiology.

Programmed neuronal death is well documented in several systems (Silver, 1978). Particularly in neurons with peripheral connections, it appears that

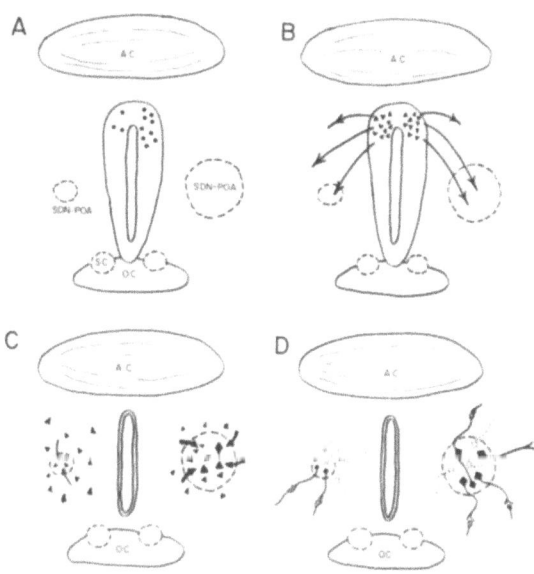

Figure 8. Highly schematic representations of four theoretical mechanisms whereby the steroid environment (right side of each panel) could determine the number of neurons within the Sexually Dimorphic Nucleus of the Preoptic Area (SDN-POA) of the adult rat. (A) Steroids might promote mitotic division of cells destined to form the SDN-POA. (B) Steroids might promote the migration of neurons from their origin (presumably in the ependymal lining of the roof of the third ventricle (V; Altman and Bayer, 1978) to the SDN-POA. (C) Steroids might promote the aggregation of neurons into the SDN-POA. (D) By promoting or maintaining the growth of neuronal processes and/or synaptic connectivity, steroids might reduce neuronal death during development. See text for discussion. Abbreviations: A.C., anterior commissure; O.C., optic chiasm; S.C., suprachiasmatic nucleus.

more neurons develop than can be accommodated by the peripheral receptive field and those neurons which fail to make or sustain appropriate synaptic contact die. Cell death has also been reported to occur following loss of afferent input (Lund, 1978). Although nothing is known about the connectivity of specific neurons to the SDN-POA, several observations are consistent with the possibility that steroid hormones prevent neuronal death. Toran-Allerand (1980) has demonstrated that estrogen stimulates and may be necessary for the growth of processes from hypothalamic explants in culture. Moreover, such neurite outgrowth appears to arise only from neurons which contain steroid receptors (Toran-Allerand et al., 1980). In vivo, estrogen treatment has been shown to increase the rate of synapse formation in the arcuate nucleus during development (Matsumoto and Arai, 1976). In unpublished experiments we have found by autoradiography that the SDN-POA in the adult does contain a high concentration of steroid-binding neurons. Thus, these data are consistent with the hypothesis that the hormone environment could stimulate the growth of processes and synapse formation by the neurons of the SDN-POA, but it remains to be determined whether or not cell death actually occurs in the region of the SDN-POA of the perinatal animal. Note from Fig. 5 that the volume of the SDN-POA in the female appears simply not to grow in comparison to that of the male over the first week or so of life. Further studies are obviously needed to determine the fate (growth, maturation or death) of individual neurons in this nucleus.

As already indicated, the discovery of morphological sex differences in the brain can be considered a valuable conceptual advance and one that could lead to a better understanding of the site of the organizational action of steroids. Moreover, these specific anatomical loci may provide model systems to study hormone action. Unfortunately, present understanding of developmental neurobiology is limited, and considerable research will be necessary before the interaction between hormonal environment and the morphological (and presumably functional) development of the brain can be explained.

In the preceding discussion we have for simplicity considered several possible mechanisms by which the steroid environment could permanently alter brain function as independent phenomena. It is important to stress that these need not be, and probably are not, mutually exclusive. For example, we have suggested that by an unknown mechanism steroid hormone action perinatally could alter steroid responsiveness in the adult. However, it is possible that the steroid responsiveness of individual neurons is normal, but that the perinatal hormonal environment determines how many steroid sensitive neurons will survive during development, or make appropriate connections so that the functional activity of these neurons can be expressed. Similarly, alterations in neural connectivity could influence neuronal chemical communication. As another example of possible overlap among these putative mechanisms, one need only assume that one result of steroid action on the neuronal genome in the adult is an alteration in the production, release or response to neurotransmitters. Thus, a permanent alteration in steroid hormone action in the adult could become manifest in altered neurochemical transmission independent of, or in parallel with, alterations in neuronal connectivity. Although the several possible mechanisms we have discussed may be complexly interactive, current levels of understanding make it imperative to consider these mechanisms as possible independent processes, at least in terms of developing testable working hypotheses.

Based on experimental evidence that the ability of exogenous steroids to exert an organizing or permanent action on the brain is limited to the perinatal period, the basic concept of a critical period has become generally accepted. Although this concept certainly defines the time when the brain is exceptionally sensitive to the organizational effects of the steroid environment, recent experimental results suggest that the brain may respond similarly to steroid hormones, at least under certain conditions, even in the adult. In fact, it is possible that steroids always have a "morphotropic" action throughout life, although other factors normally limit the expression of this action to the perinatal period of sexual differentiation. The concept that steroids may have the potential to exert an organizing effect even in the adult could have direct relevance to the process of human psychosexual differentiation (see Section 4).

Brown-Grant (1975) has reported that the injection of a large dose of EB in the adult rat can induce anovulatory persistent estrus. Although this might represent only a pharmacological response, there are two examples with more direct physiological relevance. Kawashima (1960) has reported that prolonged exposure to exogenous estrogen at a dose too low to influence the vaginal epithelium in ovariectomized rats, can induce anovulatory persistent estrus in the intact animal. It is also possible for endogenous ovarian steroids to alter neuroendocrine function permanently after puberty. We have already indicated that the injection of TP to the perinatal female rat, if the dose is adequate, will produce an animal which never ovulates and exhibits persistent vaginal estrus from the day of vaginal introitus. However, if the dose of androgen is low (10 μg TP on postnatal day five in our experiments), the animals ovulate spontaneously and regularly following puberty but within a few weeks become permanently anovulatory. Because of this period of apparently normal ovarian function prior to anovulatory sterility, we have labeled this phenomenon the Delayed Anovulation Syndrome (DAS, Gorski, 1968). It is important for our present consideration, to note that ovulatory capacity (Kikuyama and Kawashima, 1966; Arai, 1971), or the capacity to release a surge of GTH following steroid priming (Harlan and Gorski, 1978) can be prolonged by ovariectomy in such animals. In the former studies ovulatory capacity was assessed by the observation of luteinization in ovarian grafts. In our studies, we have also shown that the delay in the loss of the GTH response to positive feedback which is produced by ovariectomy, can be prevented by replacement therapy with either EB or TP. Thus, in females exposed to small amounts of androgen during the perinatal period, the exposure of the brain to steroid feedback postpubertally leads to the syndrome (anovulatory persistent estrus) typical of that of the rat with a masculinized brain. Although the precise mechanism(s) by which steroid action postpubertally leads to the DAS need not be identical to that which occurs perinatally, the possibility that the organizing action of steroid hormones is not strictly limited to the perinatal period must be considered.

In fact, it is possible that steroid hormones have the potential throughout life to alter the brain on a relatively permanent basis. Although this concept is admittedly very speculative, it would appear to merit serious consideration. Following deafferentation of the medial basal hypothalamus, estrogen has been reported to promote synapse formation in the arcuate nucleus (Arai et al., 1978). According to our current understanding of brain plasticity, we can assume that following central destruction of neurons (i.e., by lesions or transection of fibers) nerve terminals which become vacant following degeneration of this input, are rapidly reoccupied by new terminals resulting from axonal sprouting of intact cells (Raisman, 1969; Lund, 1978). Thus, it appears likely that estrogen can promote the growth of neural processes and hence, the formation of new connections, provided empty terminals are available.

We have also demonstrated an apparent permanent effect of the steroid environment on reorganization of the adult brain at least at the functional level. As described above, the genetic male normally displays lordosis behavior infrequently even when primed with ovarian hormones. Although electrolytic destruction of the lateral septum in adult females increases behavioral sensitivity to estrogen, as measured by lordosis responsiveness, this does not occur in the genetic male. However, if the genetic male is treated with EB during the first 10 days or so after destruction of the lateral septum, he now exhibits high levels of lordosis responding upon previously ineffective hormone priming, apparently on a permanent basis (Nance et al., 1975). Although we have no evidence of neural reorganization in these animals at the morphological level, these results are at least consistent with the ability of steroid hormones, even in the adult, to modify brain function on a long term basis following procedures which would permit axonal sprouting and the establishment of new connections. Thus, we suggest although only as a working hypothesis, that one action of steroid hormones on certain neurons is to stimulate the potential growth of their processes. During development when anatomical connections are being established, this action of steroids can permanently influence the connectivity of these neurons and thus, their function. In the adult, this effect of steroids may not become manifest because the environment of the neurons permits no opportunity for new connections to be established. Following degeneration of terminals and the freeing of previously occupied synaptic sites, however, the "morphotropic" action of steroids can become manifest. Note that if morphological reorganization at the level of synaptic terminals is a normal component of the functioning adult central nervous system, then this putative action of the steroid environment gains in potential significance.

3. SUMMARY OF FUNDAMENTAL CONCEPTS RELATED TO SEXUAL DIFFERENTIATION OF THE BRAIN

In the preceding sections of this chapter we have reviewed the evidence for the functional and morphological differentiation of the brain principally in the laboratory rat. In the next section we want to consider the applicability of this concept to the human being. Since the direct understanding of sexual differentiation of the human brain depends on psychological and clinical studies of several syndromes of altered development, we believe that this information can best be interpreted in terms of fundamental concepts derived from the study of animal models. Therefore, in this section we will attempt to summarize the preceding discussion in the form of a list of such concepts. Several of these are presented schematically in Fig. 9, again with the rat serving as the illustrative model.

1. For a period in development the brain, irrespective of the genetic sex of the animal, has the potential to attain functional capacities recognized as either typical of the male or female of that species.

2. The steroid environment plays a critical role in neural development: effective exposure to gonadal steroids promotes masculine differentiation. Since there are several gonadal steroids and metabolites, including estradiol, testosterone and DHT, any one or all could be involved. Although current concepts favor estrogen, the key feature is that this hormone arises at least indirectly (through the intra-neuronal aromatization of androgen) from the testes.

3. There are apparently protective mechanisms (e.g., the estrogen binding alphafetoprotein in the rat) which prevent or limit exposure of the developing brain of the female to gonadal hormones. Even though much of the process of sexual differentiation of the brain occurs postnatally in the rat, the prenatal hormone environment is also important in this species. Depending on the specific characteristic under study, the brain of the newborn male rat may

already differ from that of the female. In other mammals, the process of differentiation may be exclusively prenatal which emphasizes the need for mechanisms to protect the brain of the female from the influence of the maternal–placental hormonal environment.

4. Sexual differentiation of the regulation of individual functional processes may take place independently, in terms of time, sensitivity to hormones, site of action and possible mechanism. As a corollary, it may be assumed that this early hormone action is not limited to a specific brain locus.

5. The action of steroids during sexual differentiation of the brain is presumably mediated by cyto-

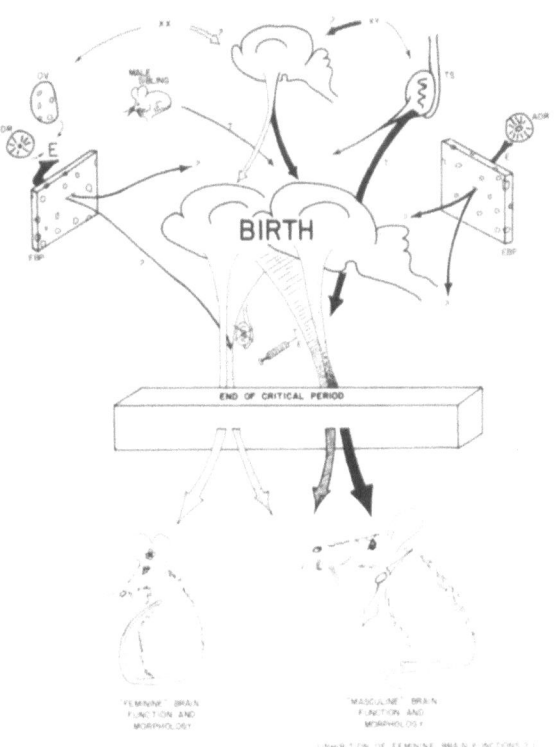

Figure 9. Schematic representation of the process of the sexual differentiation of the brain (see Fig. 1). This illustration is intended to reflect the fact that prenatal genomic and/or hormonal influences [such as testosterone (T) from the testes of the male or in the case of the female from adjacent males, or estrogen (E) which may not be bound by the perinatal estrogen binding protein (EBP)]. Thus, at birth in the rat, the brains of the male and female may already differ. In animals in which sexual differentiation is more exclusively prenatal, this figure attempts to reflect that this process may be relatively gradual. Finally, the concept that steroid action in the developing brain is terminated at the end of a critical period is also modified in this figure, although sensitivity to this influence is clearly greatest during this phase of development. For further discussion see text. Other abbreviations: Adr, adrenal gland; ov, ovary; Ts, testis.

plasmic receptors, in fact the appearance of such receptors may begin the period of differentiation.

6. Although the precise mechanism of this permanent action of steroids is unknown, in the adult it could be manifest in alterations in steroid–receptor–response coupling, in neurotransmitter or neuromodulator production-response, in the anatomical connectivity of neurons and/or in the number of neurons which ultimately comprise specific components of the adult central nervous system.

7. Because certain functional responses typical of one sex can occassionaly be elicited in the opposite sex, it may be that the process of sexual differentiation determines the accessability of a specific neural substrate to its usual stimuli. Perinatal exposure to steroids may promote the development of inhibitory systems which thus limit such accessibility.

8. Although the critical period represents the time of maximal sensitivity of the brain to the organizational action of steroid hormones, such action may not be strictly limited to development. Particularly after partial exposure to steroids during this period, subsequent hormone action may more gradually produce permanent alterations in brain function and/or morphology. It is possible that steroids exert a "morphotropic" influence in the central nervous system throughout life, an influence that can be expressed only when permitted by the local environment.

4. SEXUAL DIFFERENTIATION OF THE HUMAN BRAIN

In the preceding section we have summarized what to us appear to be fundamental concepts related to the process of sexual differentiation of the brain based on the study of laboratory animals, principally the rat. Which, if any, of these concepts can be applied to human brain development? Unfortunately, present evidence precludes our taking a firm position on this important question. Although there are notable exceptions most of the literature pertaining to sexual differentiation of the human brain is inconclusive if not controversial. Some of the reasons for this are intuitively obvious, nevertheless, they should be emphasized to put human research reports in proper perspective.

Perhaps the most significant factor is the necessary ethical restraints placed on human research. Wilson (1979) has stated, for example: "...no matter how impressive the circumstantial evidence that endocrine factors may cause a change in gender identity..., it must be noted that it is difficult to design rigorous scientific studies in human beings to prove the thesis." Even in the laboratory animal it can be difficult to distinguish the organizational effects of gonadal steroids from the activational effects necessary to evoke or facilitate a sexually dimorphic function. In the human being this potential problem is exacerbated by ethical restraints and by social, cultural and idiosyncratic factors. It is very difficult to identify significant causal factors in retrospective studies, yet virtually impossible to conduct controlled prospective studies. It should be emphasized that animal research is certainly not problem free: sampling may be too infrequent, behavioral criteria too liberal, important variables uncontrolled, and complexly interactive processes studied in misleading isolation. Nevertheless, these problems can be much more acute in research involving human beings.

Although it is certainly possible to characterize certain aspects of human neuroendocrinology in adulthood (e.g., GTH or steroid titers, response to exogenous steroids) or during development [e.g., the human male fetus between 10 and 20 weeks of age has a higher titer of testosterone than the female as measured via amniocentesis (Zondek et al., 1977)], other aspects such as sexual performance or sexual preference, in general must be obtained from questionnaires or from the personal interveiw and may be biased by feelings of guilt, defiance, or a desire to please the investigator, and by the absence of adequate controls. Given even a remote possibility that like laboratory animals, the human being passes through a developmental stage(s) when environmental factors (e.g., steroids) could have permanent or long-lasting effects, it is not possible on an ethical basis to manipulate willingly that environment. It should be pointed out, however, that the study of human differentiation has been aided inadvertently by physicians. The developing reproductive system, and perhaps the brain as well, has been disturbed accidentally by clinical procedures considered necessary or therapeutic at the time. For example, pregnant women have been treated with progestins or the potent non-steroidal estrogen diethylstilbesterol to prevent threatened abortion. In addition, premature infants have been treated with anabolic steroids in high doses in order to maintain and increase body weight. Women, thus exposed to steroids at a "prenatal" age, could constitute a human parallel to the androgenized or estrogenized laboratory rat.

There are two additional populations of human beings which have been studied in terms of possible sexual differentiation of the brain. Those individuals with various genetic abnormalities, including congenital adrenal hyperplasia, the feminizing testes syndrome of complete or partial androgen insensitivity, and genetic males with 5α-reductase deficiency, who exhibit abnormal sexual development at least in terms of genetic constitution, represent a valuable population in terms of the evaluation of the process of sexual differentiation. Finally, homosexual and transexual individuals have been studied from a retrospective point of view in an attempt to determine the etiology of their behavioral patterns.

In the following discussion we will consider briefly the relevance of the basic concepts from animal research to possible sexual differentiation of the human being. Since clinical research is beyond the scope of our expertise we shall refer, whenever possible, to critical reviews of the clinical literature. Our goal is to highlight unanswered questions which require further research.

Perhaps the most important concepts derived from animal research are that the brain of either sex has the potential, at some period in development, to attain functional capacities recognized as typical of either the male or female, and that the steroid environment plays a critical role in this process. The results of animal studies indicate that sexually dimorphic functions include the pattern of GTH secretion, reproductive behaviors and a number of additional, but less well understood parameters of brain function.

With respect to the pattern of GTH secretion, the human female and male exhibit a sexual dimorphism comparable to that seen in laboratory animals. In the intact female, a dramatic cyclic pattern characterizes pituitary, ovarian and uterine function and this is not present in the intact male. However, the degree of independence of this sex dimorphism from the activational effects of gonadal steroids is unclear. Although the genetic human male has been shown to exhibit positive feedback albeit reduced in magni-

tude (Kulin and Reiter, 1976), Dörner (see Meyer-Bahlburg, 1977) has reported that homosexual men differ from heterosexual men in this regard. Since the male rhesus monkey also exhibits positive feedback (Karsch et al., 1973), it may be that the masculinization of GTH regulation as seen in the androgenized female rat is a process relatively specific to this species (Goy and McEwen, 1980). Consistent with this view is the observation that externally masculinized women (as well as female rhesus monkeys) due to congenital adrenal hyperplasia or prenatal exposure to progestins do ovulate. However, as indicated above in the case of the monkey, to our knowledge no one has established that an ovarian graft in the castrated human male would luteinize cyclically. Without this demonstration, the presence of a positive feedback response to exogenous steroids could merely be a pharmacoligical artefact rather than an indication that a true physiological sex difference(s) does not exist.

Moreover, the phenomenon of the DAS in the rat suggests the possibility that women with adrenal hyperplasia, for example, may yet experience premature ovulatory failure as a consequence of prenatal exposure to androgen. Rothchild (1971) has summarized various classes of functional amenorrhea and suggests that hypothalamic dysfunction probably contributes to this complex syndrome. Finally, in a very provocative paper, Ichinoe and Yokota (1978) report that of four women born 2 months prematurely and exposed to methylandrostenediol, an anabolic steroid, as infants, three exhibited disturbances in their ovulatory cycles as determined by measurement of basal body temperature. Similar steroid treatment of female infants born after the eighth postconception month apparently did not disturb their ovulatory cycle as adults. These authors interpret their findings to suggest that in the human female "there might exist a critical period of cyclic center development." Although the results of this study must be confirmed, it would appear that the conclusion that the pattern of GTH secretion in the human female is not altered by prenatal hormone exposure may be premature.

The area of sex differences in human behavior and their development has received considerable attention. In this sphere of research, however, the laboratory animal model of sexual behavior, especially that of the rodent, is clearly inadequate. Note that in the laboratory situation, sexual behavior is evaluated by the quantification of specific, often reflexive, components of behavior, e.g. the lordosis reflex for feminine behavior, and mounting, intromission or ejaculatory patterns for masculine behavior. It is important to note that even among researchers there are significant differences in methods of behavioral scoring (see Gorski, 1974 for discussion). Although rodent behavior is treated qualitatively by some investigators (i.e., a single lordosis response is considered evidence of normal female behavioral potential) others utilize the level of responding (e.g., the lordosis quotient: the number of lordosis responses expressed as a percentage of a minimum of 10 mounts) to characterize sex differences. The present authors have adopted the latter system and consider a single lordosis response as a poor index of behavioral potential.

The problems in interpreting the animal literature imposed by these technical differences actually become of minimal significance when one attempts to compare animal behavior to that of the human being. A far more significant problem from the conceptual point of view is the fact that the present empirical analysis of animal behavior does not test the qualities of human behavior which have been analysed in clinical studies such as sexual preference, sexual motivation, or more cognitive qualities such as gender identity. Experiments testing sexual motivation in the rat (Meyerson and Lindström, 1973), dog (Beach, 1976) and monkey (Michael et al., 1972) are relatively rare. This is unfortunate since the results of such studies would appear to approach more closely the questions relevant to human behavior.

In spite of this difference in the conceptual approach to behavioral analysis which currently precludes the use of the laboratory animal as a model for the differentiation of sexual preference or gender identity in the human being, the results of these animal studies clearly suggest that the hormonal environment during development can alter behavioral potential. The possibility exists, therefore, that certain components of human behavior are also modified by the hormonal environment during development. Perhaps because of the strong influence of social, environmental and experimental factors in the development and expression of gender identity, it has been difficult to establish a clear role for hormones in human behavioral development.

Nevertheless, the evaluation of individuals in which development (at least of the genitalia) has been altered iatrogenically or through genetic dysfunction, clearly leaves open the distinct possibility that steroid hormones do exert an effect which could be of considerable significance in those cases where the sex of rearing has been ambiguous. The evidence for the influence of the prenatal hormone environment on psychosexual differentiation in the human being has been extensively reviewed (Goy and McEwen, 1980; Ehrhardt and Meyer-Bahlburg, 1979; Baker, 1980) and a re-review of this information is beyond the scope of this discussion. It may be helpful, however, to quote from the conclusions of Ehrhardt and Meyer-Bahlburg (1979): "The empirical evidence strongly suggests effects of prenatal hormones, albeit quite limited, on sex dimorphic behavior such as physical energy expenditure, childhood rehearsal of parenting, and related behaviors. Best established is the role of prenatal androgens, whereas the evidence for an antiandrogenic action of prenatal progesterone and related compounds seems insufficient as yet. A role of prenatal hormones for sexual orientation has not been demonstrated. The development of gender identity depends on the sex of rearing rather than on chromosomes, gonads and prenatal hormones."

However, the recent report (Imperato-McGinley et al., 1979) on the development of male gender identity at puberty in a group of genetic males from the Dominican Republic with 5α-reductase deficiency, who were raised as females because of the appearance of their genitalia at birth, has rekindled controversy concerning the importance of the hormonal environment vis-à-vis rearing. Imperato-McGinley et al. (1979) conclude: "Thus, exposure of the brain of normal levels of testosterone in utero, neonatally and at puberty appears to contribute substantially to the formation of male-gender identity. These subjects demonstrate that in the absence of sociocultural factors that could interrrupt the natural sequence of events, the effects of testosterone predominates, over-riding the effect of rearing as girls."

Although the significance of this report clearly depends on the validity of the statement that the sex of rearing of these genetic males was unambiguously female, and on other factors (Wilson, 1979), this provocative report would appear to be of great potential significance to the attempt to relate principles of sexual differentiation as obtained from animal research to the human being.

As indicated above, an evaluation of homosexual and transexual individuals might also provide a clue to the etiology of their behavioral pattern subject to the limitations of retrospective studies. Recently Meyer-Bahlburg (1977, 1979) has published two thorough and critical reviews of the literature relating sex hormones and homosexual behavior to which the interested reader should refer. In general, it would appear that although an influence of the hormone environment on the etiology of homosexuality has not been established, neither has it been precluded.

Since the animal literature supports the possibility that the reported sex differences in performance in learning tasks are also influenced during development by the hormonal environment (Beatty, 1979), and since sex differences in cognitive function may exist (Witelson, 1976), it is possible that the prenatal hormone environment plays a significant role in this aspect of human development. However, critical reviews of this field (Reinisch, 1976; Ehrhardt and Meyer-Bahlburg, 1979) again conclude that presently available data are inconclusive.

Since the significance of the steroid hormonal environment for sexual differentiation of the human brain still has not been established, it is difficult to evaluate the applicability of the remaining fundamental concepts based on animal research to human development at this time. However, it does appear likely that the various hormone sensitive aspects of human brain development which may be demonstrated in the future will differ in their sensitivity to hormones, the time course of their development, as well as the specific neural loci involved. Moreover, we consider it likely that morphological sex differences do exist in the human brain, although even

more so than in laboratory animal, the role of the hormone environment vis-à-vis genomic factors or other environmental influence will be difficult to establish. If sexual differentiation occurs prenatally in the human being, the existence of protective mechanisms would seem most probable. However, current evidence suggests that α-fetoprotein is not the mechanism since the human being this protein does not bind estrogen (Nunez et al., 1976).

Finally, the recent conclusion of Imperato-McGinley et al. (1979) that hormonal titers at puberty may influence psychosexual differentiation, is consistent with our present view that even in the rat, at least under certain circumstances, the hormone environment well beyond the perinatal period can have permanent, perhaps "morphotropic" effects.

In conclusion, the results of animal research clearly document an important role of the steroid environment in the development and differentiation of brain function and morphology. At present the application of this concept to human development is inconclusive due in part to the limitations of clinical retrospective studies and probably to the likelihood that the activity of higher neural centers can mask even a fundamental influence of hormones on brain development. Hopefully, further research both at the level of laboratory animals and the human being will elucidate the relevance of animal models to human development, and importantly, the role of the hormone environment in the differentiation of the complex brain of our own species.

ACKNOWLEDGEMENTS

The authors gratefully acknowledge the financial assistance provided by NIH grant HD-01182 and the Ford, Kroc and Grant Foundations which have supported the original investigations of the authors reviewed in this manuscript, and the secretarial assistance of Ms. Nicole Lotwin. A special acknowledgement is offered to Mr. James Shryne for the art work.

REFERENCES

Altman J, Bayer SA (1978) Development of the diencephalon in the rat. I. Autoradiography study of the time of origin and settling patterns of neurons of the hypothalamus. J Comp Neurol 182: 945.

Arai Y (1971) A possible process of the secondary sterilization: delayed anovulation syndrome. Experientia 27: 463.

Aria Y, Matsumoto A, Nishizuka M (1978) Synaptogenic action of estrogen on the hypothalamic arcuate nucleus (ARCN) of the developing brain and of the deafferented adult brain in female rats. In Dorner G, Kawakami M, eds. Hormones and brain development, pp 43–48. Amsterdam: Elsevier/North Holland Biomedical Press.

Arnold AP (1980) Effects of androgens on volumes of sexually dimorphic brain regions in the zebra finch. Brain Res 185: 441.

Attardi B, Geller LN, Ohno S (1976) Androgen and estrogen receptors in brain cytosol from male, female and Tfm mice. Endocrinology 98: 864.

132

Baker SW (1980) Psychosexual differentiation in the human. Biol Reprod 22: 61.

Barraclough CA, Wise PM, Turgeon J, Shander D, Depaulo L, Rance N (1979) Recent studies on the regulation of pituitary LH and FSH secretion. Biol Reprod 20: 86.

Beach FA (1974) Effects of gonadal hormones on urinary behavior in dogs. Physiol Behav 12: 1005.

Beach FA (1976) Sexual attractivity, proceptivity, and receptivity in female mammals. Horm Behav 7: 105.

Beach FA, Buehler MG (1977) Male rats with inherited insensitivity to androgen show reduced sexual behavior. Endocrinology 100: 197.

Beatty WW (1979) Gonadal hormones and sex differences in nonreproductive behaviors in rodents: organizational and activational influences. Horm Behav 12: 112.

Breedlove SM, Arnold AP (1980) Hormone accumulation in a sexually dimorphic motor nucleus of the rat spinal cord. Science, in press.

Brown-Grant K (1975) On "critical periods" during the postnatal development of the rat. Int Symp on Sexual Endocrinology of the Perinatal Period, INSERM, 32: 357.

Bubenik GA, Brown GM (1973) Morphologic sex differences in primate brain areas involved in regulation of reproductive activity. Experientia 29: 619.

Campbell CS, Schwartz NB (1977) Steroid feedback regulation of luteinizing hormone and follicle-stimulating hormone secretion rates in male and female rats. J Toxicol Environ Health 3: 61.

Casper R, Vernadakis A, Timaras PS (1967) Influence of estradiol and cortisol on lipids and cerebiodidis in the developing brain and spinal cord of the rat. Brain Res 5: 524.

Christensen LW, Gorski RA (1978) Independent masculinization of neuroendocrine systems by intracerebral implants of testosterone or estradiol in the neonatal female rat. Brain Res 146: 325.

Clemens LG, Gladue BA, Coniglio LP (1978) Prenatal endogenous androgenic influences on masculine sexual behavior and genital morphology in male and female rats. Horm Behav 10: 40.

Crowley WR, O'Donohue TL, Jacobowitz DM (1978) Sex differences in catecholamine content in discrete brain nuclei of the rat: effects of neonatal castration or testosterone treatment. Acta Endocrinol 89: 20.

Denef C (1974) Effect of hypophysectomy and pituitary implants at puberty on the sexual differentiation of testosterone metabolism in rat liver. Endocrinology 94: 1577.

Döhler KD (1978) Is female sexual differentiation hormone-mediated? Trends Neurosci 1: 138.

Dörner G, Staudt J (1978) Structural changes in the preoptic anterior hypothalamic area of the male rat, following neonatal castration and androgen substitution. Neuroendocrinology 3: 136.

Dörner G, Staudt J (1964) Structural changes in the hypothalamic ventromedial nucleus of the male rat, following neonatal castration and androgen treatment. Neuroendocrinology 4: 278.

Dunlap JL, Gerall AA, Carlton SF (1978) Evaluation of prenatal androgen and ovarian secretions on receptivity in female and male rats. J Comp Physiol Psychol 92: 280.

Dyer RG, MacLeod NK, Ellendorf F (1976) Electrophysiological evidence for sexual dimorphism and synaptic convergence in the preoptic and anterior hypothalamic areas of the rat. Proc R Soc Lond (Biol) 193: 421.

Ehrhardt AA, Meyer-Bahlburg HFL (1979) Prenatal sex hormones and the developing brain: effects on psychosexual differentiation and cognitive function. Ann Rev Med 30: 417.

Elsaesser F, Parvizi N (1979) Estrogen feedback in the pig: sexual differentiation and the effect of prenatal testosterone treatment. Biol Reprod 20: 1187.

Gandelman R, vom Saal FS, Reinisch JM (1977) Contiguity to male foetuses affects morphology and behaviour of female mice. Nature 266: 722.

Goldfoot DA, Feder HH, Goy RW (1969) Development of bisexuality in the male rat treated neonatally with androstenedione. J Comp Physiol Psychol 67: 41.

Gorski RA (1966) Localization and sexual differentiation of the nervous structures which regulate ovulation. J Reprod Fertil Suppl 1: 67.

Gorski RA (1968) Influence of age on the response to paranatal administration of a low dose of androgen. Endocrinology 82: 1001.

Gorski RA (1971) Gonadal hormones and the perinatal development of neuroendocrine function. In Martini L, Ganong WF, eds. Frontiers in neuroendocrinology, pp 237–290. New York: Oxford University Press.

Gorski RA (1974) The neuroendocrine regulation of sexual behavior. In Newton G, Riesen AH, eds. Advances in psychobiology, Vol II, pp 1–58. New York: John Wiley.

Gorski RA (1979) The nature of hormone action in the brain. In Hamilton TH, Clark JH, Sadler WA, eds. Ontogeny of receptors and mode of action of reproductive hormones, pp 371–392. New York: Raven Press.

Gorski RA, Harlan RE, Christensen LW (1977) Perinatal hormonal exposure and the development of neuroendocrine processes. J Toxicol Environ Health 3: 97.

Gorski RA, Gordon JH, Shryne JE, Southam AM (1978) Evidence for a morphological sex difference within the medial preoptic area of the rat brain. Brain Res 148: 333.

Gorski RA, Christensen LW Nance DM (1979) The induction of heterotypical sexual behavior in the rat. Psychoneuroendocrinology 4: 311.

Gorski RA, Harlan RE, Jacobson CD, Shryne JE, Southam AM (1980) Evidence for the existence of a sexually dimorphic nucleus in the preoptic area of the rat. J Comp Neurol, in press.

Goy RW, McEwen BS (1980) Sexual differentiation of the brain. Cambridge: MIT Press.

Greenough WT, Carter CS, Steerman C, DeVoogd TJ (1977) Sex differences in dendritic patterns in hamster POA. Brain Res 126: 63.

Gregory E (1975) Comparison of postnatal CNS development between male and female rats. Brain Res 99: 152.

Griffiths EC, Hooper KC, Jeffcoate SL, Holland DT (1976) Effect of neonatal androgen on the activity of peptidases in the rat brain inactivating luteinizing hormone-releasing hormone. Horm Res 7: 218.

Gurney ME, Konishi M (1980) Hormone induced sexual differentiation of brain and behavior in zebra finches. Science 208: 1380.

Harlan RE, Gorski RA (1978) Effects of postpubertal ovarian steroids on reproductive function and sexual differentiation of lightly androgenized rats. Endocrinology 102: 1716.

Harlan RE, Gordon JH, Gorski RA (1979) Sexual differentiation of the brain: implications for neuroscience. In Reviews of neuroscience, Vol 4, pp 31–71. New York: Raven Press.

Harris GW (1964) Sex hormones, brain development and brain function. Endocrinology 75: 627.

Henry JL, Calaresu FR (1972) Topography and numerical distribution of neurons of the thoraco-lumbar intermediolateral nucleus in the cat. J Comp Neurol 144: 205.

Ichinoe K, Yokota H (1978) Study of androgen sterility syndrome on adolescent girls. Acta Obstet Gynaecol Jpn 30: 253.

Ifft JD (1964) The effect of endocrine gland extirpations on the size of nucleoli in rat hypothalamic neurons. Anat Rec 148: 599.

Ifft JD (1972) An autoradiographic study of the time of final division of neurons in rat hypothalamic nuclei. J Comp Neurol 144: 193.

Imperato-McGinley J, Peterson RE, Gautier T, Sturla E (1979) Androgens and the evolution of male-gender identity among male pseudohermaphrodites with 5α-reductase deficiency. New Engl J Med 300: 1233.

Jacobson CD, Shryne JE, Shapiro F, Gorski RA (1980) Ontogeny of the sexually dimorphic nucleus of the preoptic area. J Comp Neurol, in press.

Josso N, Picard J, Tran D (1977) The antiMüllerian hormone. In Greep RO, ed. Recent progress in hormone research, Vol 33, pp 117–167. New York: Academic Press.

Karsch FJ, Dierschke DJ, Knobil E (1973) Sexual differentiation of pituitary function: apparent differences between primates and rodents. Science 179: 484.

Kawashima S (1960) Influence of continued injections of sex steroids on the estrous cycle in the adult rat. Annot Zool Jpn 33: 226.

Kikuyama S, Kawashima S (1966) Formation of corpora lutea in ovarian grafts in ovariectomized adult rats subjected to early postnatal treatment with androgen. Sci Papers Coll Gen Educ Univ Tokyo 16: 69.

Kulin HE, Reiter EO (1976) Gonadotropin and testosterone measurements after estrogen administration to adult men, prepubertal and pubertal boys, and men with hypogonadotropism: evidence for maturation of positive feedback in the male. Pediat Res 10: 46.

Larsson K (1979) Features of the neuroendocrine regulation of masculine sexual behavior. In Beyer C, ed. Endocrine control of sexual behavior, pp 77–163. New York: Raven Press.

Litteria M (1977) The effects of neonatal androgenization on the in vivo transport of alpha-aminoisobutyric acid into specific regions of the rat brain. Brain Res 132: 287.

Lobl RT, Gorski RA (1974) Neonatal intrahypothalamic androgen administration: the influence of dose and age on androgenization of female rats. Endocrinology 94: 1325.

Lund RD (1978) Development and plasticity of the brain. New York: Oxford University Press.

MacLusky NJ, Lieberburg I, McEwen BS (1979) The development of estrogen receptor systems in the rat brain: perinatal development. Brain Res 178: 129.

Matsumoto A, Arai Y (1976) Developmental changes in synaptic formation in the hypothalamic arcuate nucleus of female rats. Cell Tiss Res 169: 143.

McEwen BS (1978) Sexual maturation and differentiation: the role of the gonadal steroids. In Corner MA et al., eds. Maturation of the nervous system, Progress in brain research, Vol 48, pp 291–307. Amsterdam: Elsevier/North-Holland Biomedical Press.

McEwen BS, Plapinger L, Chaptal C, Gerlach J, Wallach G (1975) Role of fetoneonatal estrogen binding proteins in the associations of estrogen with neonatal brain cell nuclear receptors. Brain Res 96: 400.

Meyer-Bahlburg HFL (1977) Sex hormones and male homosexuality in comparative perspective. Arch Sex Behav 6: 297.

Meyer-Bahlburg HFL (1979) Sex hormones and female homosexuality: a critical examination. Arch Sex Behav 8: 101.

Meyerson BJ, Lindström LH (1973) Sexual motivation in the female rat. Acta Physiol Scand Suppl 389: 1.

Michael RP, Zumpe D, Keverne EB, Bonsall RW (1972) Neuroendocrine factors in the control of primate behavior. Rec Prog

Horm Res 28: 665.

Naess O, Haug E, Attramadal A, Aakvaag A, Hansson V, French F (1976) Androgen receptors in the anterior pituitary and central nervous system of the androgen "insensitive" (Tfm) rat: correlation between receptor binding and effects of androgens on gonadotropic secretion. Endocrinology 99: 1295.

Naftolin F, Ryan KJ, Daview IJ, Reddy VV, Flores F, Petro Z, Kuhn M, White RJ, Takaoka Y, Wolin L (1975) The formation of estrogen by central neuroendocrine tissues. In Greep RO, ed. Recent progress in hormone research, Vol 31, pp 295–319. New York: Academic Press.

Nance DM, Shryne J, Gorski RA (1975) Facilitation of female sexual behavior in male rats by septal lesions: an interaction with estrogen. Horm Behav 6: 289.

Neill JD, Smith MS (1974) Pituitary–ovarian interrelationships in the rat. In James VHT, Martini L, eds. Current topics in experimental endocrinology, Vol 2, pp 73–106. London: Academic Press.

Nottebohm F, Arnold AP (1976) Sexual dimorphism in vocal control areas of the songbird brain. Science 194: 211.

Nunez EA, Benassayag C, Savu L, Vallette G, Jayle MF (1976) Serum binding of some steroid hormones during development in different animal species. Discussion on the biological significance of this binding. Ann Biol Anim Biochem Biophys 16: 491.

Olsen KL (1979) Androgen-insensitive rats are defeminized by their testes. Nature 279: 288.

Olsen KL, Whalen RE (1980) Sexual differentiation of the brain: Effects on mating behavior and ³H-estradiol binding by hypothalamic chromatin in rats. Biol Reprod 22: 1068.

Peck EJ, Miller AL, Kelner KL (1979) Estrogen receptors and the activation of RNA polymerases by estrogens in the central nervous system. In Hamilton TH, Clark JH, Sadler WA, eds. Ontogeny of receptors and reproductive hormone action, pp 403–410. New York: Raven Press.

Pfaff DW (1966) Morphological changes in the brains of adult male rats after neonatal castration. J Endocrinol 36: 415.

Pfaff DW (1976) The neuroanatomy of sex hormone receptors in the vertebrate brain. Neuroendocrinol Regul Fertil, Int Symp, Simla, pp 30–45.

Pfeiffer CA (1936) Sexual differences of the hypophysis and their determination by the gonads. Am J Anat 58: 195.

Quadagno DM, Briscoe R, Quadagno JS (1977) Effect of perinatal gonadal hormones on selected nonsexual behavior patterns: a critical assessment of the nonhuman and human literature. Psychol Bull 84: 62.

Raisman G (1969) Neuronal plasticity in the septal nuclei of the rat. Brain Res 14: 25.

Raisman G, Field PM (1973) Sexual dimorphism in the neuropil of the preoptic area of the rat and its dependence on neonatal androgen. Brain Res 54: 1.

Reinisch JM (1976) Effects of prenatal hormone exposure on physical and psychological development in humans and animals: with a note on the state of the field. In Saachar EJ, ed. Hormones, behavior and psychopathology, pp 69–94. New York: Raven Press.

Rothchild IM (1971) Functional amenorrhea. In Mack HC, Sherman AI, eds. The neuroendocrinology of human reproduction, pp 171–182. Springfield: Charles C. Thomas.

Seress L (1978) The effect of the neonatal testosterone treatment on the postnatal cell formation of the rat brain. Med J Osaka Univ 28: 285.

Sheridan PJ (1979) Estrogen binding in the neonatal cortex. Brain Res 178: 201.

Sheridan PJ, Sar M, Stumpf WE (1974) Autoradiographic locali-

134

zation of ^{3}H-estradiol or its metabolites in the central nervous system of the developing rat. Endocrinology 94: 1386.

Silver J (1978) Cell death during development of the nervous system. In Jacobson M, ed. Handbook of sensory physiology, Vol IX: Development of sensory system, pp 419–436. Berlin: Springer Verlag.

Staudt J, Dörner G (1976) Structural changes in the medial and central amygdala of the male rat, following neonatal castration and androgen treatment. Endokrinologie 67: 296.

Stumpf WE, Sar M (1978) Anatomical distribution of estrogen, androgen, progestin, corticosteroid and thyroid hormone target sites in the brain of mammals: phylogeny and ontogeny. Am Zool 18: 435.

Tarttelin MF, Gorski RA (1973) The effect of ovarian steroids on food and water intake and body weight in the female rat. Acta Endocrinol 72: 551.

Toran-Allerand CD (1980) Sex steroids and the development of the newborn mouse hypothalamus and preoptic area in vitro. II. Morphological correlates and hormonal specificity. Brain Res 189: 413.

Toran-Allerand CD, Gerlach JL, McEwen BS (1980) Autoradiographic localization of ^{3}H-estradiol related to steroid responsiveness in cultures of the newborn mouse hypothalamus and preoptic area. Brain Res 184: 517.

Vértes M, King RJB (1973) Studies on (6,7-^{3}H) oestradiol binding in rat brain and other tissues. In Recent developments of neurobiology in Hungary, Vol IV, pp 33–52. Budapest: Akademiai Kiado.

Vito CC, Fox TO (1979) Embryonic rodent brain contains estrogen receptors. Science 204: 517.

Vito CC, Wieland SJ, Fox TO (1979) Androgen receptors exist throughout the "critical period" of brain sexual differentiation. Nature 282: 308.

Vom Saal FS, Bronson FH (1978) In utero proximity of female mouse fetuses to males: effect on reproductive performance during later life. Biol Reprod 19: 842.

Vom Saal FS, Bronson FH (1980a) Sexual characteristics of adult female mice correlate with their blood testosterone levels during prenatal development. Science, in press.

Vom Saal FS, Bronson FH (1980b) The estrous cycle: variation in length due to former intrauterine proximity to male fetuses in mice. Biol Reprod, in press.

Weisz J, Ward IL (1980) Plasma testosterone and progesterone titers of pregnant rats, their male and female fetuses, and neonatal offspring. Endocrinology 106: 306.

Whalen RE, Olsen KL (1978) Chromatin binding of estradiol in the hypothalamus and cortex of male and female rats. Brain Res 152: 121.

Wilson JD (1979) Sex hormones and sexual behavior. New Engl Med 300: 1269.

Witelson SF (1976) Sex and the single hemisphere: specialization of the right hemisphere for spatial processing. Science 193: 425.

Yamanouchi K, Arai Y (1977) Possible inhibitory role of the dorsal inputs to the preoptic area and hypothalamus in regulating female sexual behavior in the female rat. Brain Res 127: 296.

Yanai J (1979) Strain and sex differences in the rat brain. Acta Anat 103: 150.

Zondek T, Mansfield MD, Zondek LH (1977) Amniotic fluid testosterone and fetal sex determination in the first half of pregnancy. Br J Obstet Gynaecol 84: 714.

12. GENDER IDENTITY/ROLE (G-I/R) IN MALE HERMAPHRODITISM

EILEEN HIGHAM

1. INTRODUCTION

Until recently, male hermaphroditic conditions were differentiated on the basis of anatomical characteristics of the reproductive system. Technical advances of recent years now allow, in many cases, a differential diagnosis of the syndromes of male hermaphroditism on the basis of etiology and prognosis. The specialist in behavior and psychology is not expected to have a specialist's diagnostic knowledge of genetics and endocrinology. Thus, the necessary information is presented in this chapter.

With the discovery of hermaphroditic disorders based on chromosomal constitution or on endocrine production, metabolism, and utilization, it is possible to determine whether or not there is a relationship between any of these etiologic factors and the differentiation and development of G-I/R in cases of male hermaphroditism. Some infants born as male hermaphrodites have been assigned and reared as males, others as females. As a result, the syndromes of hermaphroditism, which are experiments of nature, provide an opportunity to assess the relative contribution of chromosomal, prenatal hormonal, pubertal hormonal and sociocultural events on G-I/R differentiation and erotosexual status. The purpose of this paper is to summarize the results of investigations of G-I/R and erotosexual status in male hermaphroditism. The secondary purpose is to discuss the methodology of investigating G-I/R status.

2. CHARACTERISTICS OF THE SYNDROMES

The syndromes of male hermaphroditism are defined in terms of an ambiguity of the genital organs and the presence of testicular tissue, typically in a 46,XY chromosomal individual. The role of the H-Y antigen explains, in part, testicular development in a 45,X or 46,XX male. Normally, the Y chromosome directs testicular organization in the fetal gonad through the action of H-Y antigen, a cell surface, or plasma membrane protein. In some instances, Y chromosomal material is detached from its normal position on cells; the H-Y antigen is expressed nonetheless, organizing testicular tissue in an individual without the expected 46,XY karyotype. The findings regarding the presence of H-Y antigen and testicular development in male hermaphroditism are sometimes inconsistent and contradictory, however (Jones et al., 1979).

In light of today's knowledge, classification according to etiology comprises: (1) chromosomal defects affecting masculinization; (2) defects in the central nervous system affecting the production of gonadotropins; (3) defects of the synthesis of testosterone in the fetal gonads; and (4) defects of the end organ utilization of testosterone. The common factor, regardless of etiology, is, in the final analysis, incomplete prenatal masculinization of the body.*

---

* Other defects of gonadal and peripheral end organ function associated with male hermaphroditism are described by Park et al. (1975); the majority of cases with a known etiology are included in the four classifications listed above. The exception is the syndrome of a male with a uterus resulting from demasculinization secondary to Müllerian inhibiting factor deficiency. This defect of prenatal male phenotypic development occurs when the fetal testes fail to secrete the Müllerian inhibiting factor, although testosterone is secreted in normal amounts. As a result, the internal and external reproductive structures, controlled by testosterone and its products, are masculinized, but the uterus and Fallopian tubes, normally suppressed by the Müllerian inhibiting factor, also develop. Individuals born with this disorder are assigned as boys since there is no indication of an abnormality of the internal reproductive structures. The abnormality may be discovered by the presence of an inguinal hernia containing the Fallopian tubes.

S.J. Kogan and E.S.E. Hafez (eds.), Pediatric andrology, 135–145. All rights reserved.
Copyright © 1981, Martinus Nijhoff Publishers bv, The Hague/Boston/London.

136

3. METHOD OF INVESTIGATION OF G-I/R AND EROTOSEXUAL STATUS

Gender identity/role is the result of a sequential process of differentiation and development from conception to maturity. The major events in that process are depicted in Fig. 1.

The procedures for investigating G-I/R status include direct observation, interviewing, oblique inquiry techniques and formal psychological testing of the subject. In addition, parents or other family members, and lover or spouse, are interviewed. Laboratory studies are also included in a complete workup.

The schedule of procedures used in the Psychohormonal Research Unit for patients with a history of birth defect of the sex organs is listed in the appendix to this paper. The information obtained from interviewing is tape-recorded and transcribed. Interview and test data and the observations of the individuals provide information regarding G-I/R, including erotosexual functioning. These methods are employed because ordinary paper and pencil tests and projective tests of personality rarely provide data pertaining specifically to G-I/R status, especially in its erotosexual aspects. Tape-recorded, transcribed interviews present the data in the subjects' own words, not in the words of the impressions or interpretations of the interviewer. Interviewer observations and impressions provide information which supplements the subject's direct personal report of feelings, imagery and cognitions. Photographs also convey information regarding the degree to which an individual conforms to the social stereotypes of masculinity or femininity.

4. SYNDROMES OF MALE HERMAPHRODITISM

4.1. Demasculinization secondary to chromosomal defect

Sex-chromosomal abnormality is rarely associated with male hermaphroditism, except in variants of Turner's syndrome in which vestigial testicular tissue is present. In these cases the presence of an enlarged clitoris, partial labial fusion, and some androgen-secreting cells in the streak gonads fulfills the criteria for male hermaphroditism. Individuals with Y chromosomal mosaicism (45,X/46,XY karyotype) or with Y chromosome abnormalities typically have malformed testes and some degree of genital ambiguity characteristic of male hermaphroditism. The degree of genital ambiguity varies, depending upon the degree of testicular dysfunction (Sohval, 1964; Park et al., 1975; Money, 1977).

In such cases assignment and rearing varies with the degree of genital ambiguity. Typically, those reared as girls differentiate a feminine gender identity, and those reared as boys differentiate a masculine gender identity complicated by incomplete virilization at puberty. Morphologically masculinized individuals with mosaic karyotypes have not been studied intensively with respect to erotosexual status.

In Klinefelter's (46,XXY) syndrome, incomplete virilization at puberty raises the possibility that some degree of covert deandronenization occurs in the fetus. These individuals are always assigned and reared as males. Erotosexual disinterest or apathy is common in adulthood, regardless of erotosexual status as bisexual, heterosexual or homosexual. Behavioral disabilities may include, in some cases, transvestism or transexualism. Whether such disabilities stem from a vulnerability to error in psychosexual differentiation, secondary to a minor degree of prenatal demasculinization, is conjectural (Money et al., 1974).

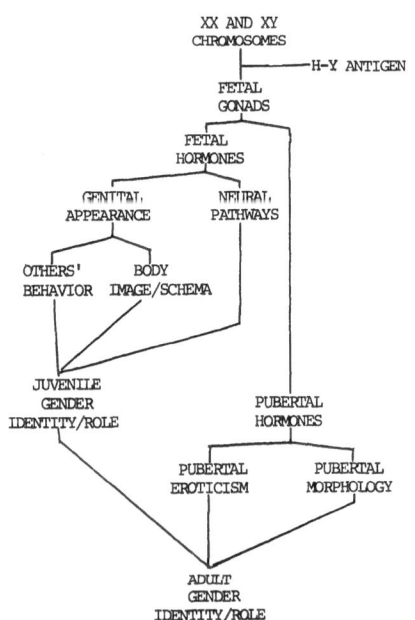

Figure 1. The sequential determinants and differentiation of gender-identity/role (G-I/R). [Reprinted, with permission, from Money and Ehrhardt (1972).]

4.2. Demasculinization secondary to central nervous system defect of gonadotropin production

There is one case report of an adult patient with minimally ambiguous genitalia attributed to failure of the fetal pituitary to secrete gonadotropins for stimulation of the fetal testes, in whom, at puberty, the testes remained inactive and the body failed to masculinize (Park et al., 1976). The individual was assigned and reared as a girl. In adulthood, an endocrine workup included stimulation by an exogenous gonadotropin and a strong hormonal masculinizing effect occurred rapidly from the androgen released from the testes.

4.3. Demasculinization secondary to impaired testosterone biosynthesis

Among the known defects in biosynthesis of testosterone are: pregnenolone synthesis defect, or lipoid adrenal hyperplasia; 3β-hydroxysteroid dehydrogenase defect; 17α-hydroxylase deficiency; 17β-hydroxysteroid dehydrogenase deficiency; 17-20 desmolase deficiency; 17-ketosteroid reductase deficiency; 5α-reductase deficiency. Each involves an enzyme deficit which blocks the synthesis of testosterone at some point in the pathway of steroid synthesis.

These defects are rare, some extremely so. Lipoid adrenal hyperplasia is incompatible with life beyond a few months. The enzyme defect occurs at the beginning of the steroid synthesis pathway so that female genitalia differentiate.

Indidivuals with a 3β-hydroxysteroid dehydrogenase defect have variable degrees of genital ambiguity because the enzyme defect blocks the synthesis of testosterone, but not the synthesis of a precursor of androgen, dehydroepiandrosterone. Affected infants are assigned as male or female, in accordance with the degree of genital defect (Bongiovanni, 1961; Park et al., 1971).

In 17α-hydroxylase deficiency, a condition in which the testes are unable to secrete androgen, the genital anatomy differentiates as ambiguous. Puberty is characterized by the absence of secondary male sexual characteristics and gynecomastia. In the single published account of a genetic male with this deficiency, gender identity is in accord with sex of rearing (New and Suvannakul, 1970; Money, personal communication). The patient evaluated by both

New and Money was not assigned as male until age 20 months. He developed a primarily male G-I/R, despite the psychic traumas of a small phallus (6 cm) bound down with chordee, and pronounced gynecomastia. He claimed a masculine erotosexual life including erections and attempted intercourse with a girlfriend, lacking only ejaculation.

Steroid 17-20 desmolase deficiency is an enzymatic defect which blocks the synthesis of testosterone precursors. Zachman et al. (1972) described this deficiency in two young children with ambiguous external genitalia. They were reared as boys, and provided with genital reconstructive surgery; outcome of the surgery was not reported. Behavioral data for this deficiency, though sparse, are compatible with the concept that G-I/R differentiates to be concordant with sex of assignment and rearing.

In 17-ketosteroid reductase deficiency, the conversion of androstenedione to testosterone in the testes is blocked, so that the latter hormone is unavailable to the cells which require it. The enzyme defect has a prenatal deandrogenizing effect, producing ambiguous external genitalia. At puberty, however, secondary sexual differentiation is virilizing. Virdis et al. (1978) summarize the previous clinical studies of this syndrome and report findings on another pubertal patient. All but one of the individuals were reared as female, but behavioral data were not reported. Another case report by Park et al. (1975) includes some behavioral data for a patient with this enzyme deficiency; detailed information regarding childhood behavior and pubertal and adult eroticism are also available (Money, personal communication). The patient was 28 years old when he requested surgery to close the opening of the urinary meatus at the base of a very small (6 cm) phallus. Three previous surgical efforts had failed to free the phallus from chordee, lengthen it, and provide a penile urethra. The patient had been born with ambiguous genitalia, and assigned as a girl. He lived as a girl with tomboy interests and activities until age 17, when puberty was masculinizing. In the following year, his family and village doctor advised him to move from his natal village to a large city and change his status to that of a male. He was able to begin living as a male for several reasons: he had always felt like a boy as well as a girl; his father had wanted his first-born to be a son, and was happy, finally, to have one; his grandmother's remarks about lumps in his groin in childhood agreed with the idea of being a boy; he recognized that males in his Moslem culture had greater freedom and more opportunities than females, and that it would therefore be relatively more advantageous to live as a man. He had, in fact, grown up with an ambiguity regarding gender status, and when confronted with a masculinizing puberty, and the social advantages of being a male, it was possible for him to begin living as a man. Some years later he married, partly for reasons of immigrant status, but was unable to maintain the relationship, complaining of the sexual inadequacy associated with a very short penis.

In the 17β-hydroxysteroid dehydrogenase deficiency syndrome, the enzyme deficiency prevents normal testosterone production prenatally, so that the infant is born with feminized, or ambiguous, external genitalia. The results on eleven individuals with this condition are summarized by Imperato-McGinley et al. (1979). The infants were assigned as girls at birth, but one was reannounced as a boy at one year. Pubertal maturation was variable. All of them virilized to some degree, but at least half also had breast development. Gender role among the ten patients reared as girls was also variable: those castrated prepubertally or in teenage continued to live as girls; of those not castrated, one continued to live as a female while two reassigned themselves to live as males in teenage. One patient, followed from age 14 to 30, lived as a girl from birth to adolescence. Masculinization at puberty prompted a medical evaluation which revealed ambiguous genitalia. Given the option to live as a boy, the patient did so, participating in athletics and dating girls. Later, he married and reported satisfactory sexual intercourse, despite the handicap of a 5 cm phallus. The authors posit a hormonal effect at puberty responsible for the patient's change in G-I/R status, neglecting the possibility that postnatal social variables were also contributing factors. The fact that not all hermaphroditic patients living as girls, with a masculinizing puberty, change gender role casts doubt upon the possibility of an exclusively hormonal determinant in G-I/R status. The patient described by Park and Money (see above) was reared ambiguously, albeit living as a girl until age 17. Then, social and cultural factors, interacting with an ambiguous rearing, and the masculinized body image, contributed jointly to the patient's ability to live as a man.

In 5α-reductase deficiency, intracellular conversion of testosterone to dihydrotestosterone in target-organ cells is prevented. The 5α-reductase deficiency could, therefore, be classified as a defect in the target organ, or as a defect in testosterone biosynthesis (Imperato-McGinley et al., 1973; Park et al., 1976). Children with this defect are born with feminized, ambiguous external genitalia. Partial secondary sexual virilization occurs at puberty. The voice deepens and the phallus and scrotum enlarge. Acne is absent. Facial hair, hairline recession and prostatic growth are insufficient.

Imperato-McGinley et al. (1974) reported a number of male hermaphrodites in a pedigree of 13 families through three generations. When the first children with ambiguous genitalia were born they were assigned as girls; later, when the condition was understood by the families and village people to be associated with a masculinizing puberty, such children were assigned as boys, and became known as "guevedoces," or children who masculinized at age 12. The social customs which governed the upbringing of children born with defects of the sex organs were not reported. The investigators claimed, however, that those children who were assigned as girls changed their gender identity from female to male at puberty, as a consequence of androgenic hormonal stimulation. To have been accurate, it should have been claimed only that they changed their social and legal status, for the investigators did not report any behavioral data regarding the differentiation of G-I/R, nor did they study the individuals at puberty. They did not support the hypothesis that some of the affected individuals were assigned and reared exclusively as female rather than as sexually indeterminate. It is quite probable that the children were reared as sexually indeterminate, with the door open, so to speak, for a masculine gender status at some future time. In hermaphroditic children reared ambiguously, self-reassignment is not unusual (Money, 1970; Money and Ehrhardt, 1972). Incomplete masculinization in the 5α-reductase deficiency syndrome is attributed, by Imperato-McGinley and her coworkers, to the lack of dihydrotestosterone, secondary to the enzyme defect. This explanation is improbable however, for boys with hypopituitarism, either idiopathic or postsurgical, also are insufficiently masculinized, and they do not have a 5α-reductase deficiency nor a testosterone deficiency in production capability (Clopper et al., 1976). The hormonal and/or neurosecretory conditions underlying the incompleteness of virilization in this, or other syndromes with defective masculinization, are not fully understood. At present, it is reasonably to suppose a hypothalamic and/or pituitary defect, but not a specific steroid hormone deficit, in cases of inadequate pubertal masculinization.

Not all children with 5α-reductase deficiency differentiate a masculine or ambiguous G-I/R. Money (personal communication) describes an 11½-year-old patient reared as female who had a feminine G-I/R, including a teenage romantic interest in a boyfriend. As a younger child this patient had somewhat tomboyish interests which were nonetheless integrated into a feminine G-I/R. Gonadectomy was performed to prevent pubertal virilization. The cases reported by Walsh et al. (1974) and Saenger et al. (1978) were also reared as girls, but the investigators do not report behavioral data regarding G-I/R. Saenger's cases are known not to have changed their gender status.

4.4. Demasculinization secondary to defects of end organ utilization of testosterone

The syndromes of complete and partial androgen insensitivity in XY individuals derive from the fact that androgen cannot be utilized by the receptor cells because androgen-binding in these cells is defective. The complete form of the syndrome is also known as the testicular-feminizing syndrome because the estrogen secreted by the testes is sufficient to produce feminization of the body at puberty. The partial androgen-insensitivity syndrome is also known as Reifenstein's syndrome. Recent findings from endocrine studies of Reifenstein's syndrome show that the defects of the reproductive system are the result of partial tissue insensitivity to androgen (Amhrein et al., 1977).

In the androgen-insensitivity syndrome, androgen is secreted in normal amounts by the fetal testes, but the internal and especially the external reproductive anlagen are unable to respond by masculinizing. The reproductive organs respond normally to the Müllerian inhibiting substance, thus inhibiting the development of the uterus, the Fallopian tubes and the proximal or innermost segment of the vagina. In all other respects, the infant is born with normal female morphology. Occasionally the gonads descend into the groins, alerting the physician to the hermaphroditic condition. Otherwise, with the gonads undescended, the condition is discovered when menstruation does not occur at the expected time, despite feminization of the body.

Children with the complete form of androgen insensitivity are, with extremely rare exception, assigned and reared as girls. A detailed study of ten adolescent or adult sexually mature patients showed that they differentiate a stereotypic feminine G-I/R, no different from that of 46,XX girls and women (Masica et al., 1971; Money et al., 1968). On the whole these women conform to the idealized stereotype of femininity in our society. In childhood these patients were not tomboys; instead, they anticipated romance, marriage and motherhood, in play activities and toy preferences. Later, they preferred marriage, domesticity and rearing a family by adoption, as opposed to a career outside of the home. Infertility was accepted realistically. Clothing and grooming styles were fashionably feminine. In both fantasy and practice sexual imagery was heterosexual, in agreement with sex of rearing. They considered themselves as affectionate, with a normal libido. While not erotically experimental, nor likely to take the initiative erotically, intercourse typically culminated in orgasm. Erotic sensitivity was typical for females and sensitivity of the vagina was not impaired by surgical lengthening. The tactile sense was more important than the senses of sight, taste or smell for erotic stimulation; erotic narratives were also stimulating.

Children with the partial androgen-insensitivity syndrome are born with varying degrees of incompletely differentiated genitalia. The degree of genital anomaly is such that some children have been assigned and reared not as boys, but as girls, or ambiguously. The effects of these three conditions of rearing for ten patients with partial androgen insensitivity is reported by Money and Ogunro (1974): one was reared as a girl, one as a hermaphroditic girl and eight as boys. Five of the eight boys had been originally assigned as girls, and later in infancy reassigned as boys. They ranged in age from six to 38 years at the initial evaluation and were followed for a period ranging from one month to 22 years. All of them had a partially feminizing puberty. All but one of those reared as boys underwent multiple cor-

140

rective or reconstructive penile surgery at various ages.

The partial androgen-insensitivity patients reared as boys differentiated a masculine gender identity. The handicaps of uncertainty of sex of assignment, genital surgery, genital anomaly, and inadequate masculinization did not interfere with a masculine G-I/R and erotosexual status. In childhood they lack the interest in vigorous and competitive activities expected in boyhood, and even in adulthood, fighting, rivalry and aggression are uncharacteristic. Interest in parentalism is not prominent in the childhood play of these patients, but an interest in fatherhood emerged in adulthood. In adulthood, all eight patients reported experiences of heterosexual romantic and erotic imagery in thought, fantasy or daydreaming, but only half reported erotic sleeping imagery; none reported wet dreams with ejaculation. Four of the patients were married and two anticipated marriage; the remaining two avoided or rejected the possibility of marriage. the frequency of erection and orgasm, from masturbation or shared erotic activity with a partner, varied extensively. Orgasm was described as a gradual peak of feeling with or without fluid discharge. While erotically responsive to both visual and tactile stimuli, the threshold of arousal corresponded more closely to that of normal females, for whom touch is the predominant sensory channel of erotic arousal. On the whole, they manifest less active erotic functioning than is reported in ordinary males, and they are less inclined to intiate sexual activity; the latter may be related to inhibitions stemming from penile inadequacies. None of these factors interfere, however, with their sense of being masculine (Money, 1973).

The two reared female underwent gonadectomy and vaginoplasty in teenage. One also had a clitorectomy. The erotic and non-erotic aspects of gender identity were concordant with rearing as feminine. Erotic imagery and experience was appropriately heterosexual except for a brief lesbian experience in early teenage in one woman. Reared as a hermaphroditic girl, she had obsessional doubts and fears about being a normal female which intensified with a romantic sexual experience and with marriage. The other woman married. In childhood, both patients were interested in doll play and maternalism, but in adulthood parenthood was avoided. The threshold for erotic arousal to visual and tactile stimuli was similar to that of normal women.

5. CONCLUDING REMARKS

The evidence from studies of male hermaphroditism indicates that G-I/R typically differentiates concordantly with sex of assignment and rearing, and that erotosexual status is in agreement with G-I/R. Prenatal demasculinization of the male fetus does not preclude functioning as a male, genital handicap notwithstanding, in individuals assigned and reared as male. The reverse applies when the individual is assigned and reared as female.

The long-term effects of prenatal demasculinization on the individual reared male include disability in the typical boyhood activities requiring high energy expenditure and competitiveness, and some degree of erotic inertia with respect to response to visual imagery, and to the frequency and intensity of erotosexual activity in adolescence and adulthood. The degree of variation from the expected gender norms for males may depend upon the degree of fetal demasculinization, as illustrated by the syndromes of complete and partial androgen insensitivity. Whether or not demasculinization secondary to the other biochemical defects differently affects G-I/R requires further study.

Male hermaphrodites reared as females are not, as a combined result of a 46,XY chromosomal constitution, of some degree of prenatal and pubertal masculinization, of infertility, and of genital feminizing surgery, significantly different from 46,XX women in their G-I/R status. Those who are tomboys in childhood, possibly as a consequence of a prenatal androgen effect on CNS differentiation, are able to integrate such behavioral traits into a postpubertal feminine G-I/R. In adolescence, and later, their feminine gender identity is manifested in heterosexual responsiveness to males, in marriage, and in an interest in rearing children. Erotically, such women do not appear to differ significantly from 46,XX women with respect to intensity of libido or to the sensory stimuli of erotosexual arousal.

The report by Imperato-McGinley et al. on male hermaphroditism in the Dominican Republic, and the followup report on a patient in the United States, do not contradict the conclusions presented above. In the absence of behavioral data, the logical assumption, with respect to the Dominicans, is that they were reared as children with a hermaphroditic birth defect, and therefore, were able to change gender status after the onset of a masculinizing puberty. In a village with no medical facilities for the treatment of hermaphroditism, rearing as sexually indeterminate or ambiguous, leaving the door open to live as a male, as a female, or as a misfit, in keeping with pubertal differentiation, may have represented the best possible solution for the upbringing of an hermaphroditic infant.

As yet, there is no evidence for a simple, straight-line relationship between sex hormones and masculine or feminine G-I/R erotosexual status in human beings. There is evidence, however, that social and cultural stimuli interact with the prenatal neuro-endocrine components of G-I/R differentiation. The findings on endocrine status in homosexuals, transexuals and the syndromes of hermaphrotism dictate extreme caution in attributing causality on the basis of correlation. Both prenatal and postnatal components must be weighed in understanding the complexities of G-I/R differentiation and erotosexual functioning. Moreover, the assessment of G-I/R status and erotosexual status requires the full participation of a behavior specialist. Assessment of psychosexual differentiation and development requires a specialist who understands socio-cultural reactions to disease and disability, who is skilled in obtaining the necessary behavioral and personal information and informed about sexual disorders.

ACKNOWLEDGEMENTS

Supported in part by USPHS Grants HD00325 and HD07111.

REFERENCES

Amhrein J, Klingensmith G, Walsh P, McKusick J, Migeon J (1977) Partial androgen insensitivity: the Reifenstein syndrome revisited. New Engl J Med, 297: 350.

Bongiovanni A (1961) Unusual steroid pattern in congenital adrenal hyperplasia: deficiency of 3β-hydroxy dehydrogenase. J Clin Endocrinol 21: 860.

Clopper R, Adelson J, Money J (1976) Postpubertal psychosexual function in male hypopituitarism without hypogonadotropinism after growth hormone therapy. J Sex Res 12: 14.

Ehrhardt A, Greenberg N, Money J (1970) Female gender identity and absence of fetal hormones. Johns Hopkins Med J 126: 237.

Imperato-McGinley J, Peterson R (1973) Male pseudohermaphroditism: the complexities of male phenotypic development. Am J Med 61: 251.

Imperato-McGinley J, G rrero L, Gautier T, Peterson RE (1974) Steroid 5α-reductase deficiency in man: an inherited form of male pseudohermaphroditism. Science 186: 1213.

Imperato-McGinley J, Peterson R, Stoller R, Goodwin W (1979) Male pseurohermaphroditism secondary to 17β-hydroxysteroid deficiency: gender role change with puberty. J Clin Endocrinol Metab 49: 391.

Jones H, Rary J, Rock J, Cummings D (1979) The role of H-Y antigen in human sexual development. Johns Hopkins Med J 145: 33.

Masica D, Money J, Ehrhardt A (1971) Fetal feminization and female gender identity in the testicular feminizing syndrome of androgen insensitivity. Arch Sec Behav 1: 131.

Money J (1970) Matched pairs of hermaphrodites: behavioral biology of sexual differentiation from chromosomes to gender identity. Engineering and Science (California Institute of Technology, Special Issue: Biological Bases of Human Behavior) 33: 34.

Money J (1973) Effects of prenatal androgenization and deandrogenization on behavior in human beings. In Ganong W, Martini L, eds. Frontiers in neuroendocrinology, p 249. New York: Oxford University Press.

Money J (1976) Gender identity and hermaphroditism. Science 191: 872.

Money J (1977) Prenatal deandrogenization of human beings. In Money J, Musaph H, eds. Handbook of sexology, p 259. New York: Elsevier/North Holland.

Money J, Ehrhardt A (1972) Man and woman, boy and girl: the differentiation and dimorphism of gender identity from conception to maturity. Baltimore: Johns Hopkins University Press.

Money J, Ogunro C (1974) Behavioral sexology: ten cases of genetic male intersexuality with impaired prenatal and pubertal androgenization. Arch Sex Behav 3: 181.

Money J, Ehrhardt A, Masica D (1968) Fetal feminization induced by androgen insensitivity in the testicular feminizing syndrome: effect on marriage and maternalism. Johns Hopkins Med J 123: 105.

Money J, Annecillo C, Van Orman B, Borgaonkar D (1974) Cytogenetics, hormones and behavior disability: comparison of XYY and XXY syndromes. Clin Genet 6: 370.

New M, Suvannakul L (1970) Male pseudohermaphroditism due to 17β-hydroxylase deficiency. J Clin Invest 49: 1930.

Park I, Aimakhu V, Jones H (1975) An etiologic and pathogenetic classification of male hermaphroditism. Am J Obstet Gynecol 123: 505.

Park I, Burnett L, Jones H, Migeon C, Blizzard R (1976) A case of male pseudohermaphroditism associated with elevated LH, normal FSH, and low testosterone possibly due to the secretion of an abnormal LH molecule. Acta Endocrinol 83: 173.

Parks G, Bermudez J, Anast C, Bongiovanni A, New M (1971) Pubertal boy with 3-hydroxysteroid dehydrogenase defect. J Clin Endocrinol Metab 33: 269.

Saenger P, Goldman A, Levine L, Karthschutz S, Muecke E, Katsumata M, Doberne Y, New M (1978). Prepubertal diagnosis of steroid 5α-reductase deficiency. J Clin Endocrinol Metab 46: 627.

Sohval A (1964) Hermaphroditism with "atypical" or "mixed" gonadal dysgenesis. Am J Med 36: 281.

Virdis R, Saenger P, Senior B, New M (1978) Endocrine studies in a pubertal male pseudohermaphrodite with 17-ketosteroid reductase deficiency. Acta Endocrinol 87: 212.

Walsh P, Madden J, Harrod M, Goldstein J, MacDonald P, Wilson J (1974) Familial incomplete male pseudohermaphroditism, type 2. Decreased dehydrotestosterone formation in pseudovaginal perineoscrotal hypospadias. New Engl J Med 291: 944.

Zackmann M, Vollmin J, Hamilton W, Prader A (1972) Steroid 17, 20-desmolase deficiency: new cause of male pseudohermaphroditism. Clin Endocrinol 1: 369.

APPENDIX: SCHEDULE OF PROCEDURES FOR GENDER IDENTITY/ROLE STATUS

Psychological tests
    Wechsler Intelligence Scale for Children-Revised
    Stanford-Binet Intelligence Scale
    Wechsler Adult Intelligence Scale
    Bender Visual-Motor Gestalt Test
    Guilford-Zimmerman Temperament Survey (300 items)
    Cornell Index, Form N2 (101 items)
    Draw-a-Person Test
        (1) Draw a person
        (2) Draw a person of the opposite sex
        (3) Draw yourself and a friend
        (4) Draw your family
    Sacks Sentence Completion
    Thematic Apperception Test
        Cards: 7BM
                  3BM
                  6BM
                  13MF
                  8BM
                  16 (blank)
Oblique inquiry techniques
    Three wishes game
    Alone; shipwrecked; choose whom?
    If I had $ 100,000...
    If I had ten years to live...
    If I were invisible...
    The cause of my condition is...
    If I were an animal, I'd be a... Why?
    If I could change just one thing about myself...
    The first thing I remember...
    The earliest thing I remember...
    Other early memories
    Self description for a penfriend
    Looking back, age seventy
    Myself ten years from now, and how it happened
    Advising young parents how to rear children; give sex education, etc.
    Advising medical student on own case
    Game of reversing roles of patient and interviewer
    Pygmalion game: statue comes to life, asks how, when, why of a number of emotions
    Define: good (bad) personality
    Define, for a friend: psychiatrist, psychologist, counselor
    Make up a daydream, eyes closed
    Free-association game: like turning on a radio, all the messages
Ten minute speech sample (for psycholinguistic research)
Interviews with patient
    (1) Past history: birth, health, school, etc.
    (2) Personal life data and function
    (3) Sex history and function
    (4) Aggression history
    Interview with lover or spouse
        Cross-validate with interview schedules (1) and (3) above
        Personal attitudes and reactions to patient's condition
    Interview with parents or next of kin
        Cross-validate with interview schedules (1) and (4) above
        Personal attitudes and reactions to patient's condition
    Photographs

Medical
Personal
Electroencephalogram
Genetic laboratory studies—chromosomal and blood
Genetic interview
Physical examination
Hospital and physician insurance data
Financial arrangements information
Police clearance

Interview Schedules
(1) Past history: birth, health, school, etc. (for use with patient, parents and other informants)
    Ordinal position plus birthdates of siblings
    Age of parents: birth and marriage dates
    Pregnancy and birth history of patient
    Childhood illnesses
    Sensitivity to light, sound, smell, temperature, touch, pain
    Developmental habits (childhood onward)

eating	fighting
sleeping-waking	impulsiveness
toilet training	overactiveness
enuresis and encopresis	crying
tantrums	moodiness
phobias	cuddliness
obsessions	stealing
irrational behavior	delinquency
"funny" habits	
nail biting	unusual mannerisms
thumb sucking	inattentiveness
head banging	fits
rocking	coughing and sneezing
hair twisting, etc.	giggling and smiling
play habits and interests	cops and robbers games
dramatics	war games
mothers and fathers	cowboys games
mother's or father's occupations	spacemen games
doctors	playing house, school
pregnancy	toys and pets
wedding	television programs and storybooks
physical energy, athletic play, sports, etc.	
hallucinations and delusions	

    Psychosexual differentiation, history of
    Pubertal history
    Family relationships
      All persons in the household
      Absent kin
      Family's reaction to patient's condition
      Sleeping arrangements
    School history
    Friendship history
    Vocational history
    Hobby and recreational history
    Military status and service
    Police history
    Genetic history
      Similar cases in immediate family and kinship family
    Health history and hospital career
    Drug and addiction history
    Previous "mental testing"
      Where
      Dates
    Referral physician and address
    Other doctors in patient's history
(2) Personal life data and function (for use with patient)
    Sex history and function (see separate schedule)

Religion and moral conceptions
Philosophy of life
Family, household and kinship dynamics (patient's version)
Heroes and idols
Supernatural and uncanny experiences
Course of a specific, typical day
(3) Sex history and function (for use with patient and, selectively, with parent, lover or spouse)
Early sex history: curiosity, theories, investigations, play
Sex education and information
Masturbation
Masturbation fantasies
Erotic and romantic daydreams
Dating, petting and love-making
Homosexuality; other paraphilias
Transexualism
    First feeling of wanting to be a girl (boy)
    First awareness that sex reassignment surgery available
    Surgery decision made
Cross-dressing
    First experience
    History
    Fetishistic use of clothing, erotically
    Present activities
    When total living/working as a girl (boy), woman (man) began
Names: female, male; name changes and associated personalities; nicknames
Parentalism: motherliness, fatherliness and child care ambitions
Marriage, etc.
Children
Menstruation: date by landmark, e.g., class, birthday; pregnancies; substitute menses (in males)
Hormones, dosage history, erotic effects
Orgasm relative to hormone history (exact dosages)
Erotic zones and orgasm
Perceptual arousal stimuli and history of changes with treatment, if any
Sleep dreams
    Love dreams (including intercourse)
    Climax dreams
    Dressing-up dreams
    Wedding dreams
    Pregnancy dreams
    Mothering dreams
    Fathering dreams
    Nightmares
    Other dreams
Body image, clothed and nude
    In dreams and daydreams
    Masturbation fantasies
    Intercourse fantasies
Intercourse: who initiates it? techniques and positions; prostheses
Phantom phenomenon
Physique and secondary sexual features
    Height
    Weight
    Hips
    Breasts
    Beard, including electrolysis and hormone effects
    Voice, on telephone and face to face talking
Knowledge of condition and causal explanation
Surgery and hormone treatment results
    Physical feelings
    Emotional changes
    Temperature changes; hot flashes; sweating
    Castration effects and hormonal control
    Was it worth it?
    Advice to others
Expectations of treatment

(4) Aggression history (for use with patient and parents or other kin)
    Sibling rivalry
    Pecking order and fighting in childhood
    Gang membership (leadership)
        Childhood
        Adolescent
    Group delinquency in childhood
        Violence
        Destructiveness
        Stealing
    Body contact sports
    Aggressive and warlike games
    Competitiveness and nonviolent rivalry
    Acquisitiveness
    Defense of property
    Sexual jealousy and nonviolent rivalry
    Sexual sadism and masochism
    Black-out spells
    Depersonalization phenomena
    Deja vu
    Spectator cruelty
    Personal experiences of fights
    Personal experiences in war
    Hormonal treatments: aggression effects

13. PATHOGENESIS OF CRYPTORCHIDISM

F. Hadžiselimović

1. EVOLUTION OF TESTICULAR DESCENT

Testicular descent is a process which is typical for mammals. Among Mammalia, three different types of descent can be distinguished, i.e. testicond (without descent), partial (epididymis descended) and complete (epididymis and testis descended). The descent is characteristic for evolutionary younger species, particularly those living on the ground and the most specialized animal forms among each species have complete descensus. Bedford postulated that the scrotal state may be linked to the sexual capacity of the male, in particular the ability to produce fertile ejaculates repeatedly within a limited period of time. The descent into the scrotum has been influenced primarily by the need for migration of cauda epididymis to the cooler location: testicular descent is seen as a merely mechanistic event, which enables the cauda epididymis to project from the body, but has no significance for the biological function of the testis as such (Bedford, 1978).

The morphology of epididymis is completely different in mammals without descent as compared to those with complete descent. In hyrax, for example, there is no testicular descent and caput and particularly cauda epididymis are rudimentarily developed. The corpus has few tubuli and the interstitium is wide. In contrast, in the mouse, where descent is complete, the epididymis is coiled, caput and cauda epididymis are fully developed and the interstitium is vestigial.

In man all three evolutionary forms of testicular descent can be found (Fig. 1A). For all these abnormal positions, the common term cryptorchidism is used.

2. ROLE OF EPIDIDYMIS IN TESTICULAR DESCENT

Normal testicular descent in the mouse takes place from the dorsal abdominal wall ventrally and caudally into the scrotum. Three different phases can be distinguished:
1. Movement along the dorsal abdominal wall between the 13th and 15th day of gestation.
2. Transabdominal movement: 15th day of gestation until birth.
3. Descent into the scrotum, accompanied by development of the processus vaginalis from birth until the 21st day post natum.

The descent of the epididymis always precedes that of the testis. There is no direct connection between gubernaculum and testis at any phase of testicular descent. Epididymis differentiation from the Wolffian duct develops in a craniocaudal direction (Hadžiselimović et al., 1980).

In 1938 Green et al. succeeded in producing cryptorchidism in the male issue of gravid rats by administration of estrogen on the 13th day of gestation. However, it was postulated that cryptorchidism in the mouse was caused by a direct inhibitory effect of estrogen on the gubernaculum (Raynaud, 1942). Our studies with the electron microscope have shown that the Leydig cells of such cryptorchid mice are atrophic (Hadžiselimović and Herzog, 1976) (fig. 2). It was possible by simultaneous administration of human chorion gonadotropin (HCG) and estradiol (E_2B) on the 13th or 14th day of gestation to prevent atrophy of the Leydig cells and cryptorchidism. Similar results have also been obtained by Rajfer and Walsh (1978), who were able to prevent cryptorchidism in estradiol-treated rats by simultaneous administration of HCG or dihydrotestosterone DHT.

148

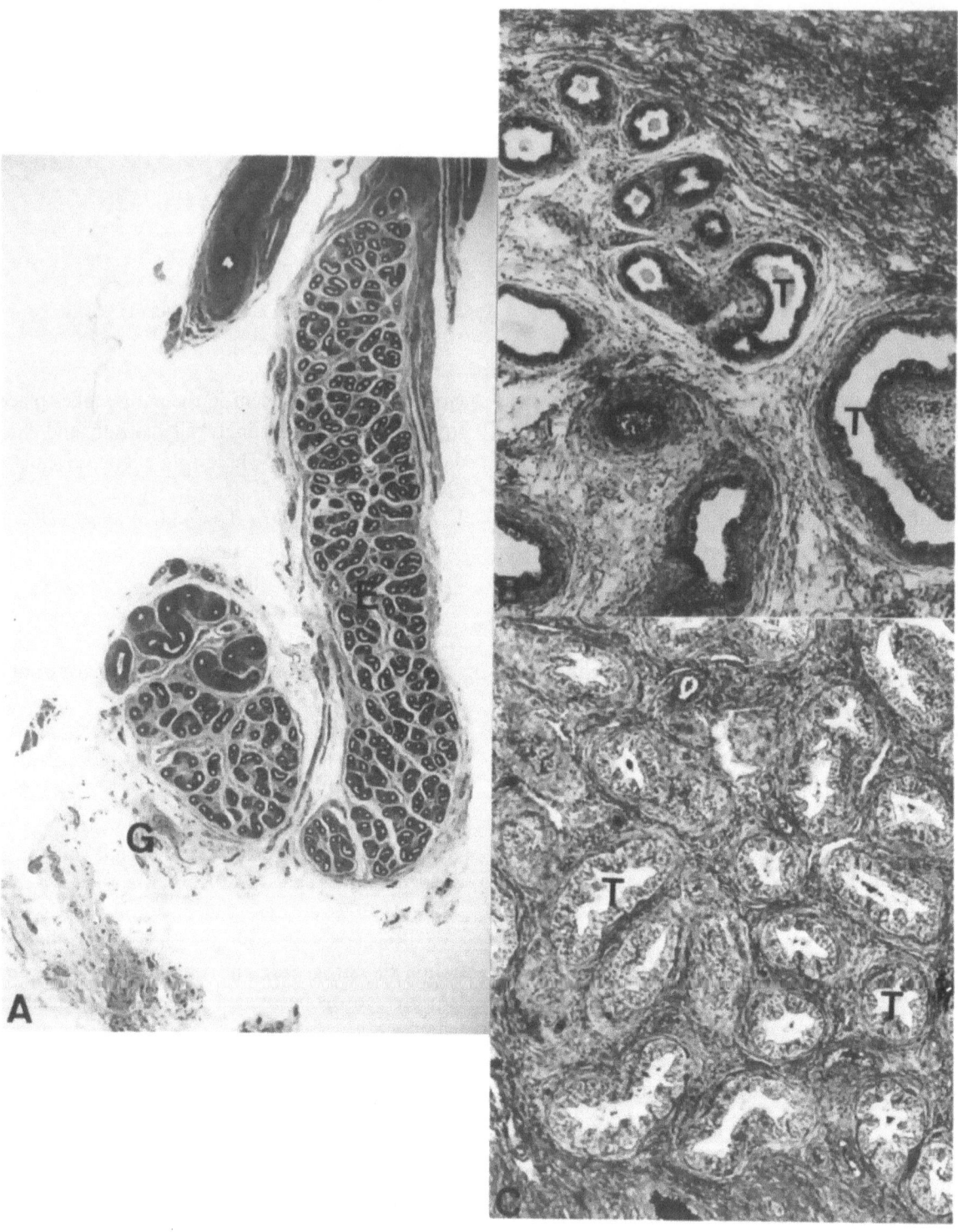

Figure 1. (A) Descended epididymis only after "unseccessful treatment" with LH-RH nasal spray (4-year-old boy). No testes were determined at operation. Note gubernaculum (G) inserts as usual into cauda epididymidis. (B) Undescended epididymis from an adult orchidectomized patient (26 years), showing broad interstitium and few tubuli (t) with underdeveloped epithelium (14.4 ×). (C) The same part of epididymis normally descended. There is a narrow interstitium and tubuli are more coiled (14.4 ×).

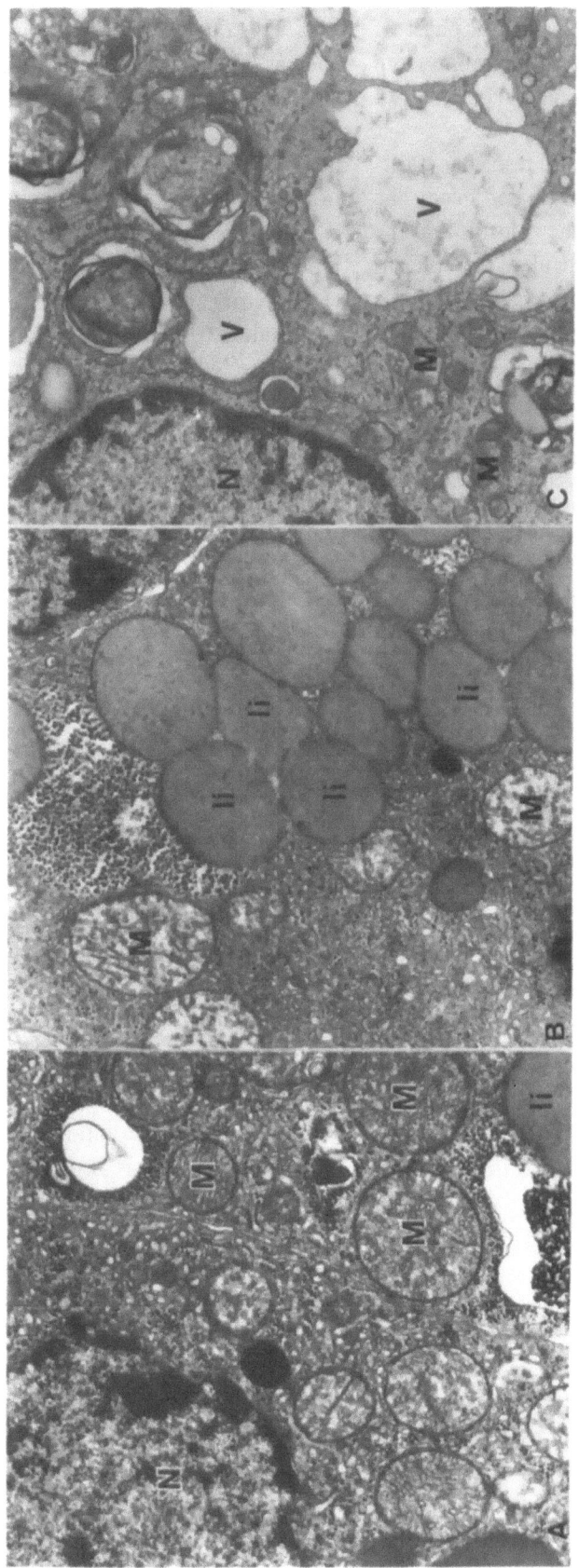

Figure 2. Electron microscopic view of mouse fetal Leydig cells. (A) Estrogen- and HCG-treated, (B) control, (C) estrogen-treated with typical appearance of atrophic Leydig cells. Li, Lipoid droplets; M, Mitochondria; N, Nucleus; V, Vacuoles in the atrophic Leydig cells (6000 ×).

The first postnatal day is particularly suitable for examination of testicular descent and any anomalies in connection with it, because the critical phase of descensus, namely intra-abdominal migration from a dorsal to a ventral position, should be completed at birth (Hadžiselimović et al., 1978).

The epididymis, which holds the testis like a forceps, is under-developed in E_2B-treated mice. The tubuli are much fewer than in the controls and the interstitium is broader. In particular, the concentrical arrangement of mesenchymal cells around the single tubuli is characteristic for cryptorchid E_2B epididymis. In HCG- and E_2B-treated mice, where descent occurs normally, the differentiation and coiling of the tubulus is advanced and similar to that of the controls (Hadžiselimović et al., 1978).

Administration of estradiol hinders the transformation of the Wolffian duct. This should not be regarded as resulting from direct effect of estradiol on the mesonephros, but rather as a consequence of the androgen deficiency brought about by insufficient stimulation of the Leydig cells by gonadotropins. Simultaneous administration of HCG and E_2B prevents atrophy of the Leydig cells, the Wolffian duct becomes transformed into the vas deferens and epididymis, and descensus takes place (Hadžiselimović et al., 1978) (Fig. 2).

In cryptorchid boys an anomaly of the epididymis is frequently observed (Scorer and Farrington, 1971; Marshall and Shermeta, 1979). In adult cryptorchids the epididymis has fewer tubuli, with infantile tubular epithelium and a broad interstitium (Fig. 1B).

3. ETIOLOGY OF CRYPTORCHIDISM IMPAIRED FETAL LH SECRETION

3.1. Experimental observations

The genetic findings in mutant mice with hypogonadism due to LH-RH deficiency suggest that the mutant is akin to Ewer's series of human subjects who have familial monotrophic pituitary insufficiency as an autosomal recessive LH-RH deficiency. These mice are cryptorchid and sterile (Cattanach et al., 1977). There is also an absence of androgen-dependent differentiation of male genitalia and organ insensitivity to androgens in testicular feminization of the mouse. Affected mice have male genotypes, female phenotypes and cryptorchid testes (Blackburn et al., 1973).

The ultrastructural appearance of the Leydig cells in cryptorchid E_2B newborn mice showed that these cells are atrophic (Fig 2C). In these mice the testicular testosterone content is significantly lower than in the normal controls and remains so even into adulthood (Tables 1 and 2). The application of

Table 1. Testicular testosterone content in newborn mice

Newborn male mice	No. of testicles	Testosterone, $\bar{x}$	pg/testis, s.d.
E_2B-treated	38	49.7	12.9
Controls	28	106.4	61.8

Table 2. Testicular testosterone content in adult mice

Adult male mice	No. of testicles	Testosterone, $\bar{x}$	ng/mg testis, s.d.
E_2B-treated	22	0.07	0.11
Controls	12	0.53	0.46

estradiol on the 13th day of gestation completely depresses embryonal testicular testosterone production (Fig. 3).

In spontaneously cryptorchid mice, the testicular testosterone content is also significantly lower than in adult controls of the same age (Table 3). Similarly, the reduced testicular testosterone content is observed in congenitally cryptorchid pigs (Hanes and Hooker, 1937) and dogs (Eik-Nes, 1966).

Table 3. Basal values for LH and FSH from 8 controls and 53 cryptorchid boys (unilateral)

	S/T control ⩾ 2	S/T = 0	S/T > 0 < 0.5	S/T ⩾ 0.5
LH mIU/ml	4.3 ± 2.2	2.5 ± 2.2	3.9 ± 1.9	4.0 ± 2.7
FSH mIU/ml	1.3 ± 0.7	1.5 ± 1.3	1.36 ± 0.89	3.4 ± 2.9
No. of patients and % of distribution	8 (100%)	12 (22%)	29 (56%)	12 (22%)

151

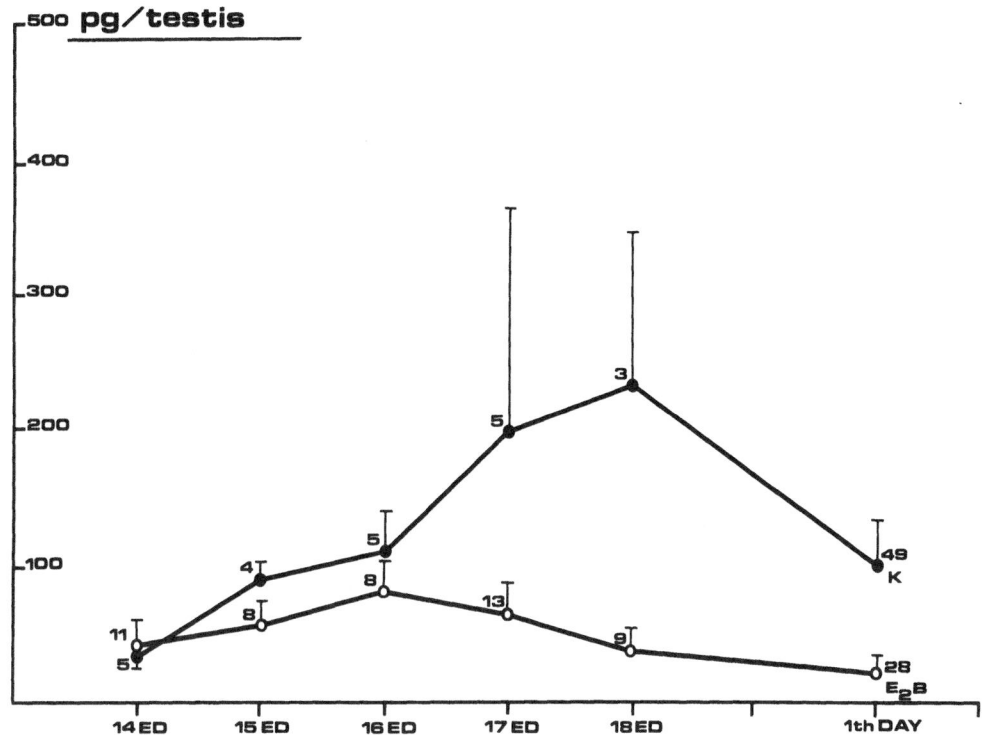

Figure 3. Longitudinal study of testicular testosterone (pg/testis) from 13th embryonal day till 1st day post natum in E_2B mice and controls. n, Number of embryos investigated; ED, Embryonal day.

4. CLINICAL OBSERVATIONS

Several clinical observations point to a connection between gonadotropin insufficiency and cryptorchidism. In the *Kallman syndrome*, a condition in which there is a deficiency of LH-RH, cryptorchidism is often observed (Bardin et al., 1969). In *congenital aplasia or hypoplasia of the pituitary gland* the testes are intra-abdominal and there is an almost complete absence of interstitial cells (Steiner and Boogs, 1965; Sedehi-Najad and Senior, 1974). In *anencephaly* the pituitary is usually hypoplastic and the testes of newborns are frequently undescended (Ch'In, 1938; Zondek and Zondek 1963). In the majority of cases, the Leydig cells are hypoplastic and the epididymis is often morphologically abnormal (Zondek and Zondek, 1963).

In newborn cryptorchid boys a lack of fetal Leydig cells is observed, in contrast to those with normally descended testicles, where these cells are present during the first year of life (Mancini et al. 1960; Hayashi and Harrison, 1971). Our observations do not conform this lack of Leydig cells in cryptorchid boys. In all biopsy studies there are always Leydig cells in the interstitium but these cells are atrophic in appearance (Figs. 4, 5 and 6). This atrophy is observed throughout childhood and is due rather to impaired stimulation (Hadžiselimović and Herzog, 1976; Lloyd et al., 1978) than to congenital malformation of the Leydig cells (Kleinteich and Schickedanz, 1976).

Plasma testosterone is also significantly lower in cryptorchid infants than in infants with physiologically delayed descent or normal testicular descent (Gendrel et al., 1978). Diminished plasma testosterone has also been reported in cryptorchid adults (Raboch and Starka, 1972). It must be stated, however, that the majority of investigators have found normal plasma testosterone levels in childhood, and almost all cryptorchid boys experience a normal puberty. It is clear, therefore, that the underlying defect must be incomplete. Growth and bone-age of cryptorchid boys also do not differ from the normal population, which in turn supports the theory that the gonadotropin deficiency is an isolated one.

5. CORRELATION BETWEEN HISTOLOGICAL AND ENDOCRINOLOGICAL DATA

In research into cryptorchidism, particular attention has always been paid to the germ cells as the most

152

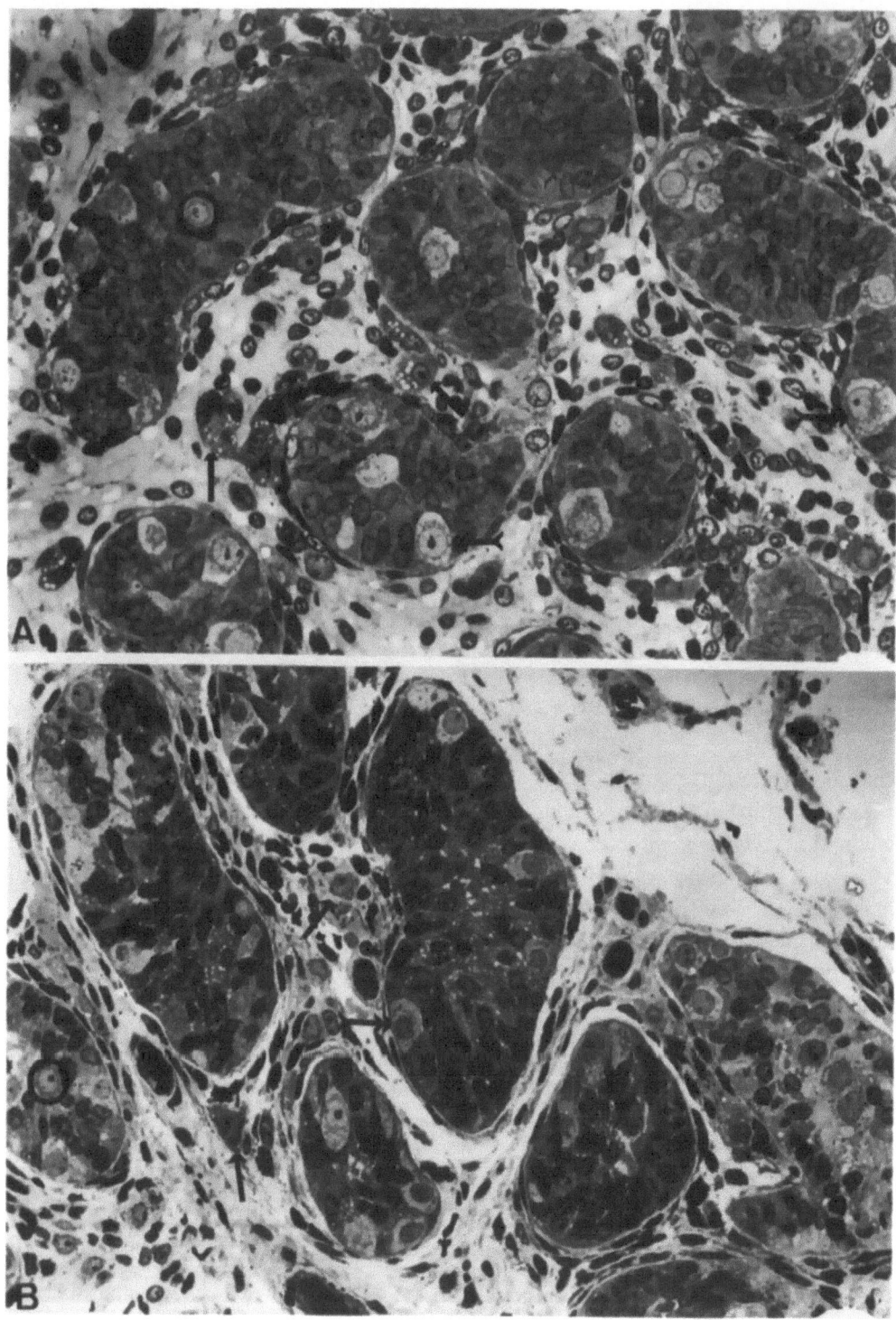

Figure 4. (A) Semi-thin sections of 2-week-old infant with normal descended testis, showing developed Leydig cells (arrow). The tubuli seminiferi contain gonocytes (circle) and fetal spermatogonia (double-arrow) (20 ×). (B) Two-week-old cryptorchid testis, which, in contrast, has only a few atrophic Leydig cells (arrow). Tubulus seminiferus contains predominantly Sertoli cells but fetal spermatogonia (double-arrow) and occasionally gonocytes (circle) are visible (20 ×).

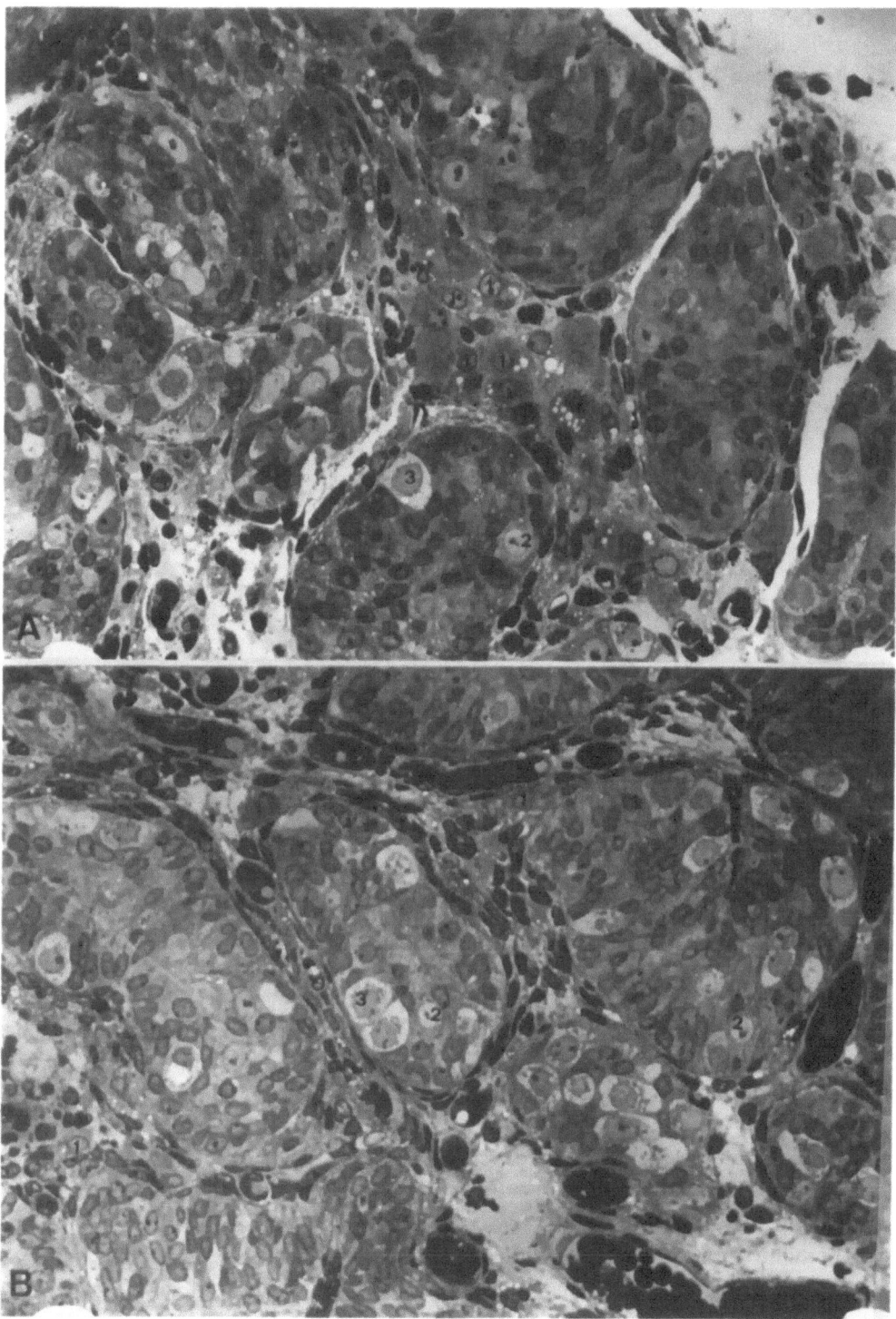

Figure 5. (A) Five-week-old normally descended testis. The interstitium is full of enlarged Leydig cells (arrow), a sign of increased stimulation. Tubuli seminiferi contain gonocytes (2) and spermatogonia (3) in addition to Sertoli cells. (20 ×). (B) Five-week-old cryptorchid testis. Note there is no physiological increase in size and number of Leydig cells. Atrophic Leydig cells are still visible (1), gonocyte (2), fetal spermatogonium (3) (20 ×).

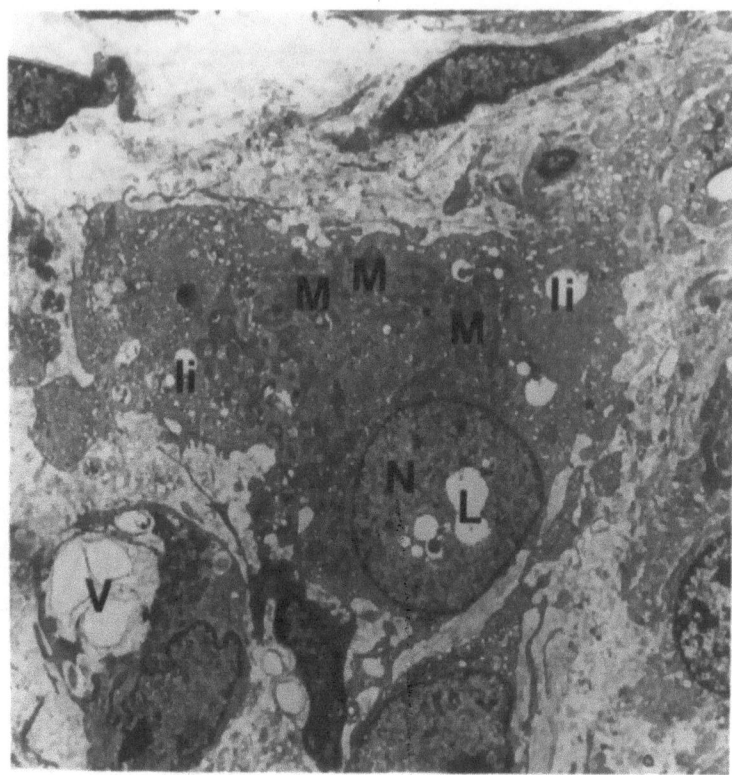

Figure 6. Atrophic Leydig cells (2-week-old cryptorchid testis) with narrow cytoplasm, containing few lipoid droplets (li) and small mitochondria (M). Nucleus (N) has a hole (L) often observed in the Leydig cells of patients with impaired fertility (4400 ×).

important parameter in assessing the quality of the tissue. However, there is still controversy about the cause of spermatogonia damage. According to Hedinger (1977), the deficiency of spermatogonia is, in some cases at least, due not to any secondary disturbance, but to congenital malformation. Scorer and Farrington (1971) observed in most cases of cryptorchidism a disturbance of the germ cells resulting from hereditary factors. In contrast, we were unable to find any signs of congenital malformation of the spermatogonia in cryptorchid testes, either with the light or electron microscope. It seems very important here to stress that within the first six months of life there is no lack of spermatogonia in cryptorchid testes. On the contrary, there is no significant difference in the spermatogonia counts of cryptorchids and controls (Fig. 7).

In the normal testis, in the first year, in addition to the fetal spermatogonia, gonocytes are also present in the seminiferous tubule. The fetal spermatogonia are ultrastructurally identical to those in cryptorchid testes of the same age (Hadžiselimović, 1977).

The gonocytes of newborns are smaller than the spermatogonia and are localised mainly in the centre of the tubule (Fig. 8). In the last months i.u. and the first weeks post natum, they migrate to the periphery. As soon as they reach the basement membrane, they give rise to fetal spermatogonia (Hadžiselimović, 1977). In semi-thin sections and with the electron microscope the typical gonocyte is easily recognizable (Figs. 4, 5 and 8). Immediately after birth, about 30% of germ cells in normal subjects are gonocytes, while in cryptorchids the percentage varies over a wide range, depending on the total number of germ cells present in the cryptorchid tubuli. The nearer to normal the number of germ cells, the more gonocytes are observed. In the 20% of cases with a low spermatogonia count, no gonocytes are observed. The transitional forms between gonocyte and fetal spermatogonia are recognizable only with the help of the electron microscope. By deducting the number of gonocytes from the total number of germ cells, it becomes clear that there is no "physiological" decrease in the number of spermatogonia in the first year of life as seen by Koch et al. (1975) and Hedinger (1977) (Fig. 7). The tubules

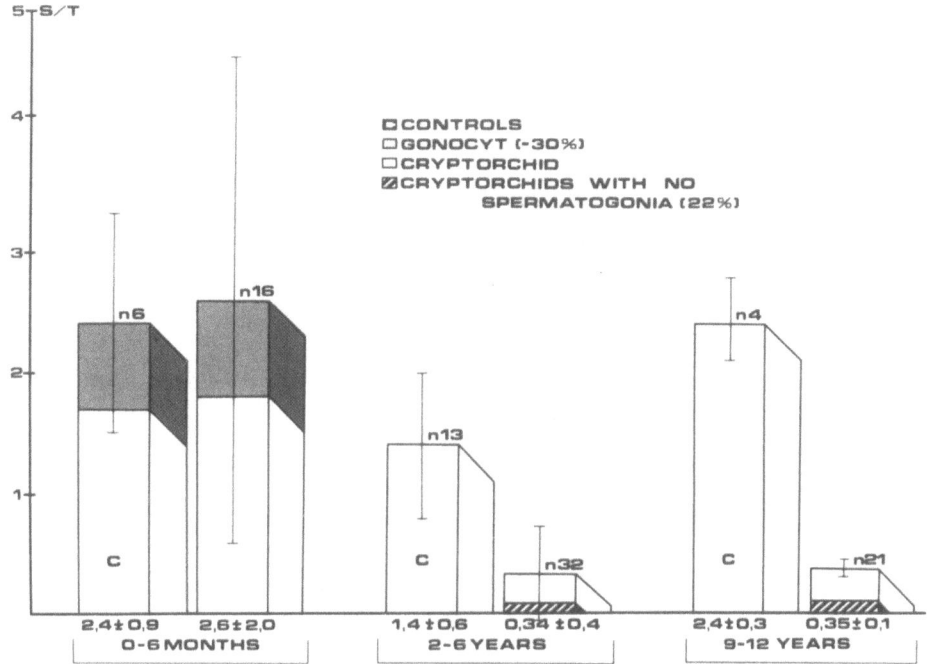

Figure 7. Spermatogonia count per tubule. (Fifty tubuli per biopsy were counted.) Note that, particularly within the first 3 months of life, there is ca. 30% gonocytes and ca. 70% spermatogonia. In this case the transient forms between gonocyte and spermatogonium were counted as spermatogonia.

diameter of biopsies fixed in glutaraldehyde is still within the normal range till the 6th year of life, even when the changes in the peritubular connective tissue are advanced (Hadžiselimović et al., 1979).

Taking into account that in the cryptorchid testis there is a clear atrophy of the Leydig cells (already visible on semi-thin sections, if the biopsy is properly fixed), then there is no question that the irregular distribution seen in the first year of life must be due to the confusion of cryptorchid testes with normal testes of somewhat "high anatomical location" (Koch et al., 1975; Hedinger, 1979).

Among the 53 cryptorchid boys at P_1 stage of puberty according to Tanner, the mean plasma values for LH (basal 3.6 ± 2.2 IU/l, peak 7.7 ± 5.0 IU/l); FSH (basal 1.85 ± 1.7 IU/l, peak 5.2 ± 3.3 IU/l) and testosterone (basal 0.42 ± 0.1 ng/ml) are in the normal range (Hadžiselimović et al., 1978).

The wide standard deviation for LH and FSH, as well as for the spermatogonia count per tubulus, may be interpreted as arising from the small number of biopsies. If histo-pathological findings are taken as parameter, a group with no spermatogonia can be recognized in the second and particularly in the third year of life. Compared to the group where the number of spermatogonia is only moderately reduced,

$S/T \geq 0.5$ ($S/T =$ spermatogonia count per 50 tubulus cross-sections). There is a considerable difference in both LH and FSH values (Fig. 9, Table 3). However, a group with $S/T = 0$ is already recognizable within the first six months of life. The mean number of spermatogonia in the first six months in cryptorchid boys is the same as in the controls, but about 20% of cryptorchids already have a low spermatogonia count of between 0.4 and 0.8 per tubulus. This group with a low number of spermatogonia lose their germ cells completely as early as the second and particularly in the third year of life. The ratio of 20% with no spermatogonia to 80% with a reduced number of spermatogonia remains the same till puberty (Fig. 9).

This is the crucial point as regards the time for cryptorchidism therapy. If we postulate that there is a physiological increase in maturation after the testis is brought down (Kleinteich and Schickedanz, 1976) even in cryptorchid boys with a hypogonadotropic axis then there is still a chance of fertility, if the testis is brought into the proper position by hormonal or surgical treatment within the first or at the beginning of the second year of life. In the first results reporting on this concept of treatment, published in 1975 by Ludwig and Potempa, over 90% of all cryptorchid

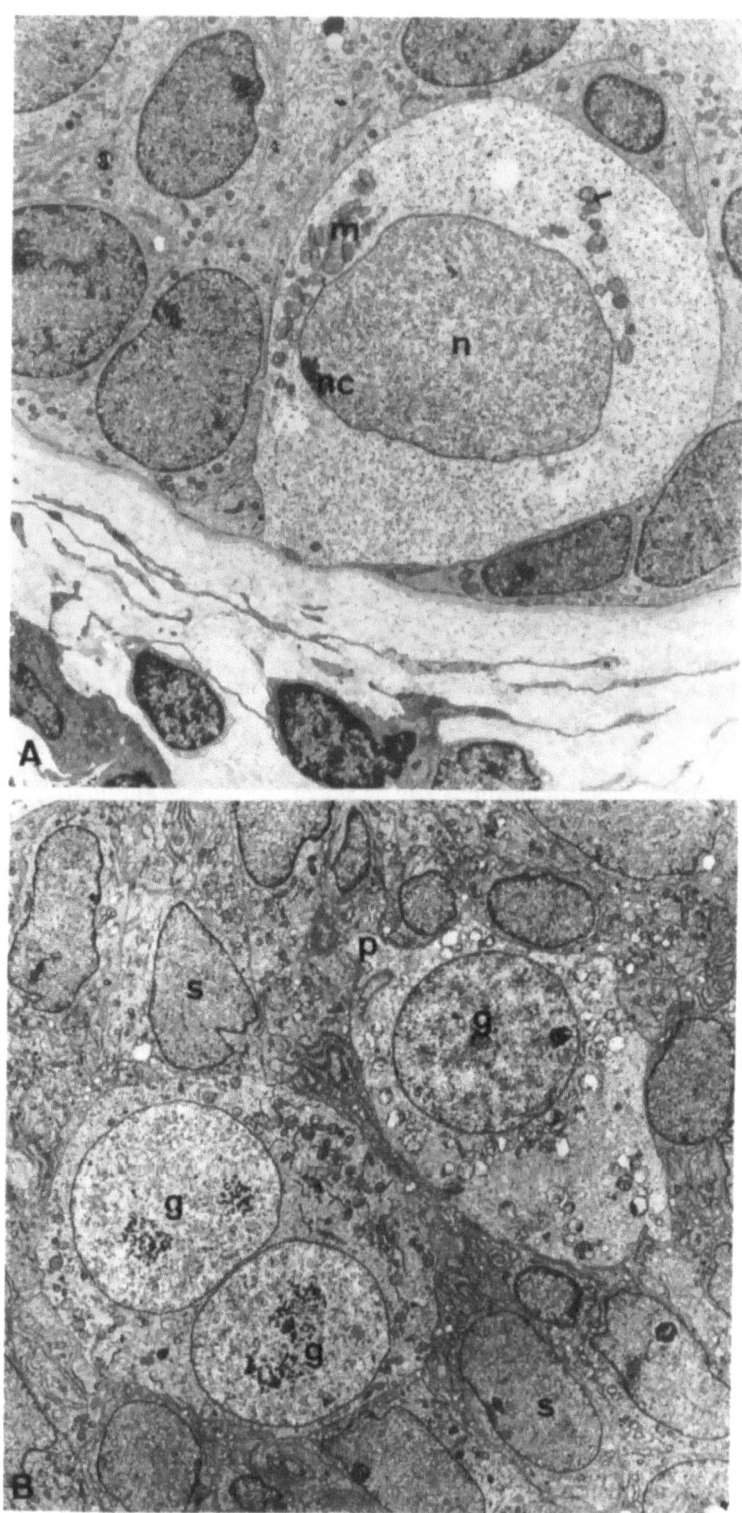

Figure 8. (A) Typical A$_p$ spermatogonium from 2-week-old cryptorchid testis. Nucleus (N) contains peripherally situated nucleolus (Nc). Mitochondria (m) hold together over intermitochondrial cement (arrow) (1450 ×). (B) Two-week-old normal testis: Gonocytes (G) dividing and moving towards basement membrane, with pseudopodia (p). Mitochondria (m). Fetal Sertoli cells (S) (2900 ×).

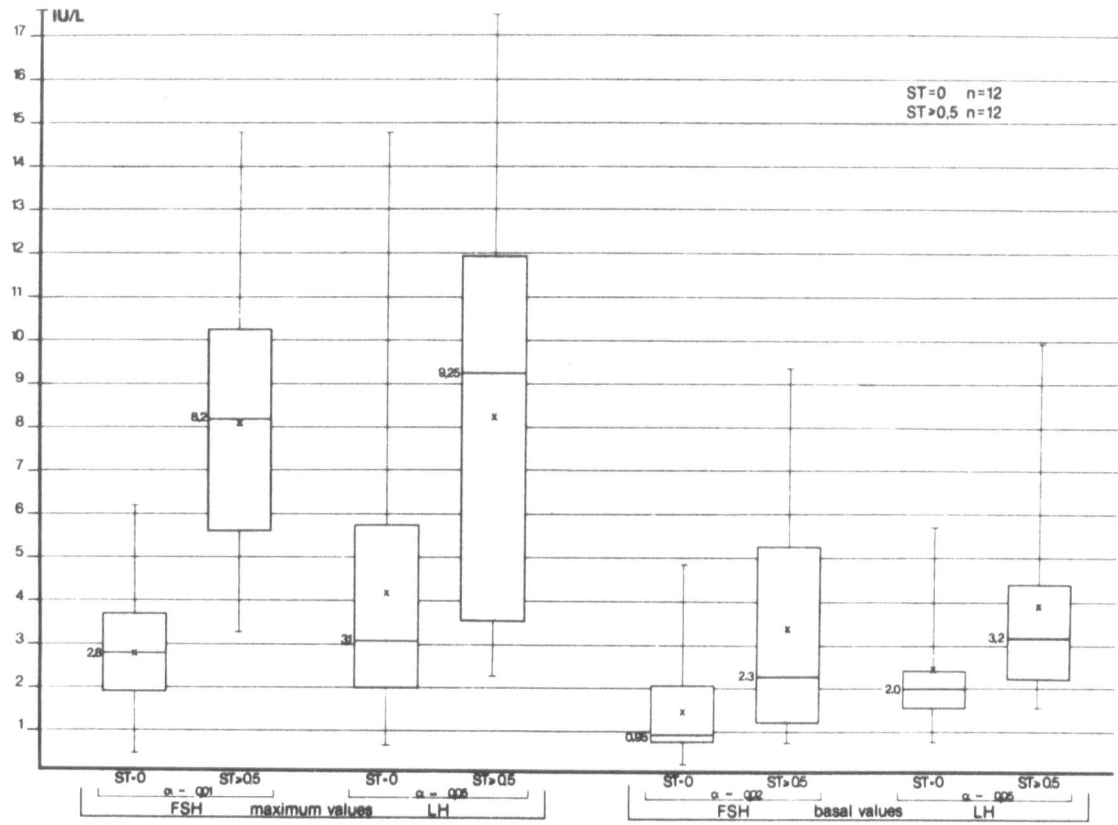

Figure 9. Basal and maximal LH and FSH plasma values after stimulation with 100μg LH-RH i.v. in 12 cryptorchid boys with S/T = 0 and in 12 cryptorchid boys with S/T ⩾ 0.5 (S/T = spermatogonia count per 50 tubulus cross-sections). Wilcoxon test (rank sum test) on TI 59 was performed.
(*) arithmetical mean, bar: interquartile range, range and median (line drawn within the bars) are given.

boys operated within the first two years of life are completely fertile in adulthood. These optimistic results certainly apply to 80% of cryptorchid boys. However, further investigation is necessary to prove whether patients with marked insufficiency of the pituitarygonadal axis require substitution therapy to achieve full fertility. A relationship between LH function and the number of spermatogonia is

Table 4. LH-RH success rate

Mode of application	No. of animals treated	No. of testes descended	No. of testes undescended
5 ng/day 17 days s.c.	10	0	20
5 ng/day 14 days s.c.	6	0	12
5 μg (3 periods of 5 days with intervals of 2 days) s.c.	6	8	4
5 μg continuously for 14 days s.c.	14	17	11

strongly suggested by both the number of spermatogonia in low LH responders and the low LH response in boys with no spermatogonia. This suggests a connection between testicular descent, the development of spermatogonia, endocrine testicular function and gonadotropin, particularly LH.

Basal FSH values are significantly higher in the group (A) where S/T is ⩾ 0.5, compared to the control group and cryptorchid groups, where spermatogonia S/T was 0 and S/T > 0 < 0.5 (Table 3).

The increased FSH in cryptorchid boys is interpreted as a cause of germinal cell deficiency (Waaler, 1976) or as a very sensitive feed-back mechanism between pituitary release of FSH and the number of spermatogonia (Sizonenko et al., 1978).

In a group of 53 patients with severely damaged spermatogonia, there was no increase in basal FSH values in 41 cases, the only increase being in the group with the best spermatogonia/tubulus ratio (S/T ⩾ 0.5) (B). It would seem, therefore, that the

158

interpretations of Waaler and Sizonenko require some modification. The increase in FSH seems to be the causative factor of the higher number of germ cells in the cryptorchid boys in group B, despite the fact that they are of the same age and that gonadal position is similar to those in group A. Since the peak FSH value group A is considerably lower than in group B, it may be assumed that in group A, as well as in the group where the spermatogonia count is $> 0 \; < 0.5$ per tubulus, no compensatory FSH excretion occurs, as a result of hypophyseal insufficiency.

These results are in contrast to those for adults with gonadal damage, where extremely high LH and FSH values are the rule. It can be conjectured from this that primary LH and FSH insufficiency disappears in later life, while the morphologically determinable damage to the testicles, arising from this deficiency and malposition, is irreversible.

6. LH-RH THERAPY FOR CRYPTORCHIDISM

If LH-RH insufficiency is postulated to be a main factor in the etiology of cryptorchidism, it seems logical that treatment with LH-RH should be successful. However, the success of the treatment is still controversial (Illig et al., 1977; Knorr, 1978). The main criticism, which also applies to HCG treatment, is that testes which descend under this therapy are retractile, with normal histology and fertility chances, and not cryptorchid. Experimental and randomized clinical studies with LH-RH therapy provide a means of resolving this controversy. The results can be summarized as follows:

6.1. Experimental studies

In spontaneously cryptorchid mice treated with 5 μg or 5 ng LH-RH, the best results are obtained with daily application of 5 μg for 14 days (Table 4). After 2 weeks' treatment, not only are the testes descended, but the scrotum is better developed and the scrotal skin has become more pigmented. The mean testicular testosterone value, which in cryptorchid mice was 2.8 ng/testis and increases after 14 days' treatment to 10.75 ng/testis (Table 5).

Table 5. Testicular testosterone in mice after LH-RH treatment

	No. of testes	ng/testis (median values)
LH-RG (5 μg—14 days s.c.)	18	10.75
Cryptorchid mice (no treatment)	12	2.8
Controls	18	7.7

Wilcoxon test for unpaired data was performed. The statistical difference between groups was: $2\alpha = 0.01$.

6.2. Clinical studies

A randomized study of 62 cryptorchid subjects aged 2-6 years was carried out. Thirty-one randomly selected patients were operated upon immediately and biopsy specimens for light and electron microscopy were obtained; a further 31 patients received 1.2 mg LH-RH nasal spray daily for 4 weeks. All the boys diagnosed as cryptorchid were examined independently by two pediatric surgeons (Hoecht, 1980). In the group operated upon, all biopsies showed typical signs of cryptorchidism, i.e. reduced number of spermatogonia, atrophy of the Leydig cells and thickening of the peritubular membrane. In 16 out of 31 patients treated with LH-RH, testicular descent had occurred by the end of the treatment. Fifteen patients treated without success were operated upon within 2 weeks of cessation of therapy and biopsied. The main histological and ultrastructural differences as compared to the untreated patients were in the appearance of the Leydig cells. Tubulus diameter, spermatogonia histology and the number of spermatogonia remained unchanged. The LH-RH-treated group (Hadžiselimović et al., 1979) had a spermatogonia count per tubule of 0.31 ± 0.5, as compared to 0.35 ± 0.5 in untreated controls. The results show that LH-RH therapy in cryptorchid boys has no further antifertility effect (Hadžiselimović et al., 1979). The most striking feature of the Leydig cells after LH-RH treatment is the marked increase in cell size and smooth endoplasmic reticulum (Figs 10 and 11). These changes are identical to those observed after HCG treatment. Apart from the stimulatory signs, there is also an increased recruitment of precursor Leydig cells from fibroblasts (Fig. 12).

Treatment with HCG of a total amount of less than 10,000 IU does not yield such good results as higher doses (Canlorbe et al., 1979), but the latter

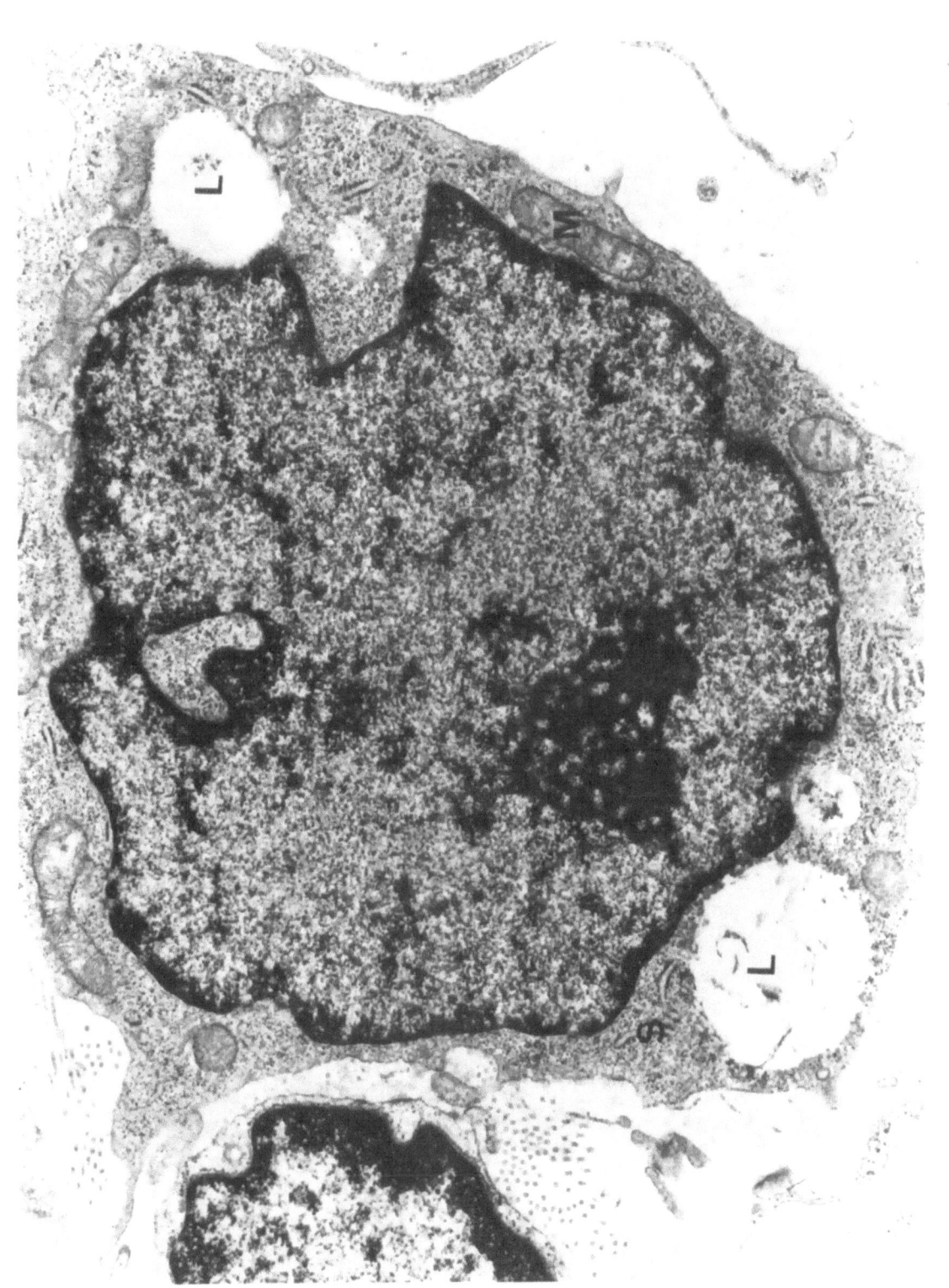

Figure 10. Transient stage of juvenile Leydig cell after unsuccessful LH-RH therapy. The round nucleus (NC) with pars amorpha and reticularis. Narrow cytoplasm has mainly rough endoplasmic reticulum (S), few lipoid droplets (L) and mitochondria (M) (7200 ×).

could be potentially hazardous. The choice therefore remains difficult. HCG treatment is successful in about 30% of all cases (Canlorbe et al., 1979). Considering the objections against HCG treatment and the 50% success rate with LH-RH treatment, as well as the mode of application, it is my opinion that LH-RH treatment is to be preferred. Only cases with manifest inguinal hernia and painful cryptorchid testes require immediate surgery.

7. CONCLUSIONS

1. Testicular descent is a process typical for evolutionary younger mammals living on the ground, with specialized body-type.
2. Three types of descent occur in mammals: testicond, descent of epididymis alone and descent of testis and epididymis.
3. In man, disturbance of testicular descent – crypt-

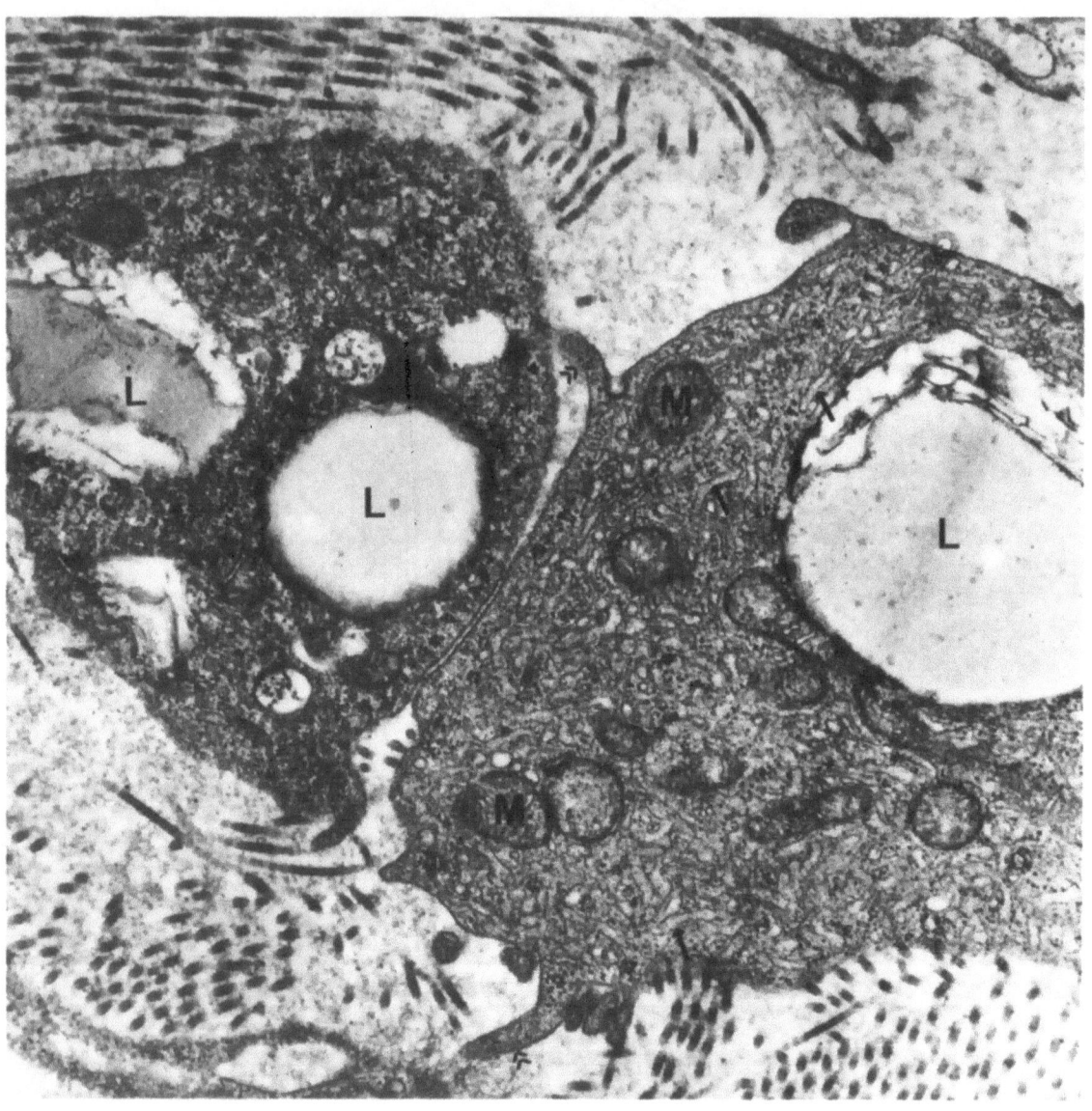

Figure 11. Cytoplasm of stimulated juvenile Leydig cells after unsuccessful treatment with LH-RH, showing abundance of smooth endoplasmic reticulum (arrow), lipoid droplets (L) and mitochondria (M). Microvilli are visible at the cell surface (double arrow) (6800 ×).

orchidism – is frequently connected with sterility. The main etiologic factor in the development of cryptorchidism is impaired gonadotropin secretion during intrauterine life and later.

4. The transformation of the Wolffian duct into epididymis and its differentiation is the prime mover responsible for descent. The gubernaculum has no active role in the process.

5. The Leydig cells play a key role in testicular descent. Impaired stimulation of the Leydig cells leads to impaired testosterone secretion and cryptorchidism.

6. Endocrine treatment of cryptorchidism should be started with LH-RH (1.2 mg LH-RH nasal spray daily for 4 weeks) or HCG (500 IU for 5 weeks) within the first year of life, but not before the sixth month. If this treatment is unsuccessful, surgery is indicated within the second year of life.

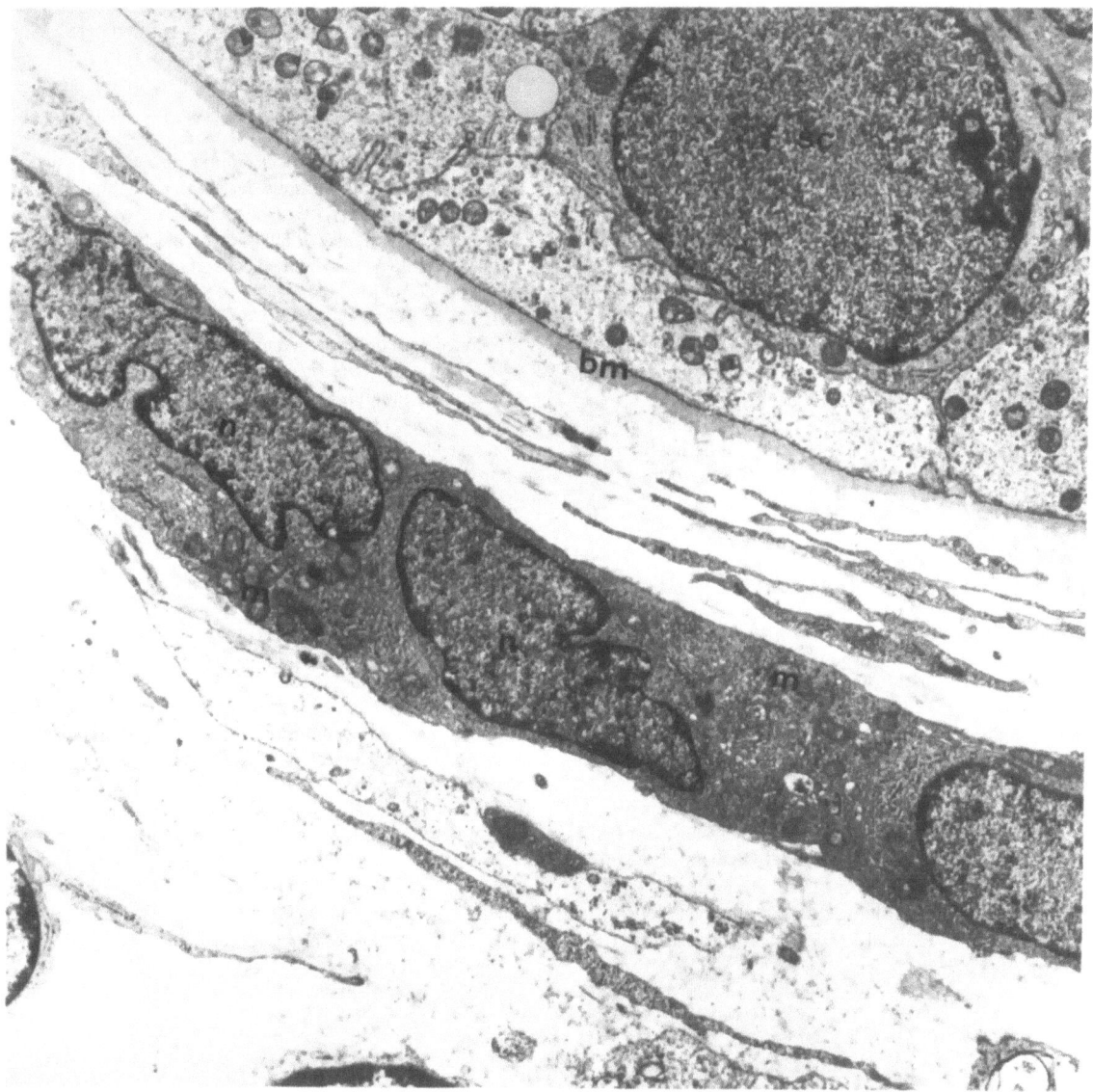

Figure 12. Precursors of Leydig cells under LH-RH therapy have been transformed from fibroblasts type II. bm. basal membrane; Sc, Sertoli cells; n, nucleus; m, mitochondria from precursor Leydig cells (1450 ×).

162

REFERENCES

Bardin CW, Ross GT, Rifkind AB, Cargille CM, Lipsett MB (1969) Studies of the pituitary-Leydig cell axis in young men, prepuberal boys and hypopituitary patients. J Clin Invest 48: 79.

Bedford MJ (1978) Anatomical evidence for the epididymis as the prime mover in the evolution of the scrotum. Am J Anat 152: 483.

Blackburn WR, Kying WC, Bullock L, Bardin CW (1973) Testicular feminization in the mouse. Studies of the Leydig cell structure and function. Biol Reprod 9: 9.

Canlorbe P, Laclyde JP, Toublanc JE, Bader JC (1979) Results of treatment with human chorionic gonadotropin in cryptorchidism. In Job JC, ed. Basel: Karger S, Cryptorchidism, diagnosis and treatment, p 167.

Cattanach BM, Iddon CA, Charlton HM, Chiappa SA, Fink L (1977) Gonadotrophin-releasing hormone deficiency in a mutant mouse with hypogonadism. Nature 269: 338.

Ch'In KY (1938) The encocrine glands of anencephalic foetuses: a quantitative and morphological study of 15 cases. Chinese Med J Suppl 2: 63.

Eik-Nes KB (1966) Secretion of testosterone by eutopic and the cryptorchid testis in the same dog. Can J Physiol Pharmacol 44: 629.

Gendrel D, Job JC, Roger M (1978) reduced post-natal rise of testosterone in plasma of cryptorchid infants. Acta Endocrinol 89: 372.

Greene RR, Burill MW, Ivy AC 1938) Experimental intersexuality. The production of feminized male rats by antenatal treatment with estrogens. Science 88: 130.

Hadžiselimović F (1977) Cryptorchidism. In Advances in Anatomy Embryology and Cell Biology, Vol 53. Berlin: Springer.

Hadžiselimović F, Herzog B (1976) The meaning of the Leydig cell in relation to the etiology of cryptorchidism. J Pediat Surg 11: 1.

Hadžiselimović F, Herzog B, Krušlin E (1978) The morphological background of estrogen-induced cryptorchidism in the mouse. Fol Anat Jugos 8: 63.

Hadžiselimović F, Girard J, Hoecht B, Baumann JB (1979) Ultrastructure of the cryptorchid Leydig-cells after LH-RH treatment. Acta Endocrinol (Copenhagen) Suppl 225: 85.

Hadžiselimović F, Herzog B, Krušlin E (1980) Estrogen induced cryptorchidism in mice. In Hafez ESE, ed. Clinics in andrology, Vol 4: Descended and cryptorchid testis. The Hague: Martinus Nijhoff.

Hanes FM, Hooker CW (1937) Hormone production in undescended testis. Proc Soc Exp Biol Med 35: 549.

Hayashi H, Harrison RG (1971) The development of the interstitial tissue of the human testis. Fertil Steril 22: 351.

Hedinger C (1977) Die Histologie des kryptorchen Hodens. In Bierich JR, Roger K, Ranke MG, eds. Maldescensus testis, p 29. Munich: Urban & Schwarzenberg.

Hedinger C (1979) Histological date in cryptorchidism. In Job JC, ed. Pediatric and adolescent endocrinology: cryptorchidism, p 2. Basel: S. Karger.

Höcht B (1979) Klinische Erfahrungen mit der LH-RH Behandlung beim praepuberalen Maldescensus Testis. Habilitationsschrift, Universität Würzburg.

Illig R, Kollmann F, Borkenstein M, Kuber W, Exner GU, Kellerer K, Lunglmayr L, Prader A (1977) Treatment of cryptorchidism by intranasal synthetic luteinising-hormone releasing hormone. Lancet ii: 518.

Kleinteich B, Schickedanz H (1976) Der Spermatogoniengehalt kongenital-dystoper und operativ verlagerter Hoden bei Kindern und Jugendlichen. Z Urol 69: 819.

Knorr D (1979) Behandlung des Maldescensus Testis. Chir Praxis 25: 100.

Koch H, Rahlf G, Köberling J, Mühlen AV et al. (1975) Endokrinologische und morphologische Untersuchungen beim Maldescensus testis. Dtsche Med Wochenschr 100: 682.

Lloyd JW III, Stecker JF, Rakestraw MG (1978) In vitro stimulation of adenosine 3', 5'-monophosphate in unilateral undescended testes of humans by follicle and luteinizing hormone. J Clin Endocrinol Metab 46: 158.

Ludwig G, Potempe J (1975) Der optimale Zeitpunkt der Behandlung des Kryptorchismus. Dtsch Med Wschr 100: 680.

Mancini RE, Rosemberg E, Cullen M, Lavieri JC, Vilar O, Bergada C, Andrada JA (1960) Cryptorchid and scrotal human testis. I. Cytological, cytochemical and quantitative studies. J Clin Endocrinol Metab 25: 927.

Marshall FF, Shermeta DW (1979) Epididymal abnormalities associated with undescended testis. J Urol 121: 341.

Raboch J, Starka L (1972) Plasma testosterone in bilateral cryptorchids in adult age. Andrology 4: 107.

Raynaud A (1942) Modification experimentale de la différentiation sexuelle des embryons des souris par action des hormones androgenes et oestrogenes. Paris: Herman et Cie.

Rajfer J, Walsh CP (1978) Hormonal regulation of testicular descent: experimental and clinical observations. J Urol 118: 985.

Scorer CG, Farrington GH (1971) Congenital deformities of the testis and epididymis. London, Butterworth.

Sedehi-Najad A, Senior B (1974) A familial syndrome of isolated aplasia of the anterior pituitary. J Pediat 84: 79.

Sizonenko P, Schindler AM, Roland W, Paunier L, Cuendet A (1978) FSH III. Evidence for possible prepuberal regulation of its secretion by the seminiferous tubules in cryptorchid boys. J Clin Endocrinol Metab 46: 301.

Steiner MM, Boogs JD (1965) Absence of pituitary gland, hypothyroidism, hypoadrenalism and hypogonadism in a 17 year old dwarf. J Clin Endocrinol Metab 25: 159.

Waaler PE (1976) Endocrinological studies in undescended testes. Acta Paediat Scand 65: 559.

Zondek HL, Zondek Th (1963) Observations on the testis in anencephaly with special reference to the Leydig cells. Biol Neonat 8: 329.

14. GONADOTROPIN THERAPY FOR THE UNDESCENDED TESTIS

J. R. BIERICH

Intensive research during the last 15 years has revolutionized our knowledge about pathogenesis and therapy of testicular maldescent. Today we know that cryptorchidism is not a uniform disorder but a syndrome, caused by a variety of conditions. The role of mechanical obstacles hampering the descent of the gonads increasingly gives way to other etiological factors. The significance of primary malformations is more clearly recognized. Evidence has, however, slowly emerged that in numerous cases initially there is an endocrine disturbance which causes the non-descent. Canlorbe et al. (1974) were the first to show the diminished LH-secretion of the infantile hypophysis resulting in an insufficient testosterone production. The morphologic correlate for this impairment has been demonstrated by Hadžiselimović et al. (1975), and Hadžiselimović and Herzog (1976). Already these discoveries suggest the rationale for treatment. If deficient LH-secretion causes maldescent then administration of preparation with LH-activity, i.e. HCG, corresponds to true replacement therapy.

Our conceptions about adequate treatment have been even more influenced by the morphologic findings of Mancini et al. (1965), Gothié et al. (1966), Toledo et al. (1970), Farrington (1969) and in particular by the group of Hedinger (Salle et al., 1968; Hedinger, 1971, 1977), i.e. that the spermatogenesis of the undescended testis is already damaged during the second year of life and not between the 5th and 10th year of life as previously believed. The findings have meanwhile been conformed by so many other competent investigators that there cannot be any reasonable doubt about their correctness. This leads to the logical conclusion that every treatment, no matter whether hormonal or surgical, should be commenced prior to the third year of life if spermatogenesis and future fertility are to be protected.

The third important experience with relevance to treatment is the realization that it is possible to manipulate the descent in more than half of the cases by giving gonadotropins alone. The surgeons and the urologists do not usually pay much attention to this therapeutic possibility, and unilateral maldescent is especially considered within the surgical jurisdiction (Deming, 1952; Dettmar, 1959; Dick, 1952). In contrast to that, the large series published by Bergadá, Bierich, Knorr and Pagliano-Sassi, unequivocally demonstrate that also in unilateral maldescent there are considerable chances of successful treatment with HCG.

The optimal prerequisites for the hormonal treatment of testicular maldescent and the therapeutical successes hitherto gained are described below. Before doing this, however, it appears to be necessary to offer a classification of the various malpositions of the testes. Only precise definitions allow a correct evaluation of the successes.

1. CLASSIFICATION

"Maldescensus testis" is the general term used for all anomalous positions of the testicles. It comprises two principally different disturbances – the dystopias and the ectopias. In the first instance the descent of the gonad is obstructed at some physiologic site on its way down, whereas in the second case it arrives at some pathologic location. By far the most frequent of the latter form is the ectopia epifascialis in which the testicle after passing the annulus inguinalis exterior (outer inguinal ring) slips upwards and is palpable as it is lying on the aponeurosis of the musculus abdominis externus directly underneath the skin. The other locations – ectopia perinealis, penilis and femoralis – are rarities. It is clearly evident that ectopias in any case have to be treated surgically. They are beyond the scope of the present discussion on hormonal treatment.

The term "cryptorchidism" is used in English as a synonym for testicular maldescent. In German, the exact translation of this term means "hidden testis", and it is reserved for those gonads which are not palpable, i.e. for abdominal testes. If the testis on its way down only reaches the inguinal canal, then we speak of "retentio testis inguinalis". Often the gonad is palpable below the externus-aponeurosis only with difficulty, especially in fat infants with small testicles. For practical reasons one can differentiate between movable and fixed inguinal testes.

"Gliding testes" is the name for gonads which are situated immediately before the outer inguinal ring and can be forced down into the scrotum only against the resistance of the too short funiculus spermaticus. When the force is withdrawn they instantly slip upwards and remain in the lowest part of the inguinal canal.

These testes have to be accurately differentiated from "retractile testicles" (testis migrans), the position of which varies from the inguinal canal to the middle or even the bottom of the scrotum. In a cold environment and upon touching they ascend upwards, drawn by the musculus cremaster. In a recumbent position and in a hot bath the cremaster relaxes and the testes move down again. Charny and Wolgin (1957) have spoken of "pseudocryptorchidism". Treatment is redundant if the gonads lie in the scrotal sac for most of the time.

2. INDICATIONS AND CONTRAINDICATIONS OF HORMONAL TREATMENT

After longstanding disputes regarding questions of whether testicular maldescent should be treated primarily hormonally or surgically, there is nowadays agreement that there are special indications for each form of therapy. Treatment by HCG is the less violent procedure and should be employed in all cases where there is a chance to achieve the aim conservatively. Surgical intervention is necessary where the anatomical situation does not permit success through hormones. Such situations are the following:
1. All ectopias.

2. Cases with accompanying hernias.
3. Retention after herniotomy with scarred fixations.
4. Children in puberty.

As mentioned earlier, unilateral maldescent has previously been considered a primary indication for operation, especially by many surgeons. Evidence now clearly emerges from the experiences of numerous investigations that the descent rate after HCG in unilateral cryptorchidism is not much worse than in bilateral maldescent. Accordingly it can be concluded that all cases not falling within the four categories quoted earlier represent primary indications for hormonal treatment.

3. DOSAGE

Until recently, the recommendations published regarding the HCG-dosage were highly heterogeneous. Very low single doses of 250 IU contrasted with doses as high as 5000 IU or more (Robinson and Engle, 1954; Hand, 1957); the proposed total amounts varied between 3000 and 50 000 IU per course in a single individual. Small doses have proved to be inadequate whereas high single doses have caused edema and painful swelling of the testes. Histologically, Charny and Wolgin (1956, 1957) and Tonutti et al. (1960) have described distinct lesions in biopsies of such testes. the injection of 2 to 3 moderate doses of HCG is preferable to the administration of one single big dose. Table 1 presents the mode and dosage of HCG-therapy as recommended by a group of experts asked by the International Health Foundation, Geneva (Bay et al., 1974). In numerous centres today treatment is carried out according to this scheme.

Table 1. HCG therapy of maldescensus testis. Doses recommended by the International Health Foundation (1974)

	IU/week	weeks
Young infants	2 × 250	5
Infants up to 6 years	2 × 500	5
Older children	2 × 1000	5

Formerly, in the case of an unsuccessful first course, a second similar series of injections has been carried out shortly afterwards. Nowadays such children are not treated again with hormones but are operated upon. If, however, a partial success is registered during the first course and the testicles can be moved down to the scrotal sac, a second course should follow. The same is true in cases where some months after hormonal treatment the testes gradually re-ascend to the groin, which occurs in ca. 20% of the patients. As a rule the testes will come down again and should then be fixed at the bottom of the scrotum by the surgeon.

Brambilla and Zanoboni (1968) have proposed the employment of menopausal gonadotropin (HMG) instead of HCG. In contrast to HCG which exhibits mainly LH-activity, HMG possesses chiefly FSH-activity. Above all it induces proliferation of the germinal epithelium, whereas the Leydig cells are scarcely stimulated. Correspondingly virilizing effects which are frequently observed under HCG are absent under HMG treatment whilst a marked enlargement of the testes is seen almost in every case. In a later publication, Brambilla and Zanoboni (1969) changed their therapeutic scheme and recommended a combination of HCG and HMG. The successes attained by the authors as well as by Bergadá and Mancini (1973) do not appear to be better than the results with HCG alone.

4. START OF TREATMENT

With respect to the start of the treatment, mainly two points are to be considered: 1) Up to which age is there a real chance for the gonads to descend spontaneously? 2) From which age on have we to take into account severe lesions of the undescended gonads?

1) As normal descent occurs only in the last three months of gestation, a physiological non-descent is observed in one third of all premature infants (Scorer, 1955). Also, in many fullterm infants the descent is not yet complete. Buemann et al. (1961) and Scorer (1955) found undescended testicles in 1 to 4% of all newborns. In two thirds of these cases a delayed spontaneous descent occurred within the first year of life. Until this limit one should wait before embarking upon any therapeutical measure.

2) The onset of puberty was formerly considered the upper limit for commencing treatment. It has been known for decades that untreated testicular maldescent causes irreversible damage of the germinal epithelium if puberty has passed by. Already in the fifties, there was a concerted postulation that discrete lesion can be observed as early as the age of 5 or 6 years (Robinson and Engle, 1954; Hinman, 1955; Weyeneth, 1956; Hecker and Braren, 1958). Employing improved histological techniques it has been elucidated during the last 15 years that the basic process causing lasting damage to germinal epithelium is the increasing loss of spermatogonia. This process can already be observed in the second year of life (Mancini et al. 1965; Gothiè et al., 1966; Salle et al. 1968; Farrington, 1969; Hedinger, 1971, 1975). Meanwhile, these observations have been confirmed by numerous other authors. Correspondingly the optimal time span for treatment must be considered as the second year of life.

5. RESULTS OF TREATMENT

The aim of the therapy is to maintain fertility or to avoid sterility, which is inevitable if the maldescent persists. The success can be judged, on the one hand according to the occurrence of the descent, and on the other hand by proving the fertility by spermatogram and fatherhood.

6. DESCENSUS

The data on the descent after HCG-treatment vary considerably in the literature. Several authors have published very poor results (Deming, 1952; Lowsley, 1959; Bergstrand and Quist, 1961; Gross and Jewett, 1956; Laron and Levy, 1965, with others having success rates of between 70 and 100% (Cernea, 1951; Webster, 1959; Baetgen, 1970). Such differences can be explained only by a different preselection of the patients. Surgeons and urologists who have experienced the worse results are as a rule treating a selective population. Frequently they deal with patients sent by pediatricians who failed to bring the testes down with conservative methods. Conversely, the children who have been successfully treated with HCG by the pediatrician are not referred to the surgeon. On the other hand the surprisingly favorable results quoted above are most probably due to erroneous inclusion of children with retractile testes in the statistics. How frequently such confusions occur emerged from a British report in which the same children were judged by different medical officers. The percentages of children diagnosed as having unilateral maldescent varied depending on the investigation in the 5th year of life between 0.7 and 14.7%, in the 8th year between 1.1 and 10.4% and by the age of 12 years or more between 0 and 5.6% (Med. Off., 1958).

In principle, a success rate of 90%, as indicated by Webster (1959), cannot be expected. On the one hand today we know that a considerable part of the undescended testes is hypoplastic and/or dysgenetic, in particular in combination with malformation syndromes. On the other hand, the number of those testes which cannot descend because of mechanical obstacles must not be disregarded. In both groups there is hardly any chance for bringing the testes down without operation. Actually, in the few large series in which HCG treatment has been statistically evaluated, successes have been reported in approximately only half of the cases. Relating the descent rate not to the number of patients treated (who may have unilateral *or* bilateral maldescent) but to the number of undescended testes, the following picture emerges:

Table 2. Therapeutic success with HCG.

Author	Number of undescended testes	Descensus under HCG	
		n	%
Bierich	612	338	55
Knorr	574	300	52
Pagliano-Sassi	213	115	54

The largest series of HCG-treated children – 1204 cases – has been reported by Bergadá (1979). The success rate appears to be lower than that reported by the European authors: 40% in bilateral, 30% in unilateral cases. Taking the large size of the populations concerned, the differences are certainly statistically significant. Most probably the difference is due to the fact that the three European authors included the gliding testicles (which must not be confused with retractile testes!) in their studies, which Bergadá did not do. It is well known that gliding testicles ideally respond to the hormone therapy.

Table 3 demonstrates the successes of HCG in different forms of testicular maldescent according to the experiences of Knorr (1970).

Table 3. Results of HCG-treatment in cryptorchidism (Knorr, 1970)

	Number of testes	Complete descent %
Abdominal retention	93	32
Inguinal retention	371	44
Gliding testicles	110	99

Gliding testicles were brought down in 99% of the cases; only in a single instance was surgical intervention needed. Our own experiences in Tübingen (Bulle et al., 1975) are in good agreement with these data. Table 4 shows the results of HCG-treatment in 114 patients. The cases are tabulated according to whether manual luxation into the scrotum was possible (movable inguinal testes and gliding testicles) or not.

Table 4. Success of HCG-treatment, related to position and mobility of testes (Bulle et al., 1975)

	Total number	HCG-therapy	
		Successful %	Without success %
Luxation into scrotum possible	75	72	28
Luxation into scrotum impossible	39	13	87

These findings permit inferences with regard to the therapeutic chances with HCG, the most significant being the response of the movable testes to the hormone therapy. If we conversely look at the material primarily from the viewpoint of the therapeutic success, then the following picture emerges:

Table 5. Mobility of testes, related to therapeutical success with HCG

	Total number	Luxation into scrotum	
		Possible %	Impossible %
HCG-therapy successful	59	91.5	8.5
HCG-therapy without success	55	38.2	61.8

Among the successfully treated cases were 91.5% movable inguinal testes and gliding testicles, whereas the therapeutic failures consisted of 61.8% of testicles which could not be brought down manually. The 55 cases of failures when scanned give the following composition: nine abdominal testes, 10 testicles which were fixed at the outer inguinal ring and 36 cases of ectopia epifascialis. In a further statistic, Bulle et al. (1975) have put together the intraoperative position of all 351 testes which were operated upon in 1973 after unsuccessful administration of HCG (Table 6).

Table 6. Intraoperative position of 351 testicles, previously treated by HCG without success

	Number	*%*
Abdominal	7	2.0
Inguinal	31	8.8
At annulus ing. ext.	38	10.9
Epifascial	262	74.6
Prescrotal	8	2.3
Anorchia	5	1.4
Total	351	100

Three-quarters of the total number were not dystopias but ectopias which never respond to conservative treatment. It is remarkable that neither the pediatrician nor the surgeon was able to make the correct diagnosis prior to operation. With abdominal testes the hormone therapy is successful in roughly one-third of the cases, as mentioned above. The majority, however, consists of hypoplastic and defective gonads which are not able to respond to HCG. Such testicles can be found in combination with other malformations, such as chromosomal aberrations and genetic disorders, e.g. Moon-Bardet-Biedl syndrome, Smith-Lemli-Opitz syndrome and Noonan's syndrome. Figure 1 demonstrates the example of an underdeveloped dysgenetic testicle of a cryptorchid infant with the chromosomal constitution XO/XYY (Bierich, 1970). In the literature the percentage of primarily dysgenetic testes is estimated to be 20-50% (Charny and Wolgin, 1957; Hecker et al., 1964; Sohval, 1953). They form a large part of the HCG-refractory cases.

In dysgenetic testes not only the structure of the germinative epithelium and the tubulus but also that of the intertubular tissue is disordered. The presence of a delayed and insufficient maturation of the interstitial cells has been unequivocally shown by De la Balze et al. (1960), Mancini et al. (1965), Hayashi and Harrison (1971) and Hadžiselimović and his co-workers (1971, 1975). In our own material, Attanasio et al. (1974) have compared the rise of plasma testosterone under HCG in 14 children after successful hormone treatment to that of 13 children who failed to respond to the therapy. Whilst the

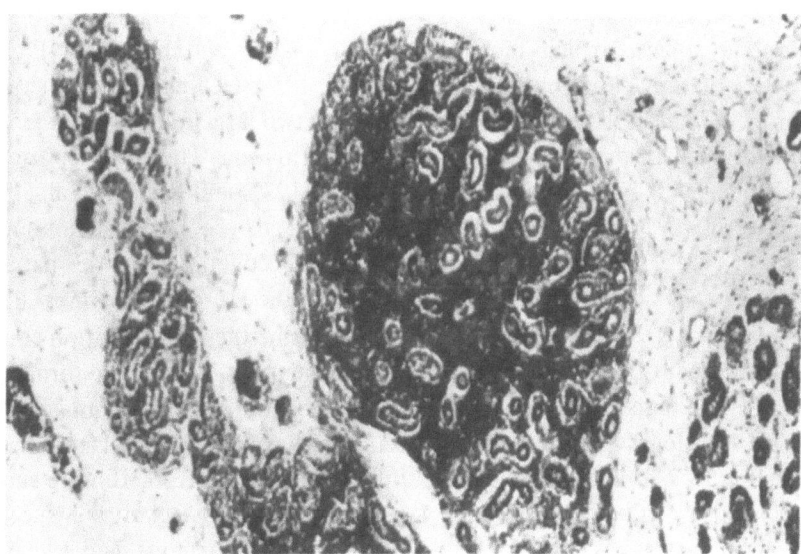

Fig. 1. Underdeveloped dysgenetic testis of a cryptorchid infant with the chromosomal constitution XO/XYY (Bierich, 1970).

first group attained a testosterone level of 302 ± 49 ng/dl, the second group showed an increase to only 176 ± 73 ng/dl ($p < 0.001$). As discussed in detail elsewhere (Bierich, 1979), testosterone which is synthesized in the interstitial cells and attains a high tissue concentration, plays an important role for the maturation of the tubular epithelium, for development and the growth of the testis as a whole and for its descent. Children with impaired testosterone synthesis, e.g. 3 β-hydroxysteroid-dehydrogenase deficiency, or with a disorder of the testosterone receptor, e.g. testicular feminization, suffer from testicular maldescent.

Among the therapeutic failures listed in Table 6, 22% were inguinal testes. Among these testicles are also included dysgenetic gonads. Above all, one finds in this position those testicles which have not descended because of mechanical obstacles, e.g. too short gubernaculum, too narrow inguinal ring, adhesions in the inguinal canal. Such obstacles are frequently found in unilateral maldescent. However, we can not agree to the proposition made chiefly by surgeons (Dick, 1952; Deming, 1952; Dettmar, 1959) that such impediments represent the majority of unilaterally undescended testes. This is not in keeping with the fact already mentioned that they can be brought down with HCG in a large percentage of cases. Nonetheless all statistics show that the successes of hormone treatment in bilateral cases are better than in unilaterals: Bergadá reports a percentage of 40% descent in bilateral cases and 30% in unilateral ones, Bierich 53 and 37%, Pagliano-Sassi (1979) 62 and 49%. In conclusion, it emerges from Table 6 that we are today able to explain most of the failures of the HCG-therapy either by primary structural defects in the gonad itself or by definite anatomical obstacles for the descent. In the absence of such defects, treatment with HCG in adequate doses is as a rule successful.

7. FERTILITY

It has been known for decades that bilateral maldescent causes sterility if the descent does not take place until puberty. The histologic alterations which during sexual maturation lead to irreversible damage have been described by numerous authors. Only in the last 15 years, however, has it been clearly shown that the pathological process sets in during the first years of life.

Microscopical investigations of the scrotal testis during orchidopexy of unilaterally undescended testicles have proved that the scrotal gonad often exhibits morphological defects equal to those in the undescended partner. Spermatological investigations have shown subfertility or sterility in a large majority of such cases (Scott, 1951, 1964; Doepfmer, 1964; Doepfmer and Nienaber, 1964; Nicole and Spindler, 1964; Giarola and Agostini, 1979). Thus, judging fertility disorders of patients previously treated because of testicular maldescent, one has to take into account not only acquired but also congenital lesions of the gonads. In an individual sterile situation, however, it can hardly be decided which of these circumstances is the causative factor. It is self-evident that follow-up studies after treatment in the first years of life as considered necessary nowadays do not yet exist.

Unfortunately only a few series without preselection are now available. The studies of Giarola (1964), Guillon and Seguy (1964), Guillon 1979), Raboch and Zahor (1955), Zahor and Raboch (1956) and Schirren (1964) concern patients from marriage advisory bureaus and out-patients on sterility problems, i.e. individuals attending the physician because of infertility. Objective information can, however, be obtained only by systematic follow-up studies of patients who have been treated as children because of testicular maldescent – without regard to the question of fertility.

Apart from some series, the material of which appears to be too small for allowing general conclusions (Zanartu and Hamblen, 1952; Charny and Wolgin, 1957; Hellinga, 1964; Bierich et al., 1965), there are two large follow-up series mediating valuable information. These are reported by Zamudio-Albescú (1979) and Richter et al. (1976). Zamudio-Albescú et al. (1971) first communicated spermatologic investigations on 43 patients previously treated at the Hospital de Niños, Buenos Aires. In the meantime their investigation could be extended to 66 patients — 34 men who formely suffered from bilateral, and 32 with previous unilateral maldescent. Twelve of the bilateral cases had been successfully treated with HCG, 18 were surgically treated, partly primarily, partly after unsuccessful hormone therapy, and 5 patients had remained untreated. Nine out of the 12 HCG-treated men were fertile, 3 infertile. Only 4 out of the 18 operated patients were fertile, while all of the untreated ones remained unfertile. In the group of the unilateral cryptorchids, HCG was successful in 11 cases; 8 of them were fertile. In the remaining 21, HCG had failed and orchidopexy had been performed. Eighteen of them proved to be fertile.

From these results the following conclusions can be drawn:

1. The frequency of fertility appears to be better in unilateral than in bilateral cases. (It can be assumed that the higher fertility rate of the unilateral cases is due to the presence of a primarily scrotal testis.)

2. Patients in whom HCG-treatment is successful have a better prognosis regarding fertility than those who do not respond to hormone therapy. (Most probably in both groups those gonads are primarily brought to descent which are functionally more or less intact. The remaining testicles presumably represent a negative selection of deficient gonads.)

The material of the follow-up study from Munich (Richter et al., 1976) is almost double that from Buenos Aires. It comprises 121 spermatological investigations of adult men who prior to puberty were treated because of testicular maldescent. Seventy-eight had successful HCG therapy, while 43 failed to respond to HCG and were operated upon. Table 7 shows the results.

The conclusion which can be drawn correspond to those from the Argentinian investigations. In both groups the unilateral cases reveal the better results — presumably on account of the intact primarily scrotal testes. The cases which respond to HCG represent in this material also constitute a positive selection. Their fertility rate is almost twice as high and their infertility half as frequent as that of the cases who had to be operated upon. Nevertheless it should be ascertained that also among the hormone-sensitive cases only 46% were fully fertile (sperm

Table 7. Fertility after exclusive HCG-therapy and after HCG-treatment and subsequent operation. Numbers in parentheses are percentages (after Richter et al., 1976)

	n = 78	Fertile	Subfertile	Infertile
	Fertility after successful HCG-treatment			
Unilateral	43	23 (53)	14 (33)	6 (14)
Bilateral	35	13 (37)	11 (31)	11 (31)
Total	78	36 (46)	25 (32)	17 (22)
	Fertility after unsuccessful HCG-treatment and subsequent operation			
Unilateral	28	9 (32)	12 (43)	7 (25)
Bilateral	15	2 (13)	3 (20)	10 (67)
Total	43	11 (25)	15 (35)	17 (40)

count above 12 million/ml). Altogether it appears to be probable that in numerous cases of maldescent the gonads are primarily qualitatively inferior. It should be emphasized that the treatment in the present series has always been performed prior to puberty — in contrast to the Argentinian series where treatment began in most but not in all cases prior to the 16th year of life. Moreover, Richter et al. divided their patients according to the age at which treatment was started (6–9 yr, 9–11 jr, 11–13 yr). The therapeutic successes of the youngest group were no better than that of the two other groups.

As the results of both of the large series prove, the prognosis regarding fertility is bad in all forms of testicular maldescent under the conditions of the therapy hitherto performed. This is also true for the HCG-sensitive cases although not as unfavorable as in the other ones.

These data are a challenge to search for an improved method of therapy. When the morphological findings of the last 15 years are taken into account they suggest early treatment. It can be hoped that the damage of the germinative epithelium which irresistibly grows from the third year on and often leads to infertility can be avoided.

REFERENCES

Attanasio A, Jendricke K, Bulle G, Flach A, Reisert I, Gupta D, Bierich JR (1974) Cryptorchidism: clinical, hormonal and histological studies. Acta Endocrinol (Copenhagen) Suppl 184: 51.

Baetgen D (1970) Behandlungsergebnisse des Testil mobils und der ein- und beidseitigen Retentio testis inguinalis mit Primo-gonyl. Med Welt I, 313.

Bay V, Bierich JR, Hecker W, Keep D van, Knorr D, Tonutti E (Editorial) (1974) Empfehlungen zur Behandlung des Hodenhochstandes. Dtsch Ärzteblatt, p. 12; Dtsch Med Wochenschr 99: 549; Méd Hyg 1119: 1629; Muench Med Wochenschr 116: 14

Bergadá C (1979) Clinical treatment of cryptorchidism. In Bierich JR, Giarola A, eds Cryptorchidism. London: Academic Press.

Bergadá C, Mancini RE (1973) Effect of gonadotropins in the

170

induction of spermatogenesis in human prepubertal testis. J Clin Endocrinol Metab 37: 935.

Bergstrand CG, Quist O (1961) Treatment of undescended testes with human gonadotropin. Acta Paediat 37: 231.

Bierich JR (1970) Über Hodenhochstand. Verh Dtsch Ges Inn Med 76: 329.

Bierich JR (1979) Clinical treatment of maldescensus testis. In Bierich JR, Giarola A, eds. Cryptorchidism. London: Academic Press.

Bierich JR, Schirren C, Schubert W (1965) Über die Behandlung des Hodenhochstandes mit HCG. Acta Endocrinol (Copenhagen) Suppl 101: 16.

Bierich JR (1977) Treatment by human chorionic gonadotropin in maldescended testes. In Bierich JR, Rager K, Ranke MB, eds. Maldescended testis. Munich: Urban & Schwarzenberg.

Brambilla F, Zanoboni A (1968) Nuova terapia del criptorchidismo: La gonadotropina muana della menopausa. Folia Endocrinol 21: 720.

Brambilla F, Zanoboni A (1969) L'Associazione gonadotropina umana della menopausa e gonadotropina corionica nel trattamento del criptorchidismo. Folia Endocrinol 22: 104.

Buemann B, Henriksen H, Villumsen AL, Westh A, Zachau-Christiansen B (1961) Incidence of undescended testis in the newborn. Acta Chir Scand 283: 289.

Bulle G, Attanasio A, Rager K (1975) Klinische Befunde zur Behandlung des Hodenhochstandes. Monatsschr Kinderheilkd 123: 354.

Canlorbe P, Borniche P, Bader JC, Vassal J, Toublanc J-E, Job J-C (1974) La cryptorchidie. Arch Franç Pédiat 31: 145.

Cernea R (1951) Zur Hormonbehandlung des Kryptorchismus. Hippokrates 22: 241.

Charny ChW, Wolgin W (1956) The management of cryptorchidism. Surg Gynecol Obstet 102: 177.

Charny ChW, Wolgin W (1957) Cryptorchidism. London: Cassell.

Deming C (1952) The evaluation of hormonal therapy in cryptorchidism. J Urol 68: 354.

Dettmar H (1959) Indikation und Zeitpunkt der hormonalen und operativen Behandlung beim Kryptorchismus. Therapiewoche 9: 334.

Dick W (1952) Über Störungen im Descensus des Hodens. Dtsch Med Wochenschr 77: 1112.

Doepfmer R (1964) Frequency of dystopias of the testis (cryptorchism) in adults and the importance of unilateral dystopia for fertility. Symp Int Fertil Assoc, Amsterdam.

Doepfmer R, Nienaber W (1964) Die einseitige Hodenektopie. Muench Med Wochenschr 106: 2096.

Farrington GH (1969) Histologic observations in cryptorchidism: the congenital germinal-cell deficiency of the undescended testis. J Pediat Surg 4: 606.

Giarola A (1964) The undescended testicle. Therapeutic aspects from the standpoint of reproductive life. Symp Int Fertil Assoc, Amsterdam.

Giarola A, Agostini G (1979) Undescended Testis and Male Fertility. In Bierich JR, Giarola A, eds. Cryptorchidism. London: Academic Press.

Gothié S, Canlorbe P, Lange J-Cl (1966) Étude histologique expérimentale et clinique du testicule cryptorchide. Ann Pédiat 42: 262.

Gross RE, Jewett TC (1956) Surgical experiences from 1222 operations for undescended testis. J Am Med Assoc 160: 634.

Guillon G (1979) Frequency and causal relationship of prepubertal cryptorchidism in male hypofertility. In Bierich JR, Giarola A, Eds. Cryptorchidism. London: Academic Press.

Guillon G, Seguy E (1964) Cryptorchidism and infertility. Symp Int Fertil Assoc, Amsterdam.

Hadžiselimović F, Herzog B (1976) The meaning of the Leydig cell in relation to the etiology of cryptorchidism: an experimental electron microscopic study. J Pediat Surg 11: 1.

Hadžiselimović F, Herzog B, Seguchi H (1975) Surgical correction of cryptorchidism at 2 years: electron microscopic and morphometric investigations. J Pediat Surg 10: 19.

Hand JR (1957) Treatment of undescended testis and its complications. J Am Med Assoc 164:

Hecker W, Chr, Braren F (1958) Zur Therapie der Hodenretention unter besonderer Berücksichtigung des Zeitfaktors. Ärztl Wochenschr 13: 83.

Hecker WChr, Daum R, Hienz HA, Haiderer (1964) Beitrag zum Kryptorchismusproblem unter besonderer Berücksichtigung der Ergebnisse von Hodenbiopsien. Dtsch Med Wochenschr 89: 2177.

Hedinger Chr (1971) Über den Zeitpunkt frühest erkennbarer Hodenveränderungen beim Kryptorchismus. Dtsch Ges Path 55: 172.

Hedinger C (1977) The histopathology of the cryptorchid testis. In Bierich JR, Rager K, Ranke MB, eds. Maldescensus testis. Munich: Urban & Schwarzenberg.

Hellinga G (1964) Fertility after hormonal or surgical treatment for bilateral cryptorchidism. Symp Int Fertil Assoc, Amsterdam.

Hinman F (1955) Optimum time for orchidopexy in cryptorchidism. Fertil Steril 6: 206.

Knorr D (1970) Diagnose und Therapie der Deszensusstörungen des Hodens. Pädiat Prax 9: 299.

Laron Z, Levy J (1965) Diagnosis, treatment and follow up of 326 cases as referred as undescended testes. Acta Endocrinol (Copenhagen) Suppl 101: 14.

Lowsley (1959) Cit. from Dettmar H: Indikation und Zeitpunkt der hormonalen und operativen Behandlung beim Kryptorchismus. Therapiewoche 9: 334.

Mancini RE, Cullen M, Rosemberg E, Lavieri JC, Vilar O, Bergadá C, Andradá JA (1965) Cryptorchid and scrotal human testes. I. Cytological, cytochemical and quantitative studies. J Clin Endocrinol Metab 25: 927.

Med. Off. (1958) Editorial 100: 379.

Nicole R, Spindler B (1964) Prognosis as to fertility following operations for cryptorchism in children. Symp Int Fertil Assoc, Amsterdam.

Pagliano-Sassi L (1979) Significance and results of medical treatment in cryptorchidism. In Bierich JR, Giarola A, eds. Cryptorchidism. London: Academic Press.

Raboch J, Zahor Z (1955) Über die Fertilität von Männern mit Kryptorchismus. Schweiz Med Wochenschr 85: 1196.

Richter W, Pröschold M, Butenandt O, Knorr D (1976) Die Fertilität nach HCG-Behandlung des Maldescensus Testis. Klin Wochenschr 54: 467.

Robinson JN, Engle ET (1954) Some observations on the cryptorchid testis. J Urol 71: 726.

Salle B, Hedinger Ch, Nicole R (1968) Significance of testicular biopsies in cryptorchidism in children. Acta Endocrinol (Copenhagen) 58: 67.

Schirren C (1964) The histology of undescended testicle and the spermatogram of hormone-treated and of surgically treated patients. Symp Int Fertil Assoc, Amsterdam.

Scorer CG (1955) Descent of the testicle in the first year of life. Br J Urol 27: 374.

Scott LSt (1951) Unilateral cryptorchidism: subsequent effects on fertility. J Reprod Fertil 2: 54.

Scott LSt (1964) Germ cell degeneration subsequent to delayed treatment of cryptorchidism. Symp Int Fertil Assoc, Amsterdam.

Toledo LA, Marambio JL, Marambio E (1970) Biopsia testicular en criptorquidia. Rev Chil Pediat 41: 209.

Tonutti E, Weller O, Schuchardt E, Heinke E (1960) Die männliche Keimdrüse. Stuttgart: Thieme-Verlag.

Webster (1959) Cit. from Dettmar H: Indikation und Zeitpunkt der hormonalen und operativen Behandlung beim Kryptorchismus. Therapiewoche 9: 334.

Weyeneth R (1956) Quand faut-il opérer un testicule ectopique? Rev Méd Suisse Rom 76: 654.

Zahor Z, Raboch J (1956) Ein Beitrag zum Problem der Hodenbiopsie bei Kryptorchismus unter besonderer Berücksichtigung des Optimalalters für die Orchidopexie. Schweiz Med Wochenschr 86: 311.

Zamudio-Albescú J (1979) Cryptorchidism and fertility. In Bierich JR, Giarola A, eds. Cryptorchidism. London: Academic Press.

Zamudio-Albescú JZ, Bergadá C, Cullen M (1971) Male fertility in patients treated for cryptorchidism before puberty. Fertil Steril 22: 829.

Zanartu J, Hamblen EC (1952) Ectopia testicular. Tratamiento y resultados observados en 132 casos. Rev Clin Espan 44: 21.

15. CONGENITAL ANOMALIES OF THE VAS DEFERENS AND EPIDIDYMIS

R. L. KROOVAND and A. D. PERLMUTTER

Congenital abnormalities of the mesonephric derivatives in males were once considered unusual, with only 74 cases of congenital vasal and epididymal anomalies recorded in urologic literature prior to 1949 (Lazarus and Marks, 1947; Michelson, 1949). More recently, with increased interest in the investigation and treatment of male infertility plus more careful observation and documentation of findings at orchiopexy, it is apparent that these abnormalities are relatively common. Their exact incidence, however, is undetermined and it is unlikely that it can be done accurately, as operative records of testicular or scrotal surgery generally do not provide detailed description of findings and hospital discharge coding is not specific enough. Also, most descriptions of anomalies of the testicular ducts are isolated case reports or are from selected populations and are therefore of limited statistical value (Badenoch, 1946; Dickinson, 1973; Emery et al., 1974; Mahboubi and Spackman, 1978; Nelson, 1950; Rosenberg and Urca, 1972; Rubin, 1975). There have been few large series (Marshall and Shermeta, 1979; Michelson, 1949; Scorer and Farrington, 1971) and until 1971, there had been little attempt at organization or classification of these anomalies (Marshall and Shermeta, 1979; Scorer and Farrington, 1971).

Existing data reflect that congenital atresia or absence of the vas deferens causes approximately 1% of all cases of azoospermia in the general population (Kaplan et al., 1968; White and Paulson, 1977) and that grossly identifiable anomalies of the vas deferens and epididymis may occur in 36% or more of undescended testicles (Marshall and Shermeta, 1979; Michelson, 1949; Scorer and Farrington, 1971), especially in those located in the mid-inguinal canal or more proximally.

These findings, combined with the observation of impaired spermatogenesis in many young adults with a unilaterally undescended testicle (Lipschultz et al., 1976), add impetus to develop a systematic, prospective method for studying these abnormalities. Furthermore, for medicolegal purposes, the incidence and implications of abnormalities of the male genital duct system should be established, as many can result in sterility.

In 1971, Scorer and Farrington, and more recently Marshall and Shermeta (1979), reviewed their experiences with epididymal and vasal anomalies associated with undescended testicles. Each group devised separate classifications which overlap. Neither is inclusive for all mesonephric derivatives. To provide a more comprehensive classification (Table 1), we have combined their descriptions and have added to them developmental anomalies of the seminal vesicles and ejaculatory ducts. While our classification is for unilateral pathology, similar or differing anomalies may also occur on the contralateral side.

A review of the normal embryology and anatomy of the testis and mesonephric derivatives will provide a sound basis for our discussion of the abnormal.

1. EMBRYOLOGY OF THE TESTIS, EPIDIDYMIS AND VAS DEFERENS

The body of the testis and its excretory duct system develop from different embryologic anlagen — the body of the testis from the genital ridge on the medial aspect of the mesonephros, and the excretory duct system from the mesonephric duct and mesonephric tubules.

During the fifth to sixth weeks of embryonic development, germ cells migrate from the yolk sac to the genital ridge. Epithelial cells covering the gonad

S.J. Kogan and E.S.E. Hafez (eds.), Pediatric andrology, 173–180. All rights reserved.
Copyright © 1981, Martinus Nijhoff Publishers bv, The Hague/Boston/London.

Table 1. Congenital anomalies of the mesonephric ducts in the male*

   I. Agenesis of all mesonephric duct derivatives
  II. Epididymis
     A. Agenesis of epididymis
     B. Failure of urogenital union: agenesis or loss of continuity[+]
        1. Nonunion between the head of epididymis and testis[+]
           a. gross
           b. microscopic
        2. Agenesis or atresia of the mid epididymis[+]
        3. Agenesis or atresia of the tail of epididymis[+]
     C. Elongated or looped epididymis
     D. Epididymal cyst, with or without loss of continuity
 III. Vas deferens
     A. Agenesis of vas deferens
        1. Complete[+]
        2. Segmental[+]
     B. Persistent mesonephric duct: ureter entering vas deferens
 IV. Seminal vesicle
     A. Agenesis of seminal vesicle
     B. Seminal vesicle cyst
     C. Ureter entering seminal vesicle
  V. Ejaculatory duct
     A. Agenesis of ejaculatory duct[+]

---

* Modified after Scorer and Farrington, 1971, 1979: Marshall and Shermeta, 1979.
[+] In some cases a fibrous band may be present in areas of loss of continuity suggesting atresia rather than agenesis. Histopathologic studies in the literature are not of sufficient detail to differentiate between atresia and agenesis.

produce cords of cells, which by the eighth week form the seminiferous tubules. These converge at the hilum of the testis to form the rete testis, a confluence of the tubules.

The excretory duct system of the testis develops from the mesonephric duct and mesonephric tubules. During the seventh to eighth week the mesonephros consists of the mesonephric duct and about 26 tubules, all in the process of degeneration. Five to twelve of the more cranial mesonephric tubules persist, remaining connected to the mesonephric duct. These form the efferent ductules of the head of the epididymis. By the ninth week the lumina of these efferent ductules unite with and become continuous with the lumen of the rete testis. The ureter separates from the mesonephric duct which differentiates into the vas deferens, ejaculatory duct and epididymis. That portion of the mesonephric duct adjacent to the testis which will form the epididymis undergoes marked convolution and folding, with separation of the epididymis into a head, body and tail.

During the third month, near where the vas joins the prostatic urethra, a localized dilation of the vas deferens forms the ampulla of the vas. The seminal vesicle evaginates from the wall of the ampulla of the vas at about the 13th week. That portion of the mesonephric duct between the origin of the seminal vesicle and its termination in the prostatic urethra becomes the ejaculatory duct. Development of the entire excretory duct system of the testis is complete by the 13th week (Gray and Skandalakis, 1972).

2. ANATOMY OF THE TESTES, EPIDIDYMIS, VAS DEFERENS AND SEMINAL VESICLE

The size and contour of the testis and epididymis, along with the attachments of the epididymis to the testis, vary slightly from one patient to another so that frequently it is difficult to decide when a normal variation becomes anomalous. The following anatomic description should serve as a guide to recognition of anomalous development (Fig. 1).

The epididymis forms an elongated structure, mainly along the posterolateral axis of the testis, tapering in size from the upper pole of the testis downward. The epididymis consists of three parts: the globus major (head), the body, and the globus minor (tail). The globus major is the largest part of the epididymis and is firmly attached to and fits like a "cap" over the upper pole of the testis. The body of the epididymis is less firmly attached to the testis

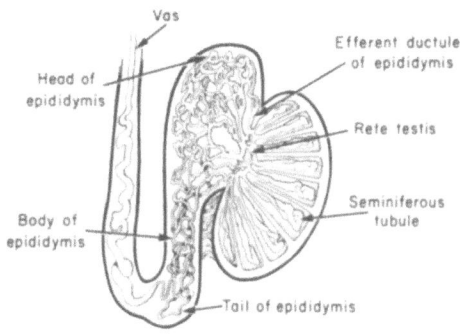

Figure 1. Normal cross-sectional anatomy, testes and epididymis.

forming a space between the testis and epididymis, the digital sinus of the epididymis. The globus minor of the epididymis is loosely attached to the testis by areolar connective tissue.

The efferent ductules within the globus major link the ductus epididymis to the rete testis. The convoluted ductus epididymis emerges from the tail of the epididymis as the vas deferens. The vas deferens ascends in the spermatic cord to the internal ring of the inguinal canal where it separates from the testicular vessels and descends behind the posterior surface of the bladder to the level of the prostate. Here it enlarges to form an ampulla and unites with the duct of the seminal vesicle to form the ejaculatory duct. The ejaculatory duct empties into the prostatic urethra.

The seminal vesicles are lobulated diverticulum-like excretory glands attached to the proximal end of the vas deferens.

3. CONGENITAL ANOMALIES OF THE MESONEPHRIC DUCT

With the separate embryologic origins of the testis and its excretory duct system, it is not surprising that a variety of developmental anomalies occur. Most of these anomalies can be diagnosed on the basis of clinical symptoms and physical examination, combined with a high index of suspicion; others may require more detailed investigation for diagnosis. This section will discuss some of the more commonly encountered anomalies of the mesonephric duct system in the male, using Table 1 as an outline.

3.1. Agenesis of all mesonephric duct derivatives

Complete absence of all mesonephric derivatives is

unusual and implies total failure of development of, or degeneration of, the mesonephric duct prior to the fourth week of intrauterine development (Dickinson, 1973; Lukash et al., 1975; Scorer and Farrington, 1971). With such early failure the ipsilateral ureter and kidney will also be absent, although the testis may be present. If the mesonephric duct degenerates after origin of the ureteral bud (fourth week), the ureter and kidney will develop. Interruption of mesonephric duct development later than the fourth but prior to the thirteenth week may produce a variety of anomalies, including a fully developed testicle and globus major of the epididymis with an underdeveloped distal duct system (Valman and France, 1969) or, more commonly, agenesis of portions of the duct system, i.e., the epididymis, vas deferens, or seminal vesicle (Marshall and Shermeta, 1979; Scorer and Farrington, 1971).

3.2. Epididymal anomalies

Epididymal anomalies (Fig. 2) vary in extent from total agenesis of the epididymis (Lazarus and Marks, 1947; Marshall and Shermeta, 1979) (Fig. 2A) to failure of union (loss of continuity in the duct system), occurring at the junction of the globus major and the testis (Fig. 2B) (Badenoch, 1946; Davis et al., 1974; Hanley, 1955; Marshall and Shermeta, 1979; Scorer and Farrington, 1971), at the mid-epididymis (Fig. 2C; D) (Marshall and Shermeta, 1979; Hanley, 1955; Scorer and Farrington, 1971), in the distal epididymis at the junction of the tail and vas (Fig. 2E) (Dean et al., 1952; Dickinson, 1973; Hanley, 1955; Hanley and Hodges, 1959; Marshall and Shermeta, 1979; Michalek and Krepp, 1972; Nowak, 1972; Scorer and Farrington, 1971), or as a microscopic nonunion of the rete testis and efferent ductules of the epididymis (Dean et al., 1952; Hanley, 1959; Marshall and Shermeta, 1979). In some cases segmental atresia or agenesis of the epididymis may occur.

While the true incidence of epididymal anomalies is unknown, an index of frequency and distribution may be drawn from data obtained at orchiopexy for undescended testis and during investigation of male infertility. In a 1949 literature review, 81% of 74 cases of vasal and epididymal anomalies involved the epididymis and 72% had associated vasal ano-

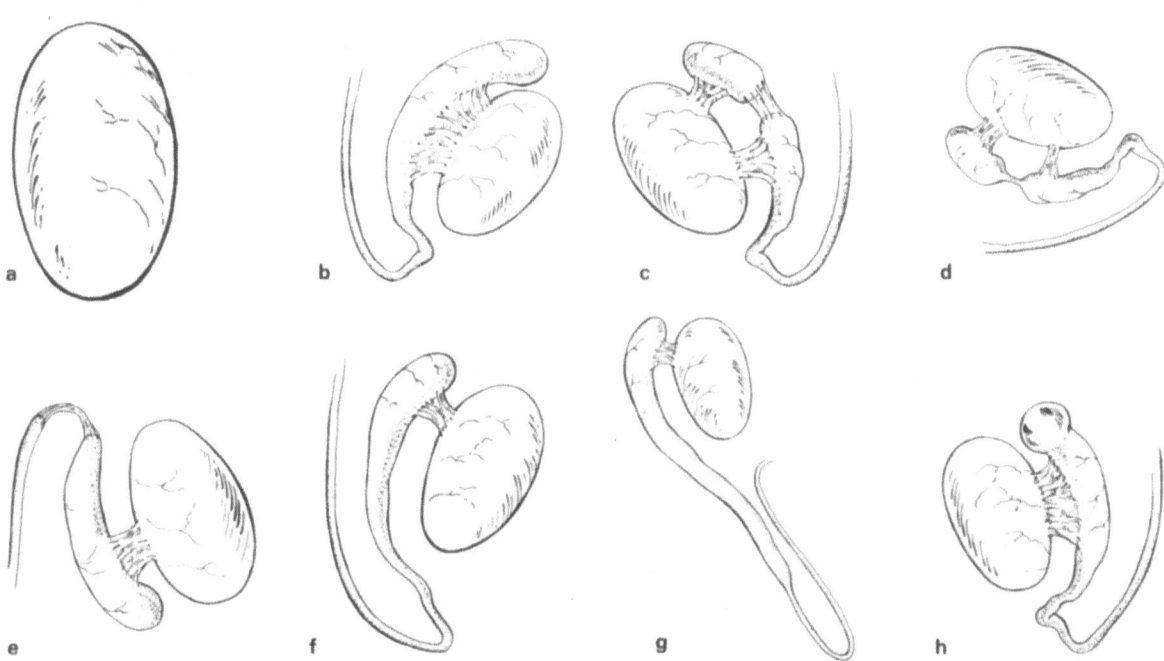

Figure 2. (A) Agenesis of all mesonephric derivatives. (B) Nonunion between the globus major of the epididymis and the testicle. (C) Agenesis at mid epididymis. (D) Atresia at mid epididymis. (E) Agenesis or atresia at tail of epididymis. (F) Extended or looped epididymis and vas deferens. (G) Extended or looped epididymis and vas deferens: more extensive anomaly than represented in (f). (H) Epididymal cyst of globus major of epididymis.

malies. 41% of these anomalies occurred in undescended testicles (Michelson, 1949). Other reports reflect a similar occurrence of epididymal and vasal anomalies with cryptorchism (Davis et al., 1974; Marshall and Shermeta, 1979; Scorer and Farrington, 1971).

Of 299 cases of obstructive azoospermia (Girgis et al., 1969), the most common anomaly involved obstruction in the tail of the epididymis or in the adjoining vas (39%) (Fig. 2E); the second most common site of obstruction was between the testis and epididymis (21%) (Figs 2B and 3A) and the least common was congenital absence of the vas deferens and epididymis (13%) (Fig. 2A). With bilateral absence of the vas deferens, the body and the tail of the epididymis are also missing; the globus major is usually intact (Hanley, 1955; Scorer and Farrington, 1971).

Microscopic nonunion of the rete testis and efferent ductules is another infrequently reported type of urogenital nonunion. This abnormality occurs in the presence of a grossly normal-appearing attachment of the globus major of the epididymis to the testis (Hanley, 1955; Hanley and Hodges, 1959; Hodges and Hanley, 1968; Olson and Weaver, 1969). The cited cases are from a series of azoospermic males with normal-appearing testes and epididymes who had excisional biopsy of one epididymis as part of the infertility investigation.

Elongated or extended epididymis (Badenoch, 1946; Lazarus and Marks, 1947; Marshall and Shermeta, 1979; Rosenberg and Urca, 1972; Scorer and Farrington, 1971) is the most common epididymal anomaly associated with cryptorchism (Figs 2F, G and 3B). Thirty-seven of 54 (68%) undescended testicles reported by Scorer and Farrington had an extended epididymis. This condition is manifest as a loosely attached, elongated and thin epididymis which may extend well beyond the retained testis into the lower inguinal canal or upper scrotum (Fig. 2G). An epididymis of normal size loosely attached to the testis by a mesentery, as is commonly seen in association with cryptorchism, is a lesser degree of extended epididymis (Fig. 2F). The vas deferens may also extend beyond the retained testis and epididymis into the lower inguinal canal or upper scrotum (Fig. 3C).

While the functional significance of these anomalies are uncertain, the surgical implication is quite evident and possibly even more important. If the

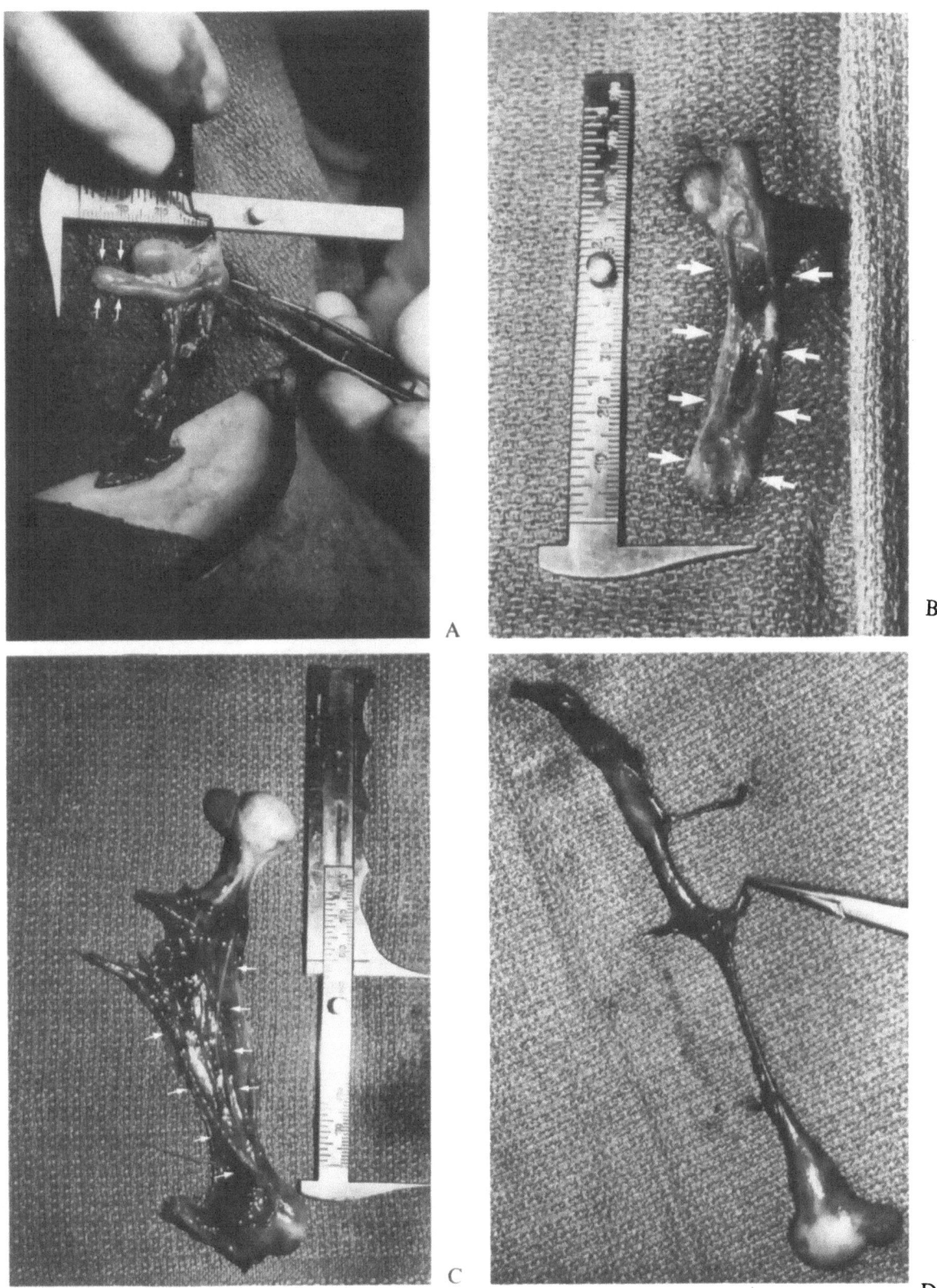

Figure 3. (A) Undescended testis with detached globus major of epididymis (arrow) and loosely attached body and tail of the epididymis. (B) Undescended testis with extended epididymis (arrows). (C) Undescended testicle with looped vas deferens (arrows). (D) Undescended testis with absence of the vas deferens and rudimentary development of the epididymis.

possibility of an extended or loosely attached epididymis or vas deferens is not considered, the descended tissue may be injured during surgical dissection, or mistaken for membranes of the tunica or for an atrophic testis and this tissue excised or placed in the scrotum, while leaving a retained testis intra-abdominally, or the testis may be considered absent with no further exploration undertaken (Dean et al., 1952; Lythgoe, 1961; Nowak, 1972).

Congenital epididymal abnormalities associated with cryptorchism are more frequent with mid-inguinal and more proximal testes (Marshall and Shermeta, 1979; Scorer and Farrington, 1971). Testes located in the lower inguinal canal and upper scrotum are less likely to have grossly abnormal mesonephric derivatives; this latter group may represent up to 25% of undescended testicles (Scorer and Farrington, 1979).

Epididymal cyst (Fig. 2H) of the globus major is an infrequently reported anomaly of uncertain embryology, possibly arising from the precursor of an efferent ductule or the most proximal epididymal duct. These cysts occur in approximately 5% of otherwise normal males. In utero exposure to diethylstilbesterol significantly increases this incidence (21%). The impact of this anomaly on male fertility is uncertain as cyst aspirates may or may not contain sperm (Gill et al., 1979).

3.3. Anomalies of the vas deferens

Data accumulated at the time of elective vasectomy and during investigation and treatment of male fertility reflect a 0.5-1% incidence of unilateral absence of the vas deferens in the general population (Benjamin and Moghaddam, 1973; Charny and Gillenwater, 1965; Dickinson, 1973; Emery et al., 1974; Girgis et al., 1968; Hanley, 1955; Hanley and Hodges, 1959; Klapproth and Young, 1973; Lukash et al., 1975; Michelson, 1949; Nelson, 1950; Schmidt, 1966; Scorer and Farrington, 1971; White and Paulson, 1977) and of bilateral absence of the vas deferens in from 1% to 10% of aspermic men in different series (Ithiri et al., 1972; O'Conor, 1960). Vasal anomalies commonly have associated abnormalities of the epididymis (Michelson, 1949) (Fig. 3D).

Congenital absence or rudimentary development of the mesonephric derivatives is an almost universal

finding in males with cystic fibrosis (Fig. 4A, B) and represents the cause of azoospermia in this population. In males with cystic fibrosis, anomalous de-

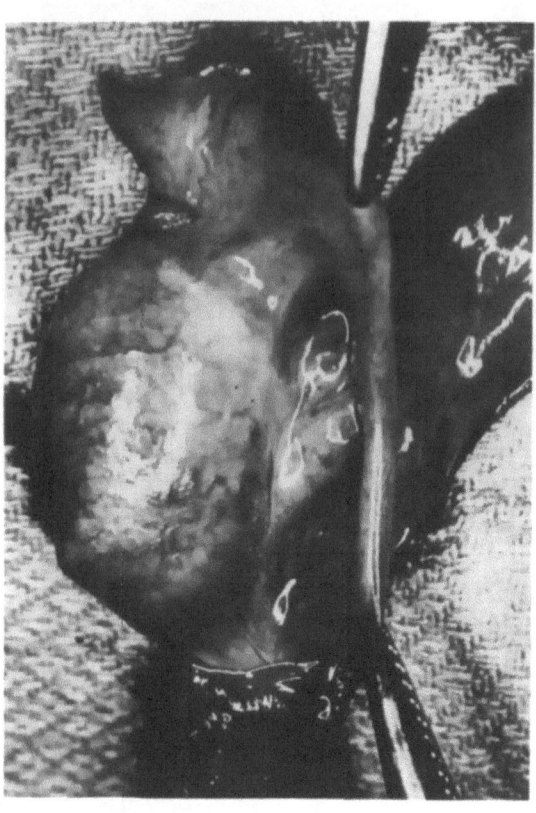

A

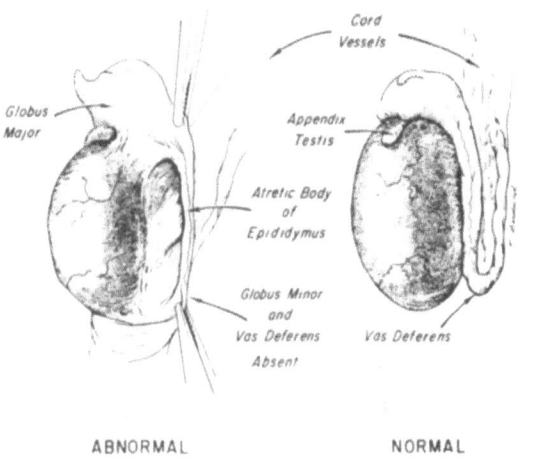

B

Figure 4. (A) Abnormal epididymis with absent globus minor and vas deferens in an 11-year-old boy with cystic fibrosis. Diagram (B) compares cystic fibrosis (abnormal) with normal. (B) Abnormal epididymis with absent globus minor and vas deferens in an 11-year-old boy with cystic fibrosis. (Reprinted with permission of the publisher of the New England Journal of Medicine.)

velopment of the mesonephric derivatives appears to be genetic, occurring either as an isolated vasal abnormality or more often accompanied by developmental abnormalities of the efferent ductules, epididymis and seminal vesicles as well (Holsclaw et al., 1971; Kaplan et al., 1968; Landing et al., 1969; Olson and Weaver, 1969; Valman and France, 1969). A growth disturbance occurring at about the 13th week of development resulting in disappearance of, or anomalous development of, the mesonephric derivatives would account for these abnormalities (Alfert and Gillenwater, 1972; Holsclaw et al., 1971; Olson and Weaver, 1969). In addition, males with cystic fibrosis have an increased incidence of inguinal hernia (15%) and cryptorchism (3.2%), as compared with the general population (1% and 0.7% respectively) (Holsclaw et al., 1971; Wang et al., 1970), further supporting the concept of altered development of the mesonephric duct-derived structures in these boys.

Persistent mesonephric duct is an unusual anomaly in which the ureter remains attached to the vas deferens, and a distal common excretory duct enters the urinary tract with its orifice situated anywhere along the migratory ectopic ureteral pathway from the trigone to the verumontanum (Alfert and Gillenwater, 1972; Boles et al., 1978; Borger and Belman, 1975; Hanley, 1955; Mahboubi and Spackman, 1978; Redman and Sulieman, 1976; Schwarz and Stephens, 1978; Seitzman and Patton, 1960; Williams and Royle, 1969). This abnormality may be accompanied by anorectal anomalies (Boles et al., 1978; Borger and Belman, 1975; Mahboubi and Spackman, 1978), although this association appears to be coincidental rather than the result of a generalized embryologic disaster (Schwarz and Stephens, 1978). Embryologically, persistent mesonephric duct appears to be the result of a more cranial origin of the ureteral bud than usual, combined with a failure of, or delayed absorption of the common excretory duct into the urogenital sinus. This results in a persistent common excretory duct with an orifice somewhere between the trigone and verumontanum. The ipsilateral seminal vesicle frequently is cystic or absent (Williams and Royle, 1969).

The clinical diagnosis of persistent mesonephric duct should be considered in any prepubertal male with recurrent or chronic epididymitis (Boles et al., 1978; Schwarz and Stephens, 1978; Williams and Royle, 1969), a rare event in that period. Because the common excretory duct is usually patulous, allowing reflux, a voiding cystourethrogram is the most useful diagnostic technique (Boles et al., 1978; Borger and Belman, 1975; Mahboubi and Spackman, 1978). The ipsilateral renoureteral unit varies in character from normal to dysplastic (Schwarz and Stephens, 1978; Williams and Roylee 1969).

3.4. Anomalies of the seminal vesicle and ejaculatory duct

Congenital anomalies of the seminal vesicles and ejaculatory duct include agenesis of the seminal vesicle or ejaculatory duct, seminal vesicle cyst (Donohue and Greenslade, 1973) and ectopic ureter entering the seminal vesicle (Brannan and Henry, 1973; Burford et al., 1949; Gordon and Kessler, 1972; Hanley, 1955; Schnitzer, 1965). An ectopic ureter entering the seminal vesicle is the most commonly reported of these anomalies. About 100 case reports of this anomaly are recorded in literature. Unfortunately, these reports are difficult to interpret, as most surgical and postmortem descriptions are sketchy and incomplete in anatomic detail. This anomaly can be explained embryologically if the ureteral bud had originated from the portion of the mesonephric duct destined to give origin to the seminal vesicle outgrowth, in which case the ureter would be included in the seminal vesicle when it developed. Whether this anomaly represents a variety of persistent mesonephric duct is uncertain; however, because ectopic ureter entering the seminal vesicle is usually associated with ipsilateral renal dysplasia while persistent mesonephric duct is not, we feel that this anomaly represents a separate, more severe expression of a similar aberrant embryogenesis.

The symptoms and signs of ectopic ureter entering the seminal vesicle are most common after puberty, and include epididymitis, painful defecation, dysuria, painful or bloody ejaculation and a tender rectal mass. The ipsilateral kidney usually does not visualize on an intravenous pyelogram. The diagnosis can be confirmed by transvesical injection of the seminal vesicle or by retrograde vasography.

Agenesis or atresia of the ejaculatory duct has been only infrequently reported (Girgis et al., 1968; Olson and Weaver, 1969).

180

REFERENCES

Alfert HJ, Gillenwater JY (1972) Ectopic vas deferens communicating with lower ureter: embryological considerations. J Urol 108: 172.

Badenoch AW (1946) Failure of the urogenital union. Surg Gynecol Obstet 82: 471.

Benjamin RB, Moghaddam A (1973) The case of the missing vas. Minnesota Med 56: 606.

Boles ET, Lobe TE, Hamoudi A (1978) Congenital vas deferens-ureteral connection. J Pediat Surg 13: 41.

Borger JA, Belman AB (1975) Uretero-vas deferens anastomosis associated with imperforate anus: an embryologically predictable occurrence. J Pediat Surg 10: 255.

Brannan W, Henrr HH II (1973) Ureteral ectopia: report of 39 cases. J Urol 109: 192.

Burford CE, Glen JE, Burford EH (1949) Ureteral ectopia: review of literature and two case reports. J Urol 62: 211.

Charny CW, Gillenwater JY (1965) Congenital absence of the vas deferens. J Urol 93: 399.

Davis EL, Shpall RA, Goldstein AMB, Morrow JW (1974) Congenitally uncoiled epididymis in a cryptorchid testicle. J Urol 111: 618.

Dean AL, Major JW, Ottenheimer EJ (1952) Failure of fusion of the testis and epididymis. J Urol 68: 754.

Dickinson SJ (1973) Structural abnormalities in the undescended testis. J Pediat Surg 8: 523.

Donohue RE, Greenslade NF (1973) Seminal vesicle cyst and ipsilateral renal agenesis. Urology 2: 66.

Emery CB, Goldstein AMB, Morrow JW (1974) Congenital absence of vas deferens with ipsilateral urinary anomalies. Urology 4: 201.

Gill WB, Schumacher GFB, Bibbo M et al. (1979) Association of Diethylstilbestrol exposure in utero with cryptorchidism, testicular hypoplasia and semen abnormalities. J Urol 122: 36.

Girgis SM, Etriby A et al. (1968) Aspermia: a survey of 49 cases. Fertil Steril 19: 580.

Girgis SM, Etriby A et al. (1969) Testicular biopsy in azoospermia. A review of the last ten years experience of over 800 cases. Fertil Steril 20: 467.

Gordon HL, Kessler R (1972) Ectopic ureter entering the seminal vesicle associated with renal dysplasia. J Urol 108: 389.

Gray SW, Skandalakis JE (1972) Embryology for surgeons. Philadelphia: W. B. Saunders.

Hanley HG (1955) The surgery of male subfertility. Ann Roy Coll Surg 17: 159.

Hanley HG, Hodges RD (1959) The epididymis in male sterility: a preliminary report of microdissection studies. J Urol 82: 508.

Hodges RD, Hanley HG (1968) Microscopic failure or urogenital union. Fertil Steril 19: 442.

Holsclaw DS, Perlmutter AD et al. (1971) Genital abnormalities in male patients with cystic fibrosis. J Urol 106: 568.

Itrihi A, Abulfadl MAM et al. (1972) Bilateral congenital absence of the vas deferens. Diagnostic features of seminal picture in 42 new cases. J Egypt Med Assoc 55: 184.

Kaplan E, Shwachman H, Perlmutter AD et al. (1968) Reproductive failure in males with cystic fibrosis. New Engl J Med 279: 65.

Klapproth HJ, Young JD (1973) Vasectomy, vas ligation, and vas occlusion. Urology 1: 292.

Landing BH, Wells TR, Wang C (1969) Abnormality of the epididymis and vas deferens in cystic fibrosis. Arch Pathol 88: 569.

Lazarus JA, Marks MS (1947) Anomalies association with undescended testis. Complete separation of a partly descended epididymis and vas deferens and an abdominal testis. J Urol 57: 567.

Lipschultz LI, Caminos-Torres R et al. (1976) Testicular function after orchiopexy for unilaterally undescended testis. New Engl J Med 295: 15.

Lukash F, Zwiren GT, Andrews HG (1975) Significance of absent vas deferens at hernia repair in infants and children. J Pediat Surg 10: 765.

Lythgoe JP (1961) Failure of fusion of the testis and epididymis. Br J Urol 33: 80.

Mahboubi S, Spackman TJ (1978) Ectopic vas deferens: a report of two cases and review of the literature. Am J Roentgenol 130: 1093.

Marshall FF, Shermeta DW (1979) Epididymal abnormalities associated with undescended testis. J Urol 121: 341.

Michalek HAL, Krepp J (1972) Failure of urogenital union with secondary amputation of the epididymal tail: a case report with complete review of the literature. J Urol 107: 436.

Michelson L (1949) Congenital anomalies of the ductus deferens and epididymis. J Urol 61: 384.

Nelson RE (1950) Congenital absence of the vas deferens: a review of the literature and report of three cases. J Urol 63: 176.

Nowak K (1972) Failure of fusion of epididymis and testicle with complete separation of the vas deferens. J Pediat Surg 7: 715.

O'Conor VJ (1960) Surgical correction of male sterility. Surg Gynecol Obstet 110: 649.

Olson JR, Weaver DK (1969) Congenital mesonephric defects in male infants with mucoviscidosis. J Clin Pathol 22: 725.

Redman JF, Sulieman JS (1976) Bilateral vasal-ureteral communications. J Urol 116: 808.

Rosenberg V, Urca I (1972) A rare congenital malformation: non-union of the testicle with the epididymis and the spermatic duct. Br J Urol 44: 499.

Rubin S (1975) Congenital absence of the vas deferens. Scand J Urol Nephrol 9: 94.

Schmidt SS (1966) Techniques and complications of elective vasectomy. Fertil Steril 17: 467.

Schnitzer B (1965) Ectopic ureteral opening into seminal vesicle: a report of four cases. J Urol 93: 576.

Schwarz R, Stephens FD (1978) The persisting mesonephric duct: high junction of vas deferens and ureter. J Urol 120: 592.

Scorer CG, Farrington GH (1971) Congenital deformities of the testis and epididymis, p. 136. New York: Appleton-Century-Crofts.

Scorer CG, Farrington GH (1979) Congenital anomalies of the testis: cryptorchidism, testicular torsion, and inguinal hernia and hydrocele. In Harrision JH, Gittes RF, Perlmutter AD, Stamey TA, Walsh PC, eds. Campbell's urology, 4th edn, Chap 44. Philadelphia: W. B. Saunders.

Seitzman DM, Patton JF (1960) Ureteral ectopia: combined ureteral and vas deferens anomaly. J Urol 84: 604.

Valman HB, France NE (1969) The vas deferens in cystic fibrosis. Lancet ii: 566.

Wang C, Kwok S, Edelbrock H (1970) Inguinal hernia, hydrocele, and other genitourinary abnormalities in boys with cystic fibrosis and their male siblings. Am J Dis Child 119: 236.

White RD, Paulson DF (1977) Obstruction of the male reproductive tract. J Urol 118: 266.

Williams DI, Royle M (1969) Ectopic ureter in the male child. Br J Urol 41: 421.

16. LEYDIG CELL TUMORS AND THEIR DISTINCTION FROM TESTICULAR TUMORS ASSOCIATED WITH CONGENITAL ADRENAL HYPERPLASIA

J. WACKSMAN

Endocrine active testicular tumors pose interesting management problems in children. The distinction between an isolated Leydig cell tumor of the testis and endocrine active testicular tumors associated with congenital adrenal hyperplasia may sometimes be difficult. In addition, the cellular origin of both of these clinical entities has been debated. In order for clinicians to accurately treat both of these disorders, a clear understanding of the distinguishing features is necessary. This chapter will review these points as well as provide speculation as to the origin of bilateral testicular tumors associated with congenital adrenal hyperplasia.

1. LEYDIG CELL TUMORS

Leydig cell tumor of the testis is a non-germinal neoplasm accounting for 1–2% of all testicular tumors. During the past 20 years, much has been written concerning the differences in clinical presentation and endocrine function tests of the isolated Leydig cell tumor as opposed to the testicular tumor associated with congenital adrenal hyperplasia. Savard et al. (1968) provided an extensive review citing 22 prior examples of individual case reports with respect to both types of virilizing tumors of the testes. Their case displayed many clinical abnormalities attributable to androgen overproduction as is usually seen in this disorder.

Most children manifest premature phallic enlargement, pubic hair, deepened voice and hirsutism. Other findings include early skeletal and muscular development, facial acne and a history of frequent erections. Savard's review revealed that precocity began between ages three and six years. In addition, the tumor was unilateral and benign in all but one case. Gynecomastia was also observed in three cases.

Biochemically, serum testosterone concentration is usually elevated. Naranjo found that the serum testosterone concentration fell following orchiectomy. The 24-hour urinary excretion of 17-ketosteroids may be variable. The testicular androgens testosterone and Δ4-androstenedione are highly potent biologically but yield only a small amount of 17-ketosteroids. On the other hand, the adrenal steroids are relatively weak androgens, and therefore to cause virilization, a large production of adrenal androgens and thus excretion of 17-keto-steroids would be necessary. Wilkins reviewed 15 cases and found the 17-ketosteroid excretion to vary from 2.9 to 520 mg/24 hours (normal pre-pubertal male less than 10 mg/24 hours), but most cases were normal or just slightly elevated. In Savard's case, the 17-ketosteroid excretion was 13 mg/24 hours. Savard further studied tumor tissue slices and demonstrated 11β-hydroxylase activity. This finding suggested the tumor possessed some adrenal tissue characteristics, but Martin et al. (1962) showed minimal amounts of 11β-hydroxy-lase activity when tissue slices were examined from their case of Leydig cell tumor. This finding is consistent with a normal adult testis. Mostofi and Price (1973) have summarized much of the work done on the hormonal activity of the Leydig cell tumor. His review 'shows that sometimes no hormones can be identified; sometimes only androgenic hormones are found; sometimes androgenic, estrogenic and progestational hormones are found; and in some tumors corticosteroids are also demonstrated.' These studies attest to the multipotential endocrine ability of the Leydig cell.

With regard to gonadotropins, it is known that serum FSH and LH levels are low in normal prepubertal males (Faiman and Winter, 1974). Patients with sexual precocity secondary to an endocrine active tumor also usually have normal

182

or low levels (Ward et al., 1960).

Pathologically, the testis may be diffusely enlarged or have several nodules. The tumor itself may vary in size from less than 1 cm to more than 10 cm (Mostofi and Price, 1973). Cross sections of the tumor are mahogany-brown in color; hemorrhage and necrosis are infrequent. Because of the brown to tan nature of the tumor, it has been described pathologically as a "brown tumor" (Fig. 1). Microscopically, the tumor consists of nests of closely packed eosinophillic cells with granular cytoplasm resembling mature Leydig cells (Fig. 2). Mostofi and Price (1973) reported the finding of Reinke's crystals (Reinke, 1896) in 40% of the cells and therefore the absence of these crystalloids (cigar shaped cytoplasmic inclusion bodies) does not exclude the Leydig cell tumor. In addition, Mostofi and Price (1973) describe four different types of cells but the clinical significance of these findings is unknown.

The management of this clinical entity requires prompt evaluation. In order to fully evaluate patients, distinction from testicular tumor of the adrenogenital syndrome should be attempted. Blood for serum testosterone, FSH, LH, ACTH, cortisol, 17-hydroxyprogesterone and Δ4-androstestenedione should be obtained. In addition, 24-hour urinary 17-KS, 17-OHCS and pregnanetriol excretion should be measured. X-ray examination includes a skull series as well as a detailed bone age. If, after all the data are analyzed, there still exists a doubt as to the diagnosis, a Dexamethasone suppression test can be performed. Once the diagnosis of a suspected Leydig cell tumor is established, orchiectomy is indicated. Because of possible mal-

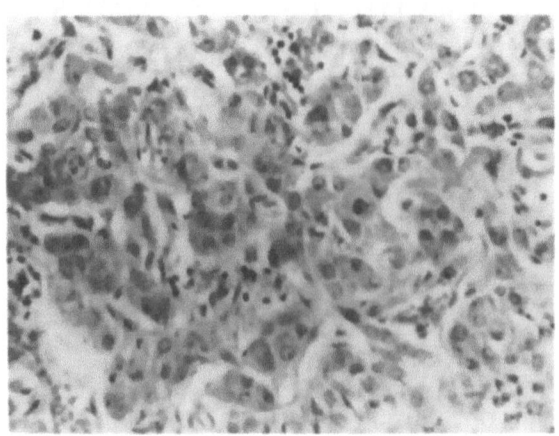

Figure 2. Microscopic appearance showing clusters of granular cells resembling Leydig cells.

ignancy, an inguinal approach is usually performed. This allows the surgeon to control the vascular pedicle of the testicle before manipulation of the tumor. Mostofi and Price (1973) reported 15 acceptable cases of malignancy in 150 Leydig cell tumors and further stated that malignancy is rare in the child, but does occur. Because of this possibility, the tumor should be considered malignant until proven otherwise. Occasionally, only demonstration of metastasis during subsequent evaluation can establish the malignant potential of the tumor (Coe and Schor, 1963; Mahon, 1973).

Followup evaluation includes repeat endocrine studies (serum FSH, LH, testosterone, 24-hour urinary, 17-KS, 17-OHCS excretion), close observation of the remaining testis and general growth patterns of the patient (bone age) (Wilkins, 1965). Savard et al. (1968) stated that no further growth occurred in the children whose epiphysis had already closed while in those patients with a height less than 127 cm and a bone age less than 12 years, a deceleration of growth rate and genital development was specifically noted. They further reported on three patients with gynecomastia and found that breast enlargment disappeared in two, but did persist in one.

Three examples of Leydig cell tumors in children, with their endocrine findings are summarized below:

1. C.S. was referred at age 2 with virilism and accelerated growth. At 6 months of age, he was in the 10th percentile for height, and over the next 18 months gradually grew to over the 90th percentile

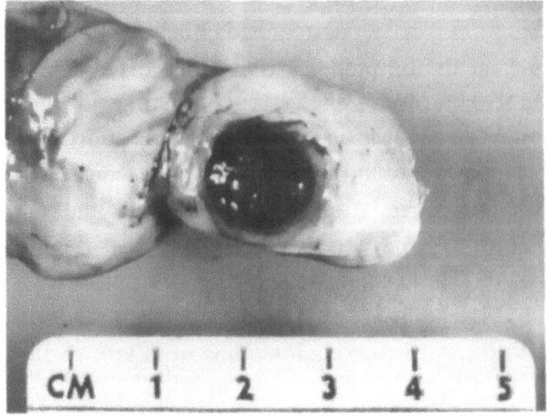

Figure 1. Gross appearance of typical Leydig cell tumor.

with a height of 36.8 inches and weight of 34 pounds. Physical examination revealed prominent signs of virilism including an enlarged phallus and large well-developed body habitus characteristic of "infant Hercules." Pubic hair was well developed but the testes were small compared to penile size. The left testis was firm with a small mass in the lower pole while the right appeared normal. Radiological evaluation revealed a bone age of 28 months. Endocrine studies yielded a serum testosterone value of 305 ng/100 ml (normal prepubertal male less than 10 ng/100 ml). Serum luteinizing hormone (LH) was 4.6 MIU/ml (normal prepubertal male less than 5 MIU/ml). Urinary 17-ketosteroid excretion revealed a baseline level of 1.3 and 1.7 mg/24 hours (normal prepubertal male less than 10 mg/24 hours), and values of 1.5, 1.1 and 1.0 mg/24 hours during three consecutive days of Dexamethasone treatment. With these studies accomplished, a left inguinal orchiectomy was performed, as well as a right testis biopsy. Histologic examination revealed an interstitial cell tumor of the left testis with no crystalloids of Reinke, while the right testicular biopsy revealed an immature testis. Following surgery, endocrine studies revealed serum testosterone of less than 10 ng/100 ml, FSH less than 1 MIU/ml, and LH of 4.6 MIU/ml, consistent with normal endocrine function.

2. T.B. presented at age 7 for evaluation of precocious puberty characterized by accelerated muscle development, voice change, facial acne, pubic hair and an enlarged phallus. Physical examination confirmed these findings. In addition, the right testis was markedly enlarged and firm, but no discrete mass was palpable. The left testis was normal to palpation. Laboratory studies revealed a serum testosterone concentration of 400 ng/100 ml, urinary 17-ketosteroids were 2.5 mg/24 hours, and bone age equivalent to 12.5 years. FSH and LH levels were not obtained. The patient underwent a right orchiectomy. Histologically, the tumor was a Leydig cell tumor and postoperatively serum testosterone decreased to 34 ng/100 ml.

3. R.F., a 9-year-old male, presented with accelerated muscular development, facial hair, acne and phallic enlargement. Physical examination revealed a well developed young "man" appearing older than his stated age. Positive findings were a penis measuring 9 cm in length and a 1.4 cm nodule at the base of the left testis; the right testis was normal. Preoperative serum testosterone concentration was 335 ng/100 ml, serum FSH 3.9 MIU/ml, serum LH 9.0 MIU/ml, urinary ketosteroid excretion of 6.9 mg/24 hours, urinary 17-hydroxysteroid excretion of 3.4 mg/24 hours, and a bone age that was 11.5 years. The left testis was removed and a histologic diagnosis of Leydig cell tumor was made. Postoperative endocrine studies revealed a serum FSH 25.7 MIU/ml, LH 15 MIU/ml and serum testosterone of 162 ng/100 ml, six months after tumor removal. Explanation of the persistent gonadotropin elevation was not evident.

2. CONGENITAL ADRENAL HYPERPLASIA

Patients with bilateral testicular tumors associated with congenital adrenal hyperplasia present in a different manner. Usually they have a history of vomiting and salt wasting during infancy. Occasionally, later presentation is manifested by phallic enlargement and bilateral testicular tumors. In reviewing Table 1, it can be seen how an enzymatic defect such as 21-hydroxylase deficiency will cause an accumulation of the precursors, progesterone and 17-hydroxyprogesterone. This in turn may result in an increase in androgenic hormones, Δ4-androstenedione, which will lead to an elevation of the urinary excretion of 17-ketosteroids. In addition, the elevation of 17-hydroxyprogesterone will also lead to a rise in the excretion of pregnanetriol. The lack of cortisol production as well as aldosterone will lead to a decreased excretion of 17-hydroxysteroids and aldosterone. This accounts for the salt wasting and failure to thrive while the increase in androgenic activity is responsible for virilization. Wilkins (1965) noted that endocrine evaluation showed an elevation of serum 17-hydroxyprogesterone with normal or slightly elevated serum testosterone concentration, elevated urinary excretion of 17-ketosteroid and pregnanetriol, and decreased serum cortisol levels and urinary excretion of 17-hydroxysteroid. Urban et al. (1978) reviewed 52 male patients with congenital virilizing adrenal hyperplasia. Fifty-one had 21-hydroxylase deficiency, while one patient had 11-hydroxylase deficiency. The patients with the salt losing form which corresponded to a complete 21-hydroxylase

Table 1. Steroid production in both adrenal and testis.

CHOLESTEROL			
↓			
Δ5-PREGNENOLENE			
↓			
PROGESTERONE→	17-HYDROXYPROGESTERONE→	Δ4 ANDROSTENEDIONE→	TESTOSTERONE
21-Hydroxylase	21-Hydroxylase		
↓	↓	↓	↓
DEOXYCORTICOSTERONE (DOC)	DEOXYCORTISONE	ESTRONE	ESTRADIOL
11-HYDROXYLASE	11-HYDROXYLASE		
↓	↓		
CORTICOSTERONE	CORTISOL		
↓	↓		
ALDOSTERONE	17-Hydroxysteroids	17-Ketosteroids	
(Mineralocorticoids)	(Glucocorticoids)	(Androgens-Estrogens)	

deficiency were seen in infancy because of failure to thrive and vomiting. In those patients with a partial 21-hydroxylase deficiency, the diagnosis was made somewhat later. These children presented with simple virilization, but had no evidence of salt wasting. The one patient with an 11-hydroxylase deficiency showed signs of premature pseudopuberty and hypertension. When this constellation of findings occurs with bilateral testicular tumors, congenital adrenal hyperplasia is likely.

Having established the diagnosis, management involves replacement therapy with glucocorticoids and mineralocorticoids together with close monitoring of adrenal function, as well as serum sodium and potassium. Wilkins (1965) stated that testicular tumors occur in patients with poorly controlled congenital adrenal hyperplasia and elevated ACTH production. Kirkland et al. (1977, 1978) showed that patients with testicular tumors and CAH can be adequately monitored by obtaining 24-hour urinary excretion of 17-KS, 17-OHCS, pregnanetriol, as well as serum FSH, LH, testosterone and

ACTH. Burke et al. (1973) found seven previously reported cases of testicular tumors and CAH which were managed successfully by replacement hormone therapy; but, as pointed out by Glenn and Boyce (1963) and Kirkland et al. (1977) occasionally bilateral orchiectomy is necessary despite adequate replacement therapy.

3. LEYDIG CELL TUMORS AND THEIR DISTINCTION FROM THE TESTICULAR TUMOR ASSOCIATED WITH CONGENITAL ADRENAL HYPERPLASIA

Non-germinal gonadal tumors that produce hormones pose interesting management problems in children. The differences between these two clinical diseases are summarized in Table 2, however sometimes the distinctions may be blurred and the exact diagnosis difficult to determine. Newell et al. (1977) reported on a 9-year-old male with poorly controlled congenital adrenal hyperplasia. This patient

Table 2. Clinical and hormonal findings in Leydig cell tumors and testicular tumors associated with congenital adrenal hyperplasia.

	History	Physical exam	Serum testosterone	24 hour urine 17-KS	24 hour urine 17-OH	Response to glucocorticoid replacement therapy
Leydig cell tumor	Gradual onset	Unilateral testicular mass	Increased	Normal	Normal	None
Bilateral testicular tumors, C.A.H.	History from infancy	Bilateral testicular masses	Normal or increased	Increased	Decreased	Decrease in testicular size

developed a unilateral right-sided testicular tumor. Pathological examination revealed an interstitial cell testicular tumor; but, five months following right orchiectomy, serum testosterone concentration rose and further studies suggested a diagnosis of congenital adrenal hyperplasia. Historically, Leydig cell tumors present later in childhood as a unilateral testicular mass, elevated serum testosterone concentration, but normal or slightly elevated 17-KS and normal 17-OHCS (Wilkins, 1965). On the other hand, patients with testicular tumors and congenital adrenal hyperplasia usually have involvement of both testes. Often there is a history of salt wasting and failure to thrive during infancy. Endocrine evaluation reveals normal or increased serum testosterone concentration, increased 24-hour urinary excretion of 17-KS, pregnanetriol with decreased serum cortisol and urinary excretion of 17-OHCS. Management also differs as Leydig cell tumors require a unilateral inguinal orchiectomy (Mostofi and Price, 1973) while bilateral testicular tumors associated with CAH are given a trial of replacement glucocorticoid therapy (Burke et al., 1973; Kirkland et al., 1977).

Data from extensive endocrinological examination of adult males with bilateral testicular tumors and congenital adrenal hyperplasia suggest an interrelationship with inadequate ACTH suppression and LH secretion. Radfar reported on a 19-year-old male with the above clinical findings. Evaluation of testicular function after ACTH suppression with Dexamethasone illustrated a normal diurnal fluctuation of plasma testosterone, but serum LH and FSH appeared elevated after ACTH suppression. Adrenal evaluation after ACTH suppression showed decreased 17-OH progesterone and plasma cortisol. In addition, both spermatic and peripheral vein cortisol, 17-OHP and testosterone increased following ACTH stimulation. The light and electron-microscopic examination of the tumors was consistent with "Leydig Cells." Radfar went on to suggest: "1) that the functional capacity of 'Leydig cell' tumors in congenital adrenal hyperplasia may not correlate with the morphological appearance; 2) such tumors may secrete cortisol and demonstrate ACTH dependence; 3) endogenous suppression of LH secretion may occur during periods of inadequate ACTH suppression." Kirkland et al. (1977) also examined a 22-year-old male with CAH and

bilateral testicular tumors. Their data clearly documented that these tumors responded to ACTH stimulation by producing an increase in testosterone, 17-OH progesterone, as well as androstenedione. In addition, Kirkland found a high serum LH concentration in association with incomplete suppression of adrenal steroid secretion. Both of these reports suggest that LH may also have contributed to the growth of these testicular tumors.

Recent debate centers around the cellular origin of both clinical conditions. Several authors (Glenn and Boyce, 1963; Burke et al., 1973) attribute the testicular enlargement to hyperplasia of adrenal rest cells of the testicle. Dahl and Bahn (1962) studied 200 testes in 100 male infants under one year of age and found no adrenal cortical tissue within the testicular parenchyma. However, adrenal cortical tissue was found in 7.5% of the examinations but located outside the testicle along the cord and adjacent to the epididymis. A similar finding was noted by Mostofi and Price (1973), stating that "histologic differentiation between Leydig cell tumor and adrenal rest tumor may be difficult. Adrenal rests usually occur on the surface of the spermatic cord or in the region of the rete testis, not in the substance of the testicle."

The cellular origin of unilateral testicular tumors associated with the symptom complex of precocious puberty appears to be the Leydig cell. Although Glenn and Boyce (1963) questions this concept, several authors including Naranjo et al. (1973), Martin et al. (1962) and Wilkins (1965) believe the origin of this unilateral endocrine active tumor to be the Leydig cell. In Mostofi and Price's extensive review, they relate multiple examples of the multipotential ability of the Leydig cell to elaborate androgenic as well as estrogenic and progestational hormones. With this evidence, it seems likely that the cellular origin of this unilateral endocrine active non-germinal tumor associated with sexual precocity is, as stated by Wilkihs (1965), the Leydig cell. On the other hand, the debate over the cellular origin of bilateral testicular tumors associated with CAH continues. Many authors including Glenn and Boyce (1963), Savard et al. (1968), and Burke et al. (1973) believe the cellular origin of these tumors to be from adrenal rests within the testis; but the data from Dahl and Bahn (1962), as well as Mostofi and Price (1973), show that adrenal rest cells usually occur outside the substance of the testis. This finding, together with the observations of Radfar et al. (1977) and Kirkland et al. (1977, 1978), which imply an interrelationship between LH and ACTH in the generation of these tumors, seems to support the concept that these tumorous cells have a multipotential ability to respond to ACTH as well as LH. In light of the interrelationship of LH, ACTH and testicular enlargement, further study will be needed to define the exact origin of bilateral testicular tumors in patients with congenital adrenal hyperplasia.

ACKNOWLEDGEMENT

We wish to thank Mark Sperling, M.D., Director of Pediatric Endocrinology and Professor of Pediatrics, University of Cincinnati for his help in reviewing this manuscript.

REFERENCES

Bishop PH, ven Meurs DP, Wilcox DR, Arnold D (1960) Interstitial cell tumor of testes in a child; report of a case and review of the literature. Br Med J 1: 23.

Burke EF, Gilbert E, Uehling DT (1973) Adrenal rest tumors of the testes. J Urol 109: 649.

Coe JI, Shor H (1963) Malignant interstitial cell tumor of the testes: a case report. J Urol 89: 851.

Dahl EV, Bahn RC (1962) Aberrant adrenal cortical tissue near the testes in human infants. Am J Pathol 40: 587.

Faiman C, Winter JSD (1974) Gonadotrophins and sex hormone patterns in puberty: clinical data. In Grumback MM, Grave GD, Mayer FE, eds. Control of the onset of puberty. New York, John Wiley.

Glenn JF, Boyce WH (1963) Adrenogenitalism with testicular adrenal rests simulating interstitial cell tumor. J Urol 89: 456.

Herwig KR, Vinson RK (1978) Interstitial cell tumor-profile of hormone-producing tumor. Urology 9: 283.

Huffman CF (1978) Interstitial cell tumor of the testicle, report of one case. J Urol 45: 692.

Jones HW, Scott WW (1971) Endocrine tumors of the testis, in hermaphrodism, genital anomalies and related endocrine disorders, p 1558. Baltimore: Williams & Wilkins.

Kirkland RT, Kirkland JL, Keenan BS, Bongiovanni AM, Rosenberg HS, Clayton GW (1977) Bilateral testicular tumors in congenital adrenal hyperplasia. J Clin Endocrinol Metab 44: 369.

Kirkland RT, Keenan BS, Holcombe JH, Kirkland JL, Clayton GW (1978) The effect of therapy on mature height in congenital adrenal hyperplasia. J Clin Endocrinol Metab 47: 1320.

Mahon FB, Gosser F, Trinity RG (1973) Malignant interstitial cell testicular tumor. Cancer 31: 1209.

Martin MM, Canary JP, Balsamo PA (1962) Virilizing tumor of the testis in one twin. J Clin Endocrinol 22: 345.

Mostofi FK, Price EB Jr (1973) Tumors of male genitalia: an atlas of tumor pathology, Fascicle 8, 2nd series, p 98. Washington, D.C.: A.F.I.P.

Naranjo CA, Kandzari SJ, Klingberg WG (1973) Interstitial cell tumor of the testicle in children. Urology 2: 49.

Newell ME, Lippe BM, Ehrlich RM (1977) Testis tumors associated with congenital adrenal hyperplasia: a continuing diagnostic and therapeutic dilemma. J Urol 117: 256.

Radfar N, Bartter FC, Easley R, Kolins J, Javadpour N, Sherins R (1977) Evidence for endogenous LH suppression in a man with bilateral testicular tumors and congenital adrenal hyperplasia. J Clin Endocrinol Metab 45: 1194.

Reinke F (1896) Betrage zur Histologie des Menschen über Krystalloidbildungen in den interstitiellen Zellen des menschlichen Hoders. Arch Mikrosk Anat 47: 34.

Savard K, Dorfman RL, Baggett B, Fielding LL, Engel LL, McPherson HT, Lister LM, Johnson DS, Hamblen EC, Engel FL (1968) Clinical, morphological and biochemical studies of a virilizing tumor in the testis. J Clin Invest 39: 534.

Urban MD, Lee PA, Migeon CJ (1978) Adult height and fertility in men with congenital virilizing adrenal hyperplasia. New Engl J Med 299: 1392.

Ward JA, Krantz S, Mendeloff F, Holtwagner E (1960) Interstitial cell tumor of the testis; report of two cases. J Clin Endocrinol Metab 20: 1622.

Wilkins L (1965) The diagnosis and treatment of endocrine disorders in childhood and adolescence, 3rd edn. Springfield: Charles C. Thomas.

17. LOWER URINARY TRACT MORPHOLOGY IN PATIENTS WITH HYPOSPADIAS

L. GONZALEZ-SERVA, J. F. STECKER, JR., C. J. DEVINE, JR. and C. E. HORTON

1. HYPOSPADIAS: ETIOLOGIC CONSIDERATIONS

Hypospadias is a relatively common anomaly of the lower urinary tract seen in 8 children per 1000 male births (Sweet et al., 1974). Developmental arrest during fetal organogenesis produces a fusion defect in the urethral tube. The fusion of the urethral folds is induced by fetal testicular androgen, therefore the occurrence of hypospadias is caused by incomplete masculinization of this target structure. This may be a result of either a decline in stimulation caused by diminution in circulating hormones, partial tissue insensitivity or improper chronologic correlation between the hormonal level and the critical time for this tissue to respond to androgens (Horton and Devine, 1972). In the great majority of cases, hypospadias occurs as a single defect with no apparent or demonstrable genetic or endocrine disturbance at birth or later in life (Aarskog, 1970). However, it may also be a manifestation of more permanent genetic and endocrine derangements, especially if there is ambiguity of external genitalia or the presence of another disorder of male sexual differentiation such as cryptorchidism or well-developed Müllerian duct structures. In practice, most of the patients with hypospadias do not exhibit these features and, therefore, there are no uncertainties regarding their sex; these patients should not be categorized as having an intersex problem (Aarskog, 1970).

Due to the fact that hypospadias of varying degrees will be one of the external manifestations of many intersex conditions, and because hypospadias may be produced by procedures in experimental embryology that affect testicular function after initial phase of male differentiation (Goldman, 1971), several authors have regarded hypospadias

as the mildest form of male pseudohermaphroditism (Campbell, 1963; Jost, 1971). Moreover, the association of hypospadias, cryptorchidism and an enlarged prostatic utricle has been regarded as sexual ambiguity (Arnold, 1869). A direct relationship between the degree of hypospadias and increasing size of the prostatic utricle has been reported with the conclusion that all hypospadias is a form of male pseudohermaphroditism (Howard, 1948).

The presence of developed remnants of Müllerian ducts in a phenotypic male, with or without hypospadias, indicates failure of the fetal testis to suppress these female structures; the direct implication would be that this is a form of male pseudohermaphroditism (Brook et al., 1973). However, pseudohermaphrodites or hermaphrodites who exhibit partial or complete Müllerian duct development will be found to have evidence of a well-structured uterovaginal canal and tubes, albeit infantile. All normal males will have vestiges of regressed Müllerian ducts represented by the appendix testis and the cranial vault of the prostatic utricle, and the presence of these structures by no means indicates an intersex problem (Fig. 1). But less than expected involution suggests either incomplete Müllerian duct regression caused by failure of the effectiveness of the Müllerian duct regression factor or incomplete masculinization of the urogenital sinus caused by one of the factors noted above or both together.

2. GROSS AND ENDOSCOPIC MORPHOLOGY IN PATIENTS WITH HYPOSPADIAS AND INTERSEXUALITY

The clinical material presented here was evaluated in an attempt to determine the incidence of enlarge-

188

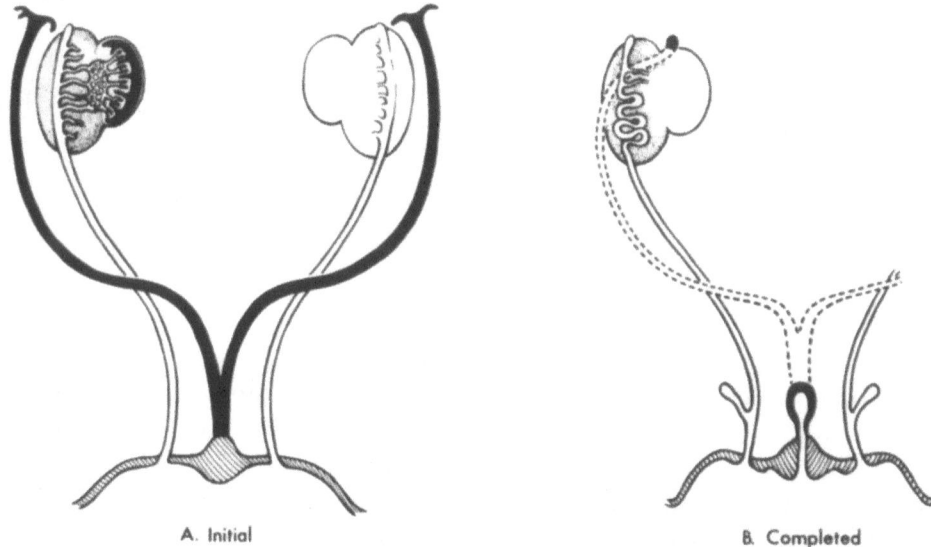

A. Initial   B. Completed

Figure 1. Normal differentiation of Müllerian and Wolffian ducts in the male as influenced by Müllerian regression factor and androgens. Müllerian remnants are the appendix testis and the dome of the prostatic utricle.

ment of the prostatic utricle in patients with hypospadias. To evaluate significance of utricular enlargement we have compared these findings with those in a series of patients with known intersex conditions. Because of the confusion in understanding the terminology, we will refer to the enlarged prostatic utricle and only use the term vagina masculinus when other unregressed Müllerian duct structures are present in continuity.

The charts of the last 100 hypospadias patients operated upon were reviewed. In 44 patients whose meatus was located in the proximal two-thirds of the penis, penoscrotal junction and perineal area, cystourethroscopy was performed immediately prior to surgery. The remainder of the patients of this series whose meatus was more distal in the penis were not cystoscoped due to the low yield of finding abnormalities in the past. Only the patients with endoscopic data will be analyzed. In addition, 8 patients found to have hypospadias and ambiguous genitalia as a manifestation of intersex were evaluated in regards to the location of the meatus, the presence of Müllerian duct derivatives and the degree of masculinization of the urogenital sinus.

During endoscopy, the presence of the verumontanum and prostatic utricle and their position in relation with the external sphincter were noted. The degree of development of the prostatic urethra and the presence of other anomalies were also

recorded. A prostatic utricle was considered enlarged when it allowed the cystoscope to be introduced into it for at least 2 cm (Howard, 1948) or more in order to examine its cranial portion searching for a cervix. Otherwise, the prostatic utricle was considered not enlarged when it appeared as a small dimple in the verumontanum and did not allow passage of the instrument.

There were 17 patients with penile hypospadias, normally descended testes and no evidence of ambiguity. One of these patients was found to have posterior urethral valves and another had an ectopic ureter. Otherwise, 16 patients had completely normal posterior urethras without evidence of abnormalities of the verumontanum or prostatic utricle (Table 1).

Among 20 patients with penoscrotal hypospadias, 18 were found to have normally descended testes, and only one of these 18 was found to have an enlarged prostatic utricle. One patient with bilateral cryptorchidism and bifid scrotum was found to have a normal posterior urethra. One patient with unilateral cryptorchidism was found to have an enlarged prostatic utricle without associated cervix. In both of these patients, the verumontanum was prominent and located proximal to the sphincter.

There were seven patients with perineal hypospadias. Five of these had normally descended testes. Among this sub-group, two exhibited an enlarged prostatic utricle, one was found to have posterior urethral valves, and two had normal posterior urethras. Two patients with perineal hypospadias had bilaterally undescended testes and small penis but no other clinical or laboratory evidence of intersex. Both exhibited abnormal posterior urethras with large utricles. In one of these patients, the verumontanum appeared to be distal to the external sphincter (Table 1).

Analysis of the patients with intersex conditions and hypospadias was also done (Table 2). Three patients had perineal hypospadias. Two of these had familial incomplete male pseudohermaphroditism (presently classified as Reifenstein's syndrome). In both of these patients the prostate was very small in size, the verumontanum prominent and the prostatic utricle was significantly enlarged. Close examination of the utricle failed to reveal a cervix. Both patients had undergone previous exploratory laparotomies which revealed no uterus or tubes. Another patient has mixed gonadal dysgenesis and was found to have a vagina joining the urethra at the level of the verumontanum and a cervix which was well visualized. Four patients with penoscrotal

hypospadias and ambiguous genitalia underwent endoscopy. There were two cases of mixed gonadal dysgenesis and two cases of familial incomplete male pseudohermaphroditism. In the mixed gonadal dysgenesis cases, urethroscopy revealed a vagina and uterus which joined the prostatic urethra at the level of the verumontanum and proximal to the external sphincter. One patient with male pseudohermaphroditism was found to have an enlarged prostatic utricle and another patient had a normal posterior urethra. Two patients in this group did not have cystoscopy, so they are not included in this analysis (Table 2).

On rectal examination, prostatic size was significantly reduced in the three patients with hypospadias and familial incomplete male pseudohermaphroditism who were found to have enlarged prostatic utricles. Also the verumontanum appeared quite prominent in contradistinction to those patients with mixed gonadal dysgenesis where the verumontanum appeared generally flat. It is interesting to note that in the intersex group, the enlarged vagina masculinus always joined the urethra proximal to the external sphincter and at the level of the verumontanum.

Table 1. Incidence of enlarged prostatic utricle in hypospadias.

| | No. patients | Cryptorchidism | | Enlarged prostatic utricle | Incidence enlarged utricle (%) |
		Unil.	Bil.		
Penile	17	0	0	0	0%
Penoscrotal	20	1	1	2	10%
Perineal	7	0	2	4	57%
Total	44			6	14%

Table 2. Intersex patients presenting with hypospadias.

Location meatus	Condition	Scrotum at birth	Müllerian derivatives	Prostatic utricle	Urogenital sinus
Perineal	MGD	Empty	Vagina + uterus	—	
Perineal	MPSH	Empty	None	Enlarged	Small prostate
Perineal	MPSH	Empty	None	Enlarged	Small prostate
Penoscrotal	MGD	Empty	Vagina + uterus	—	
Penoscrotal	MGD	Empty	Vagina + uterus	—	
Penoscrotal	MPSH	Empty	None	Enlarged	Small prostate
Penoscrotal	MPSH	Empty	None	Normal	

Abbv.: MGD - mixed gonadal dysgenesis; MPSH - male pseudohermaphroditism

3. UTRICULAR ENLARGEMENT: ITS INCIDENCE AND SIGNIFICANCE

To have any meaning, a significant number of hypospadias patients should demonstrate enlargement of the prostatic utricle, this enlargement being most frequent and more marked in patients with most proximal degrees of hypospadias.

Among 44 patients with proximal penile, penoscrotal and perineal hypospadias who underwent urethroscopy, six exhibited an enlarged prostatic utricle (14% incidence) (Table 1). Fifty-seven per cent of patients with perineal hypospadias, 10% of those with penoscrotal hypospadias and no patients with penile hypospadias had an enlarged prostatic utricle (Table 2). If patients with penile hypospadias are excluded the incidence is 22%. Of the six patients with an enlarged prostatic utricle, one who had penoscrotal hypospadias also had unilateral cryptorchidism and two with perineal hypospadias were bilaterally cryptorchid. The other three of these patients had normally descended testes. On

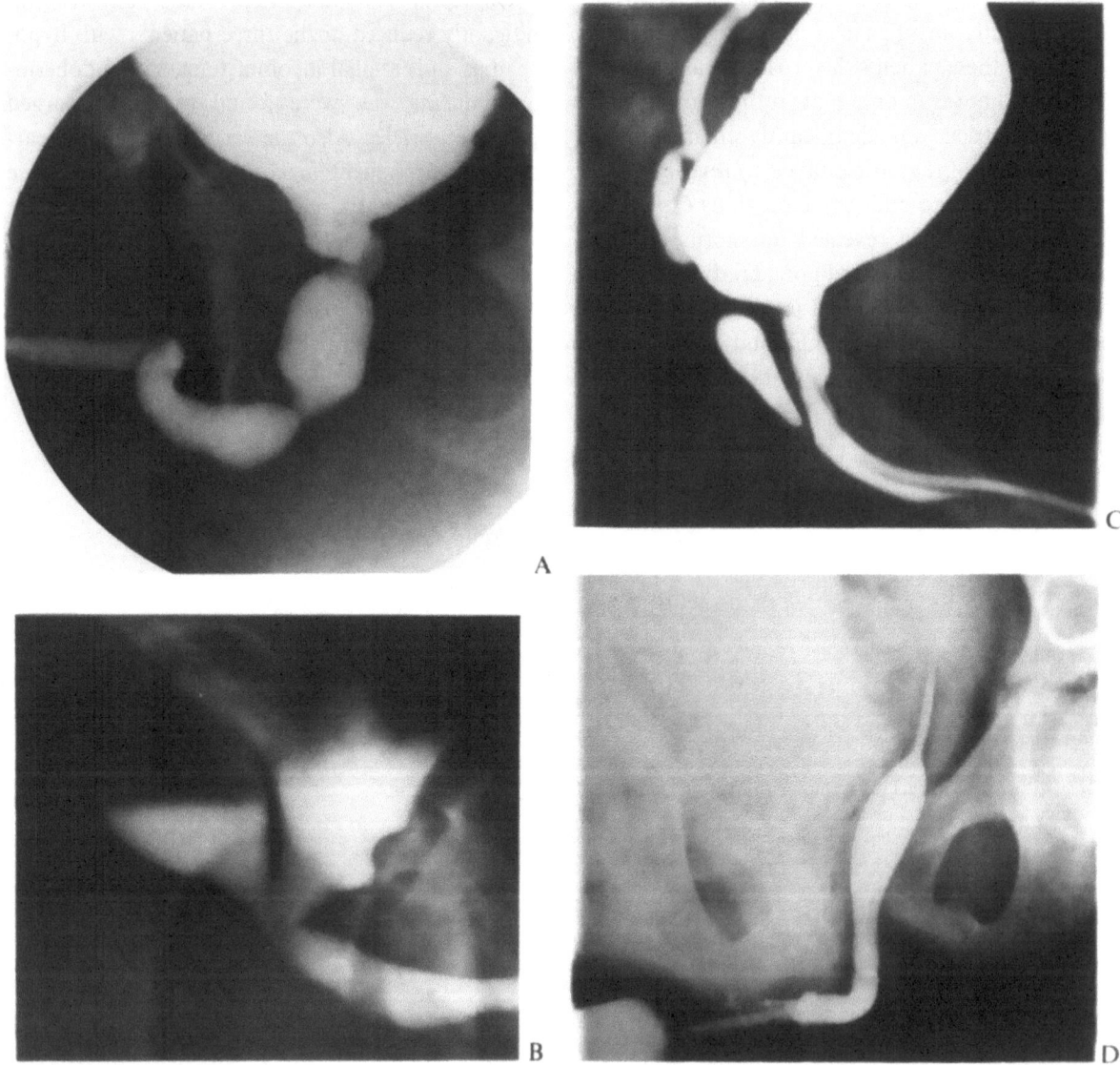

Figure 2. (A) Normal utricle. A tiny wisp of dye is seen posterior to the prostatic urethra in a patient with coronal hypospadias. (B) Larger utricle in a patient with penoscrotal junction hypospadias. Vesicoureteral reflux is also present. (C) Very large utricle in a patient with perineal hypospadias. (D) Vagina masculinus with Müllerian structures in continuity in a patient with mixed gonadal dysgenesis.

the other hand, one patient with severe hypospadias and bilateral cryptorchidism had a normal posterior urethra. In these patients penile hypospadias was not associated with utricular anomalies.

In a series of patients, some with known intersex problems and some reared as hypospadias males who were referred to us for reconstructive surgery and were found here to have intersex problems (Stecker et al., 1978), we also noted a very high incidence of posterior urethral anomalies which included either a hypoplastic prostate and enlarged prostatic utricle, or a vagina masculinus with definite Müllerian duct derivatives (Table 2). Significantly, none of the eight patients had had gonads present in the scrotum at the time of birth. When the utricle was abnormal the prostate seemed to be smaller than would be expected; and the utricle and vagina masculinus joined the urethra at the level of the verumontanum proximal to the external sphincter.

From these data one may infer that the possibility of finding an enlarged prostatic utricle increases with the severity of the hypospadias; and that in patients with penoscrotal and perinal hypospadias, especially if associated with cryptorchidism, the presence of an abnormal saccular cavitation arising from the verumontanum may be an enlarged prostatic utricle or a vagina masculinus. Differential diagnosis would include severe hypospadias without associated intersex, male pseudohermaphroditism, mixed gonadal dysgenesis and true hermaphroditism. The vagina in cases of female pseudohermaphrodites with adrenogenital syndrome, except for those with complete fusion, is located distal to the external sphincter (Jones and Jones, 1954; Rosenberg et al., 1969). Therefore in patients with hypospadias the posterior urethra should be examined carefully with endoscopy and retrograde urethrograms. The presence of a cervix suggests the presence of other unregressed Müllerian duct structures indicating the necessity for exploratory laparotomy.

We will review some concepts about the prostatic utricle, its clinical implications and its embryologic origin. The prostatic utricle is a rudimentary structure present in all males. It is a midline sinus located inside the prostate behind the middle lobe which opens in the prostatic urethra at the top of the verumontanum between the orifices of the ejaculatory ducts. Normally its walls are coapted and it is a virtual cavity which is rarely filled by contrast medium during urethrography or ample enough as to introduce the panendoscope. Usually it is visualized as a dimple which represents its narrow neck. It may have a tubular or saccular configuration and may vary widely in size in normal conditions. As measurement of the prostatic utricle has very rarely been done in a live patient, most of the reports have been done from autopsies. Autopsies of male infants have shown the prostatic utricle to measure 1/2–2/3 the distance from the verumontanum to the base of the prostate (Springer, 1898). Other authors who have examined prostatic utricles in adult patients, both alive and in autopsies, have found a variation of from 6 mm to 20 mm in length (Howard, 1948; Moore, 1937). The width of the utricle as determined by radiologic examination ranges from 4 to 6 mm at the cranial portion and 1 to 2 mm at its opening (Edling, 1949). One researcher found that 4% of newborn male infants and 1% of adult males have enlarged prostatic utricles (Slocum, 1954). Others found seven enlarged prostatic utricles in 678 adult male autopsies (1% incidence) (Moore, 1937) and five enlarged utricles in 70 neonatal autopsies (7%) (Englisch, 1873). The association of hypospadias, incomplete testicular descent and an enlarged prostatic utricle has been recognized for many years (Arnold, 1869; Howard, 1948; Paquin et al., 1957; Shopfner, 1964). However, most of these series report not only patients with simple hypospadias but a significant number of hypospadiac patients with associated cryptorchidism or frank intersex features which seem higher than what one would expect in the unselected hypospadiac population. Cryptorchidism, another relatively frequent disorder of sexual differentiation, occurs in 0.7% of the adult male population (Scorer and Farrington, 1971). When this condition occurs alone it is very rarely associated with an intersex problem. However, the association of hypospadias-cryptorchidism occurs more frequently than expected and is associated with a higher incidence of intersexuality. An incidence of 39% of intersexuality has been found in patients with both conditions (Aarskog, 1970). More recent reports show an incidence of 27% of intersexuality when this association is not accompanied by other evidence of ambiguity and 53% if there is ambiguous genitalia (Rajfer and Walsh, 1976). A series of 280 patients with hypospadias showed eight patients with associated intersex (2.9%). Cryptorchidism was present in 13 of these hypospadiac patients (4.6%), and all eight intersex patients belonged to this group (8/13 = (62%) (Table 3) (Stecker et al., 1978). This series revealed that problems are more likely to be found if cryptorchidism is bilateral rather than unilateral. Severe cases of hypospadias and cryptorchidism may be expected to be associated with intersex in a higher proportion; however, there are cases where the hypospadias is distal in location (Rajfer and Walsh, 1976). In at least 89 reported cases of enlarged prostatic utricles and Müllerian duct cysts, 14 patients (20%) were found to have hypospadias and cryptorchidism and five patients hypospadias alone, 89% of the hypospadias were of a severe degree (Schuhrke and Kaplan, 1978).

Enlarged prostatic utricles are usually asymptomatic unless they achieve a very large size or their communication with the urethra is obliterated. In these cases, symptoms result from compression on the urethra, bladder neck or ureterovesical junctions, or from pooling of urine with subsequent urinary tract infection or calculus formation. Of all the reported cases of utricular and Müllerian duct anomalies, there are many who represent a symptomatic enlarged prostatic utricle and some definite cases of Müllerian duct cysts (Schuhrke and Kaplan, 1978). Most likely this compilation represents cases of two different entities which demonstrate clear clinical and pathologic differences and should be considered separately. Enlarged prostatic utricles are usually seen very early in life and communicate with the urethra through a relatively wide neck. Utricles that have attained large proportions are easily excised, while Müllerian duct cysts usually present in the third or fourth decade of life

as large cystic cavities filled with fluid containing no spermatozoa. They are generally extra prostatic and in most cases do not communicate with the urethra. Moreover these large cysts occur as isolated anomalies in men with otherwise normal external genitalia in contradistinction to enlarged prostatic utricles which are more frequently seen and associated with hypospadias (Myers et al., 1969).

Although some studies have shown a higher incidence of upper urinary tract anomalies in patients with hypospadias (Fallon et al., 1976), not much information can be found on the incidence of lower tract anomalies associated with hypospadias, as routine endoscopy or urethrograms are not done in patients with hypospadias. Urethrograms should be done in all cases of hypospadias, especially to assess the posterior urethra and detect any degree of enlargement of the prostatic utricle or disclose the presence of a vagina (Shopfner, 1964).

4. UTRICULAR ENLARGEMENT: DEVELOPMENTAL CONSIDERATIONS

The importance of the association between hypospadias and an enlarged prostatic utricle resides in two major questions: 1. Does the presence of an enlarged prostatic utricle in a hypospadias patient indicate intersexuality? 2. Is an abnormal cavitation in the prostatic urethra an enlarged prostatic utricle or is it a vagina masculinus? In order to answer these two questions it is necessary to review the embryologic origin of the prostatic utricle and its chronologic relationship with other hormonal and morphologic events in the fetus (Fig. 3). Testicular hormonal synthesis begins at about the eighth week of fetal life when epitheloid interstitial cells (Leydig) containing 3β-hydroxysteroid dehydrogenase appear (Jirasek, 1977). There is a peak in testosterone production at the 12th week correlated with the period of maximal activity of these cells and then a decline as a result of Leydig cell involution until the 20th week when androgen concentration reaches a level similar to that seen in female fetuses (Winter et al., 1977). Differentiation of the Wolffian ducts into male internal genitalia begins at about the eighth week of fetal age. This early virilization represents a local, rather than a systemic effect of testosterone (Jost, 1971), a finding consistent with the observa-

Table 3. Incidence of intersex in hypospadias. Cryptorchidism associated with hypospadias.

No. patients	Testicular maldescent	Intersex	Intersex incidence (%)
272	5	0	
8	8	8	
Total 280	13	8	2.9%

tion that testosterone appears in the testes one to two weeks before serum concentrations begin to rise. Differentiation of the urogenital sinus and the external genitalia depends upon circulating testosterone which is reduced to dihydrotestosterone in these tissues by 5α-reductase. This converting capacity is acquired by these tissues prior to initiation of male differentiation (Siiteri and Wilson, 1974). Testicular secretion during organogenesis is initiated by chorionic gonadotropin (Frawein and Engel, 1974). During the later stages of genital differentiation (12-16 weeks) pituitary luteinizing hormone secretion begins to influence Leydig cell function while chorionic gonadotropin declines. Müllerian-regression factor (MRF) is also secreted by the testicular Sertoli cells (Josso et al., 1977) and this secretion begins immediately after testicular differentiation anteceding both appearance of Leydig cells and the first histologic signs of Müllerian duct regression. This hormone is nonsteroidal and does not have androgenic activity. Production of this hormone is not influenced by chorionic or fetal pituitary gonadotropin, and it persists until late pregnancy with a sharp decline at the time of birth (Donahoe et al., 1976). Responsiveness of a Müllerian duct to this hormone is restricted to a short "critical" period at the end of the undifferentiated stage (Josso et al., 1977).

Müllerian ducts appear in the undifferentiated stage as clefts lined by coelomic epithelium between the gonadal and mesonephric portions of the urogenital ridge at approximately 6 weeks of embryonic development (10 mm). These clefts grow caudally as solid buds of epithelial cells which burrow in the mesenchyme lateral and parallel with the Wolffian ducts. As these buds lengthen, a lumen appears in its cranial part in continuity with the abdominal ostium and extends toward the caudal

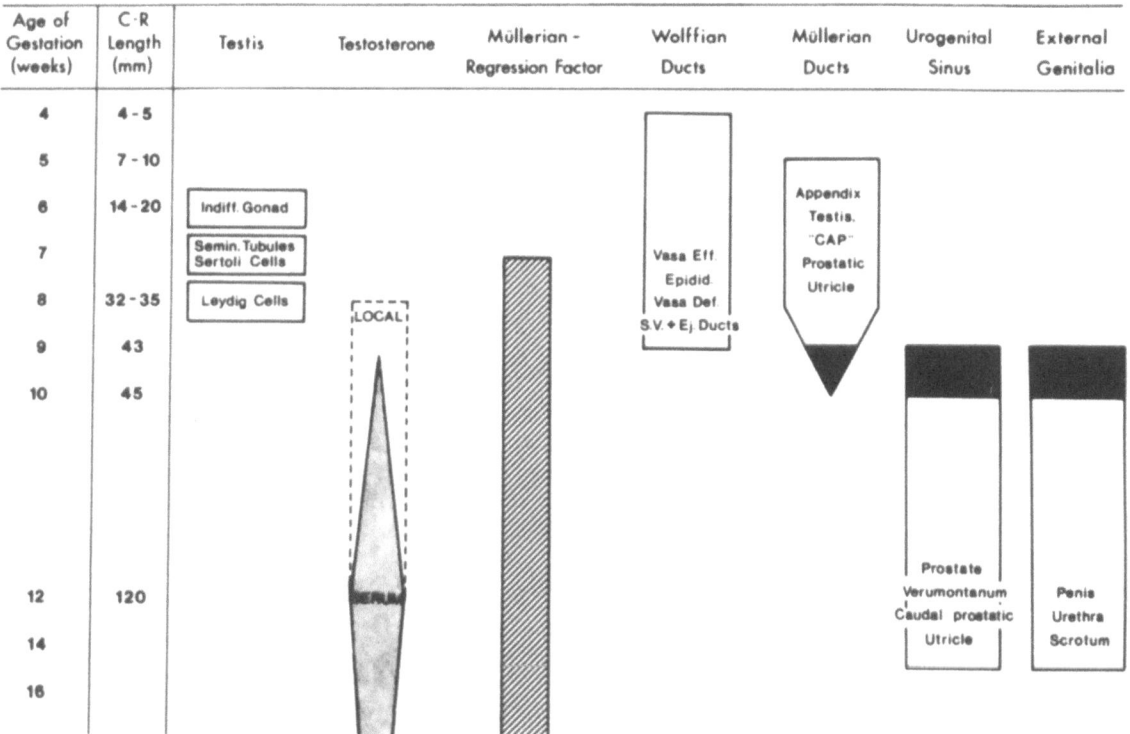

Figure 3. Fetal testicular hormones and male sexual differentiation. The two columns at the left show the age and size of the fetus. Under testis is indicated the sequential development of that organ. Under testosterone, the open column indicates the presence of locally active testosterone, beginning on the eighth week, and the stippled wedge represents increasing serum levels of circulating testosterone. The hatched bar indicates the continuing presence of Müllerian-regression factor from the seventh week on. Under Wolffian ducts, the bar indicates the period of development of the male structures as enumerated. The pointed bar under Müllerian ducts column indicates the regression of the Müllerian duct structures. The bars under urogenital sinus and external genitalia indicate the period of time during which male development takes place. The black areas in the last three columns point out the critical period of overlap where a disorder in development can lead to a large prostatic utricle in association with hypospadias.

194

tip. Both Müllerian ducts curve medially and cross the Wolffian ducts ventrally until they meet in the midline and undergo fusion. At this stage both ducts are separated by a septum which gradually disappears forming a single cavity called the utero-vaginal canal. Although there is a lumen in the cranial portion of this structure, its tip remains solid. In fetuses 30-35 mm C-R length (56-60 days), this tip reaches the entodermal epithelium of the posterior wall of the urogenital sinus causing an elevation known as the Müllerian tubercle (Jirasek, 1977; O'Rahilly, 1977). At the same time there is cellular proliferation in this portion of the urogenital sinus which forms a solid cord and grows cranially until it meets end-on with the tip of a fused Müllerian duct; it is then called the vaginal plate in the female or utricular plate in the male.

In the male embryo regression of the Müllerian ducts is closely related to the development of the ipsilateral testis (Jost, 1971). Degeneration begins at the crossing of the Müllerian duct with the caudal gonadal ligament and extends cranially as well as caudally, never reaching the cranial or caudal ends of the ducts. The cranial end forms the appendix testis; the caudal portion, the utricular plate, re-

mains attached to the proliferation of the urogenital sinus and will contribute to the formation of the prostatic utricle. At stage 43 mm or more all other portions of the Müllerian duct in a male totally disappear (Edling, 1949). The prostatic utricle had been considered a pure Müllerian duct derivative for a long time (Lowsley, 1912), but currently it is thought to be of mixed origin. Careful embryologic studies in male human embryos have recognized the "utricular plate" as a solid epithelial cord arising from the fused tips of the Müllerian ducts. At four months of fetal age there is development of two solid cords of urogenital sinus epithelium which grows into the utricular plate (65 mm). These structures eventually meet, fuse and join the utricular plate of Müllerian origin. A lumen appears in this cord at 5 months forming a hollow structure which is clearly of mixed origin with its cranial portion being from the Müllerian duct and the caudal segment of urogenital sinus origin. Enlargement of the lumen occurs during the fifth month of fetal life shortly followed by hyperplasia of the epithelium and establishment of a stratified squamous pattern (Glenister, 1962).

In the female embryo absence of Müllerian-

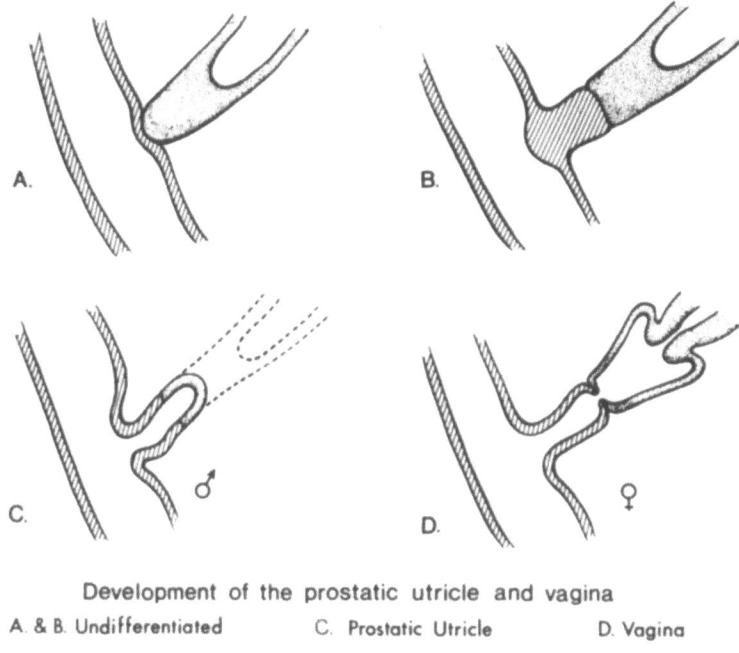

Development of the prostatic utricle and vagina

A. & B. Undifferentiated   C. Prostatic Utricle   D. Vagina

Figure 4. (A) The tip of the fused Müllerian ducts have made contact with the urogenital sinus. (B) A proliferation of urogenital sinus epithelium develops at the site of this contact forming the Müllerian tubercle. (C) Development of the utricle in the male demonstrating the parts derived from Müllerian duct substance and that from the urogenital sinus. (D) Formation of the vagina in the female.

regression factor allows the Müllerian ducts to develop into tubes, uterus and the upper portion of the vagina. There has been considerable controversy about the origin of the female vagina. However, it is currently thought that most of the vagina is a derivative of the urogenital sinus and its cranial portion of the Müllerian ducts (O'Rahilly, 1977; Bulmer, 1957). This theory appears to be corroborated clinically in cases of complete testicular feminization syndrome, and in other cases of severe male pseudohermaphroditism due to defects in androgen synthesis or action where anatomic vaginas or "pseudo-vaginas" can be found in the presence of otherwise completely regressed Müllerian systems (Imperato-McGinley and Peterson, 1976; Wilson et al., 1974; Glenn, 1976) (Fig. 4).

Due to this mixed origin, hormonal imbalances or purely morphogenetic events could influence the formation of the prostatic utricle. There are two hypothetical possibilities: 1. There is a critical embryologic period at the end of the undifferentiated stage when Müllerian ducts begin to regress and Wolffian ducts begin to differentiate as a result of ipsilateral secretion of testicular hormones (testosterone and MRF) which act locally. Müllerian ducts have completely regressed at the ninth to tenth week while male differentiation of the urogenital sinus and urethral groove has started approximately one week before. Thus, there is an overlap in this critical period where any adverse stimulus to the fetal testis may produce a decline or a delay in its hormonal output. When this transient event subsides, the most distal portion of the Müllerian ducts may be insensitive to MRF while the prostate and a portion of the proximal bulbous urethra have had some time left to masculinize but still not enough to close the entire groove. This theory is supported by the chronologic correlation between hormonal and morphogenic events in the fetus, possibly due to a primary testicular problem or delay, and is not related to placental or fetal pituitary deficiency, as in this stage testosterone formation is dependent on chorionic gonadotropin while MRF is not.

2. MRF and Müllerian ducts regression has nothing to do with this event, and the enlarged prostatic utricle in hypospadias is a result of poor androgenic stimulation which fails to fully masculinize the urogenital sinus (prostate) and the urethral groove. Without a well developed prostatic stroma, the prostatic utricle might develop larger than usual. This second theory might be supported by the fact that the male pseudohermaphrodite usually has a small prostate, an enlarged utricle arising from the verumontanum, variable degrees of hypospadias and a lack of Müllerian duct derivatives (uterus and tubes) (Wilson et al., 1974). Also, the higher incidence of utricular enlargement in patients with prune belly syndrome in whom the prostate is hypoplastic and composed of loose mesenchyme would tend to support this second theory. Perhaps both events may be operative in the formation of an enlarged utricle in severe degrees of hypospadias (penoscrotal and perineal) with variable contribution of each one for every individual case. In either case, both events are brought about by a transient decline in fetal testicular function during the critical period of urethral formation. As most hypospadias patients have normal testicular function after birth, are fertile, and do not have pure Müllerian duct derivatives (uterus and tube), these patients could hardly be considered male pseudohermaphrodites. The presence of an enlarged prostatic utricle per se does not mean intersexuality but reflects the severe degree of lack of androgenic stimulation of the urogenital sinus and the urethral groove.

5. CONCLUSIONS

The incidence of enlarged prostatic utricle is higher in patients with penoscrotal or perineal hypospadias than in the general population (22%), especially if there are associated anomalies in testicular descent. Minor degrees of hypospadias are less frequently associated with this anomaly. Although enlarged prostatic utricles are seen frequently in patients with male pseudohermaphroditism, the presence of utricular enlargement in itself does not indicate intersexuality. In patients with hypospadias of any degree, especially if associated with cryptorchidism, the presence of an abnormal cavitation in the prostatic urethra may be due to an enlarged prostatic utricle or a vagina masculinus in continuation with other Müllerian duct derivatives. The presence of a utricle without a cervix would preclude exploratory laparotomy as it would be unlikely that any other Müllerian duct derivatives would be present. Enlarged prostatic utricles, seen in patients with simple hypospadias and male pseudohermaphroditism as well as vagina masculinus found in mixed gonadal dysgenesis, join the prostatic urethra through the verumontanum proximal to the external urinary sphincter in the great majority of cases. Conversely, the vagina in cases of female pseudohermaphroditism, secondary to congenital adrenal hyperplasia, is usually found distal to the external sphincter unless there is complete masculinization (fusion) of the urethra or severe clitoromegaly where it may be proximal.

REFERENCES

Aarskog D (1970) Clinical and cytogenetic studies in hypospadias. Acta Paediat Scand Suppl 203: 1.

Arnold J (1869) Ein Fall von Uterus Masculinus, Angeborner Strictur der Harnrohre und hochgradiger Dilatation der Harnblase and Harnleiter. Virchows Arch Pathol Anat 47: 7.

Brook CGD, Wagner H, Zachmann M, Prader A, Armendares S, Frenk S, Aleman P, Najjar SS, Slim MS, Genton N, Bozic C (1973) Familial occurrence of persistent Müllerian structures in otherwise normal males. Br Med J 1: 771.

Bulmer D (1957) The development of the human vagina. J Anat 91: 490.

Campbell MF (1963) Anomalies of the genital tract. In Campbell MF, ed. Urology, 2nd edn. Philadelphia: W.B. Saunders.

Donahoe PK, Ito Y, Marfatia S, Hendren WH III (1976) The production of Müllerian inhibiting substance by the fetal, neonatal and adult rat. Biol Reprod 15: 329.

Edling NPG (1949) The radiological aspects of the utriculus prostaticus during urethrocystography. Acta Radiol 32: 28.

Englisch J (1873) Zur Pathologie der Harn- und Geschlechtorgane. Med Jahrbucher-Wien.

Fallon B, Devine CJ, Horton CE (1976) Congenital anomalies associated with hypospadias. J Urol 116: 585.

Frawein J, Engel W (1974) Constitutivity of the HCG-receptor protein in the testis of rat and man. Nature 249: 377.

Glenister TW (1962) The development of the utricle and of the so-called "middle" or "median" lobe of the human prostate. J Anat 96: 443.

Glenn JF (1976) Testicular feminization syndrome: current clinical considerations. Urology 7: 569.

Goldman AS (1971) Production of hypospadias in the rat by selective inhibition of fetal testicular 17α-hydroxylase and C-17-20-lyase. Endocrinology 88: 527.

Horton CE, Devine CJ (1972) Hypospadias and epispadias. CIBA Clin Symp 24: No. 3.

Howard FS (1948) Hypospadias with enlargement of the prostatic utricle. Surg Gynecol Obstet 86: 307.

Imperato-McGinley J, Peterson R (1976) Male pseudohermaphroditism: the complexities of male phenotypic development. Am J Med 6: 251.

Jirasek JE (1977) Morphogenesis of the genital system in the human. Birth Defects: Orig Art Ser XIII (2): 13.

Jones HW Jr, Jones GES (1954) Gynecological aspects of adrenal hyperplasia and allied disorders. Am J Obstet Gynecol 68: 1330.

Josso N, Picard JY, Tran D (1977) The anti-Müllerian hormone. Birth Defects: Orig Art Ser XIII (2): 59.

Jost A (1971) Embryonic sexual differentiation (morphology, physiology, abnormalities). In Jones HW Jr, Scott WW, eds. Hermaphroditism, genital anomalies and related endocrine disorders, 2nd edn. Baltimore: Williams & Wilkins.

Lowsley OS (1912) The development of the human prostate gland with reference to the development of other structures at the neck of the urinary bladder. Am J Anat 13: 299.

Moore RA (1937) Pathology of the prostatic utricle. Arch Pathol 23: 517.

Myers GH Jr, Lynn HB, Kelalis PP (1969) Giant cyst of the utricle. J Urol 101: 369.

O'Rahilly R (1977) The development of the vagina in the human. Birth Defects: Orig Art Ser XIII (2): 123.

Paquin AJ Jr, Baker DH, Finby N, Evans JA (1957) The urogenital sinus: its demonstration and significance. J Urol 78: 796.

Rajfer J, Walsh PC (1976) The incidence of intersexuality in patients with hypospadias and cryptorchidism. J Urol 116: 769.

Rosenberg B, Hendren WH, Crawford JD (1969) Posterior urethrovaginal communication in apparent males with congenital adrenocortical hyperplasia. New Engl J Med 280: 131.

Schuhrke TD, Kaplan GW (1978) Prostatic utricle cysts (Müllerian duct cysts). J Urol 119: 765.

Scorer CG, Farrington GH (1971) Congenital deformities of the testis and epididymis, p 19. London: Appleton-Century-Crofts.

Shopfner CE (1964) Genitography in intersexual states. Radiology 82: 664.

Siiteri PK, Wilson JD (1974) Testosterone formation and metabolism during male sexual differentiation in the human embryo. J Clin Endocrinol Metab 38: 113.

Slocum RC (1954) Müllerian duct cysts. Trans SE Sect Am Urol Assoc, pp 26-33.

Springer C (1898) Zur Kenntnis der Cystenbildung aus dem Utriculus Prostaticus. Z Heilk 19: 459.

Stecker JF, Devine PC, Horton CE, Devine CJ (1978) The incidence of underlying intersex in hypospadias. Read at the Mid-Atlantic Section, A.U.A., The Greenbriar, White Sulphur Springs, West Virginia.

Sweet RA, Schrott HG, Kurkland R, Culp OS (1974) Study of the incidence of hypospadias in Rochester, Minnesota, 1940-1970, and a case-control comparison of possible etiologic factors. Mayo Clinic Proc 49: 52.

Wilson JD, Harrod MJ, Goldstein JL, Hemsell DL, MacDonald PC (1974) Familial incomplete male pseudohermaphroditism, Type I: evidence for androgen resistance and variable clinical manifestations in a family with the Reifenstein Syndrome. New Engl J Med 290: 1097.

Winter JSD, Faiman C, Reyes FI (1977) Sex steroid production by the human fetus; its role in morphogenesis and control by gonadotropins. Birth Defects: Orig Art Ser XIII (2): 41.

18. MICROPENIS: ETIOLOGIC AND MANAGEMENT CONSIDERATIONS

S. J. KOGAN

1. INTRODUCTION

The finding of a minute, but otherwise normally formed penis at birth may be seen in a diversity of clinical conditions. Common to all these disorders are abnormalities in the fetal production or handling of testosterone. Examination of normal fetal penile morphogenesis as well as normal fetal hormonal development offers insight into the pathogenesis of micropenis.

2. NORMAL PENILE DEVELOPMENT MAY BE DIVIDED INTO TWO PHASES: EARLY MORPHOGENESIS AND SUBSEQUENT PENILE GROWTH

The embryonic genital tubercle is situated anterior to the urorectal septum in 10–15 mm embryos (5–6 weeks) and becomes surrounded by the labioscrotal swellings. The glans becomes evident, and the genital membrane disintegrates revealing the terminal opening of the urogenital sinus at the phallic base (20 mm, 7-week stage). This indifferent appearance of the phallus remains through the 9th week. The subsequent 4–5 weeks represent a critical period for male penile morphogenesis, during which time masculinization occurs. The phallic urethra forms by fusion of the urethral folds, progressing from the base towards the phallic tip and is completed by approximately 12 weeks (100 mm stage) (Jirasek et al., 1968). At this point, the external genitalia of the male and female fetus are distinguishably different and the fetus may be "sexed" by external observation. Though ventral chordee has been described as a normal phase of phallic development (Kaplan and Lamm, 1975), chordee is absent from normal individuals after birth and

from patients with micropenis.

The size of the penis and clitoris remain approximately equal during the first trimester of human development, measuring between 3.0 and 3.5 mm in length. During the second and third trimester, whereas the clitoris grows slowly, the penis grows at an accelerated rate and undergoes a tenfold increase in size, reaching 35 mm at term (Feldman and Smith, 1975) (Fig. 1).

This marked discrepancy in growth is due to stimulation of the phallus by androgens, mainly testosterone secreted by the fetal testis. Examination of the endocrine causes of this exaggerated growth reveals insights into the pathogenesis of micropenis.

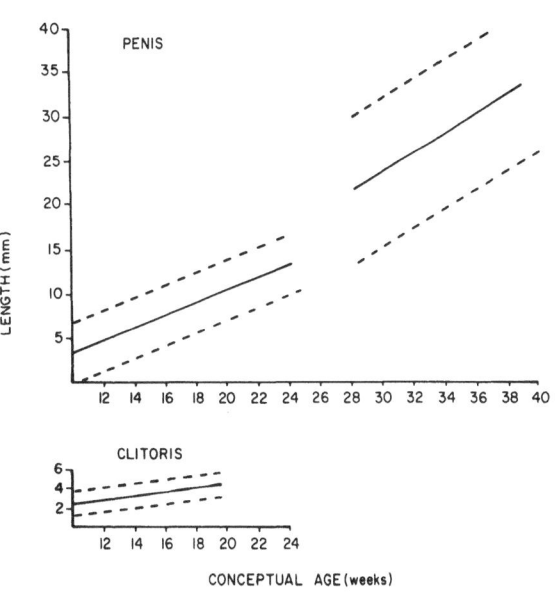

Figure 1. Phallic length of normal formalin-fixed male and female fetuses to 28 weeks, and stretched penile length of newborn premature and term male infants. (Redrawn from Feldman and Smith, 1975, with permission.)

S.J. Kogan and E.S.E. Hafez (eds.), Pediatric andrology, 197–207. All rights reserved.
Copyright © 1981, Martinus Nijhoff Publishers bv, The Hague/Boston/London.

198

3. TESTOSTERONE SECRETED BY THE FETAL TESTIS IS THE STIMULUS FOR NORMAL PENILE FORMATION AND GROWTH

During the first trimester of pregnancy, serum levels of maternal chorionic gonadotropin (CG) peak at 8–10 weeks (Marshall et al., 1968). Fetal serum CG levels closely follow maternal levels, peaking at 8–12 weeks, and slowly declining thereafter to their lowest levels at 17 weeks gestation. During this early critical time of penile organogenesis, fetal pituitary gonadotropins are not yet detectable in significant quantities. Fetal serum LH appears at 11–12 weeks, peaks at 12–16 weeks and declines thereafter (Clements et al., 1976) (see also chapter 2 of this book).

As a result of gonadotropin stimulation, the fetal Leydig cells are noted to differentiate and become hyperplastic (8–9 weeks), and shortly thereafter fetal testicular testosterone levels peak (12 weeks) and fetal serum levels rise, reaching maximum levels

at 13–16 weeks gestation (Winter et al., 1977). Thereafter, fetal testosterone secretion falls to low levels but continues through the last trimester, acting as a continued stimulus to penile growth (Fig. 2).

4. DEFECTIVE HORMONAL SECRETION IS THE CAUSE OF ABNORMAL PENILE DEVELOPMENT AND GROWTH

Both the periods of penile morphogenesis and subsequent growth are dependent on the presence and stimulation of testosterone. Defects in the production or action of testosterone, as well as disorders in the timing of normal endocrine events may affect both morphogenesis and size of the developing penis. Defective testosterone production or action during the first trimester can affect penile morphogenesis, resulting in a small, incompletely formed penis with hypospadias and chordee, and if continued into subsequent trimesters, often continues

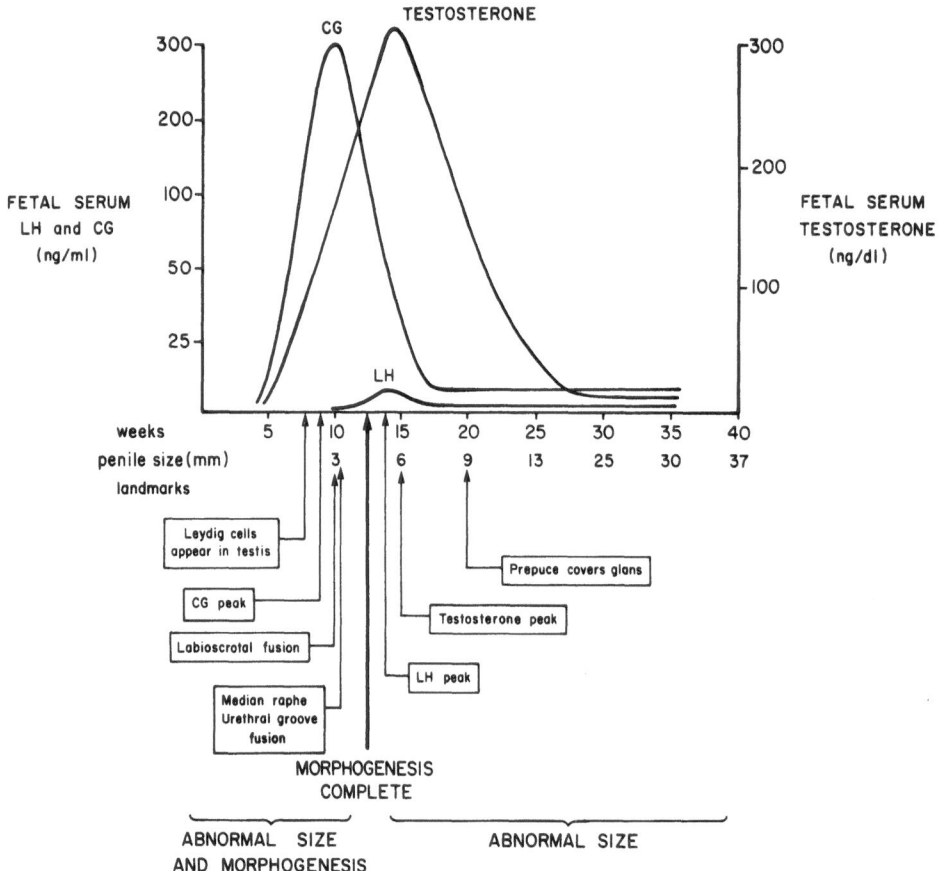

Figure 2. Endocrine and morphogenetic landmarks in penile development. (Data from Winter et al., 1977; Feldman and Smith, 1975, with permission.)

to affect growth as well. Defects in testosterone production or action during subsequent trimesters results in failure of growth of a morphologically normally-formed penis resulting in a micropenis (Fig. 3A, B).

Testosterone levels remain elevated for 2–3 months after birth, then decline to low levels until puberty onset when a second period of increased secretion occurs. There is little penile growth occurring during these earlier years other than that accompanying general body growth. Nevertheless, the penis remains sensitive to androgens as can be seen in situations where androgen excess results in exaggerated penile growth (Fig. 3C).

The necessity of fetal testosterone for normal penile morphogenesis and growth is further substantiated by both animal experimental data as well as observation of various human clinical endocrine disorders. In the rat, an animal in which the late phases of male sexual differentiation, including penile growth, occur in the neonatal period rather than ante-natally, administration of antigonadotropic antiserum during this period results in micropenis formation (Goldman et al., 1972). Similarly, neonatal castration in the rat without testosterone supplementation results in a micropenis (Rajfer et al., 1977; see also chapter 6 of this book). In the human, developmental disorders such as anencephaly, pituitary aplasia, and hypopituitarism may result in a diminutive, but normally formed penis, and conversely in syndromes where other morphogenetic defects occur, micropenis is usually absent. These observations would seem to further substantiate the separate nature of testosterone induced morphogenesis independent of fetal pituitary LH, and testosterone-induced growth, which occurs when CG levels are declining and fetal pituitary LH secretion is operative. Thus, penile size is directly related to the timing and amount of androgen elaborated and the ability to utilize this androgen, and the finding of a micropenis at birth results from misfunction of a complex set of endocrine events resulting in a net fetal deficiency of testosterone.

5. DEFINITIONS, MORPHOMETRIC DATA AND PHYSICAL FINDINGS

Though microphallus (from Greek *mikros*, small; *phallos*, penis) has been more commonly used (Hinman, 1972), *micropenis* is a more descriptive term for this disorder. The objection that "micro" is derived from the Greek, and "penis" is derived from the Latin, hardly seems justified in that "phallus," by general usage has been applied to the male and female organs, and *penis* more accurately describes the male organ.

Micropenis may be defined as a small, but normally formed organ falling beyond 2 standard deviations from the mean size, as described first for older boys (Schonfeld and Beebe, 1942), and thereafter for newborns (Feldman and Smith, 1975). Additional penile morphometric data has been published for normal Israeli (Flatau et al., 1975), East German (Kleintich et al., 1979), and Bulgarian children (Troshev, 1969); and for boys with growth hormone deficiency (Laron and Sarel, 1970) and idiophatic gonadotropin deficiency (Laron et al., 1977). These data are summarized in Table 1. Since the normal newborn stretched penis measures about 3.5 cm with a range of 2.8–4.2 cm (3rd–97th percentile) (Feldman and Smith, 1975), micropenis at birth may be defined as any value falling beyond 2 standard deviations from this measurement, i.e., 2.5 cm or less. Little growth occurs through subsequent years till early puberty where a second accelerated growth period is seen. At this time, it is more difficult to distinguish the "small prepubertal" penis of the boy who may have not yet begun puberty and has a small organ from a true micropenis, and a wider range of "normal" values exists in this age group. In boys whose stage of pubertal development lags behind their chronologic age after the expected time of puberty, comparison of penile length should be made to the prepubertal norms rather than norms for that chronologic age (Lee et al., 1980). These observations may be better understood by reference to a cumulative percentage distribution graph (Fig. 4), which demonstrates the wide range of variation in length seen at the time of puberty.

Measurements based on these data have been summarized in Table 1. Though these values are arbitrary, they would seem to set aside those individuals who would have future problems with gender identity, sexual function, etc. Additionally, it should be re-emphasized that micropenis by definition is restricted to subjects with *normally-formed*

200

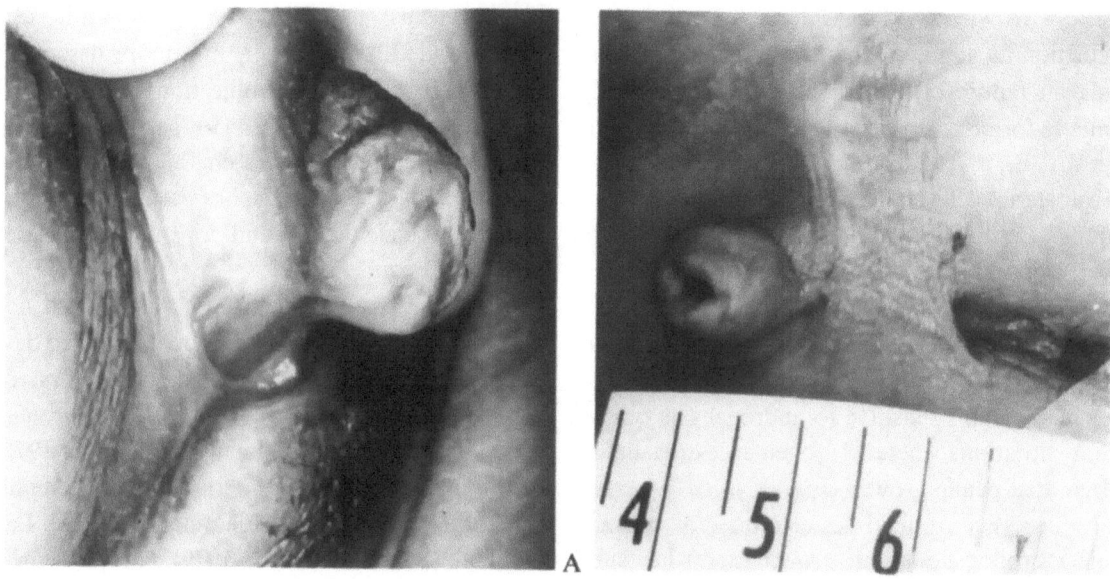

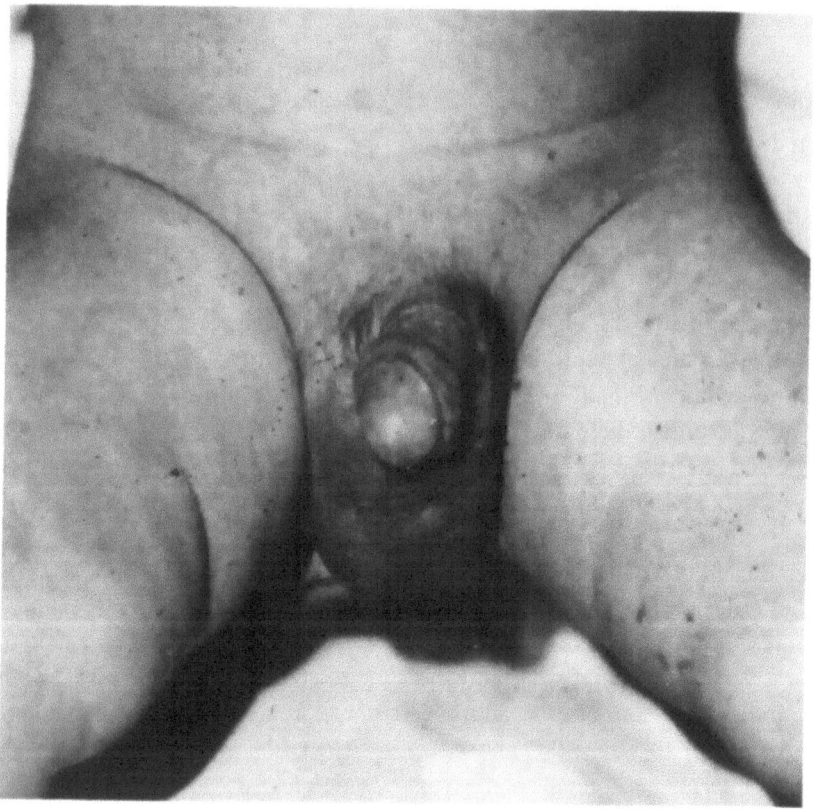

Figure 3. Genital appearance in boys with abnormal penile development. (A) Abnormal morphogenesis (hypospadias, chordee) and abnormally small penis in a boy with male pseudohermaphroditism. (B) Abnormally small, normally formed penis in newborn with micropenis. (C) Abnormal enlarged penis in 2-year-old boy with hamartoma of IIIrd ventricle (LH = 11.8 mIu/ml, testosterone = 236 ng/dl).

Table 1. Mean normal stretched penile length and estimated micropenis length for boys at various ages. Estimated stretched length has been rounded to nearest 0.5 cm to allow for clinically useful scale of measurement. For exact scale of measurement, refer to Schoenfeld and Beebe (1942) and Lee et al. (1980).

Age	Normal	Micropenis	Source
Prepubertal			
Premature (34 weeks)	3.0	2.0	Feldman and Smith (1975)
Birth	3.5	2.5	Feldman and Smith (1975)
Birth	3.5	2.5	Flatau et al. (1975)
Birth	3.11	—	Troshev (1969)
	(? Stretched)		
2 months	3.7	2.5	Schonfeld and Beebe (1942)
1 year	4.3	2.5	Schonfeld and Beebe (1942)
2 years	4.7	3.0	Schonfeld and Beebe (1942)
3 years	5.1	3.5	Schonfeld and Beebe (1942)
5 years	5.7	4.0	Schonfeld and Beebe (1942)
10 years	6.3	4.0	Schonfeld and Beebe (1942)
10 years	5.13	4.0	Kleintich et al. (1979)
Pubertal	see cumulative frequency curve (Fig. 4)		Schonfeld and Beebe (1942)
11-16 years,			
Postpubertal			
Adult	13.3	10.0	Schonfeld and Beebe (1942)

organs, thereby excluding patients with other anatomic abnormalities, i.e., male pseudohermaphrodites with chordee, hypospadias, etc.

The stretched length of the flaccid penis (SPL) offers the most convenient means of reference for penile size and for comparison between subjects. This measurement has been shown to closely correlate with the erected penile length in 150 boys between 3 and 16 years (Schonfeld and Beebe, 1942). Occasionally, the circumferential measurement is important as well, as in cases where the penis may have a visual appearance of length due to the enveloping skin and foreskin, but the corpora are markedly diminished in size. In extreme cases, the penis may consist of nothing more than a skin covered neurovascular bundle. The SPL is determined by direct measurement of the organ from the root of the penis at its junction with the pubis to the tip of the glans, with the penis maximally stretched by traction on its body. Facility with this procedure usually allows for reproducible measurements to be made with no more than a 10% error incurred.

Abnormalities of testicular location and size may be seen in association with micropenis. Undescended testes are quite frequent. In addition, testes may be diminished in size, whether fully or only partially descended. In patients with underlying hypothalamic-pituitary disease associated with their micro-

penis, testicular volume is often no more than 2–3 ml, even in adolescent-aged boys. In the extreme situation, testes may be *minute* in size (the syndrome of "rudimentary testes," Najjar et al., 1974). In virtually all cases, testicular biopsy material examined by conventional microscopy shows immature testes, without other specific abnormalities seen. Peri-tubular hyalinization and interstitial fibrosis, often seen in primary testicular failure, are usually absent (Allen, 1978).

The scrotum is usually normally formed, though diminished in size in these patients, secondary to generalized diminished androgenization as well as the lack of scrotal contents. Scrotal malformation (bifid scrotum, scroto-penile transposition, etc.), are not seen in this disorder, rather they occur in association with various intersexual states, i.e., male pseudohermaphroditism, mixed gonadal dysgenesis, etc. Similarly, Müllerian ductal remnants (vaginal out-pouching) are not seen in patients with micropenis. Vasae and epididymi are usually normally formed, even in extreme cases of testicular hypoplasia (Bergada et al., 1962; Najjar et al., 1974; Grant et al., 1976). These findings re-emphasize the apparently normal function of the fetal testis through the first trimester, and further support the concept that micropenis is a growth-failure related occurrence secondary to later testosterone insufficiency.

202

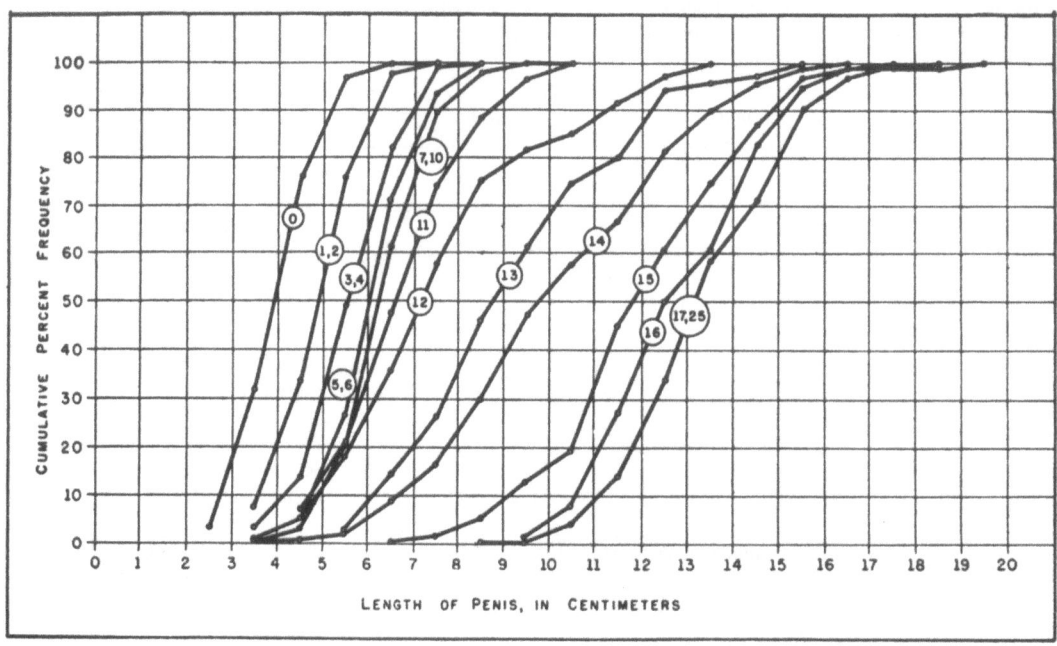

Figure 4. Cumulative percentage frequency curve of length of stretched flaccid penis for each age group from birth to maturity. (From Schonfeld and Beebe, 1942, with permission.)

6. MICROPENIS MAY BE CLINICALLY SEEN AS A MANIFESTATION OF A HETEROGENOUS GROUP OF DISORDERS

A useful clinical means of classification is to group these disorders into those where structural and/or endocrine abnormalities of the hypothalamic-pituitary axis can be identified on the one hand, those having testicular disorders, and those having other isolated sporadic situations resulting in micropenis. It may in fact be that all these have a common denominator of abnormal testosterone production or action but many of these clinical conditions have not been so evaluated. Some of the published syndromes in which micropenis has been described are tabulated in Table 2.

7. CLINICAL ENDOCRINE CHARACTERIZATION OF MICROPENIS PATIENTS HAS AFFORDED CONFIRMATION OF THE PREVIOUSLY DESCRIBED ETIOLOGY OF FETAL ANDROGEN INSUFFICIENCY

Grant et al. (1976), in studying the testosterone response to HCG in prepubertal males with various disorders, found that in his 10 micropenis patients,

all of whom had undescended testes, two groups could be identified: one responsive to short course HCG challenge with a normal rise in plasma testosterone, and another in which the serum testosterone rise was poor (Grant et al., 1976). Allen's patients all showed low plasma testosterone and

Table 2. Clinical syndromes involving micropenis.

Central nervous system disease
Anencephaly
Kallmann's syndrome
Prader-Willi syndrome
Robinow syndrome
Meckel's syndrome
Dwarfisms (Laron and other)
Pituitary aplasia
Hypopituitarism (gonadotropin deficiency, growth hormone deficiency)
Fanconi anemia

Testis
Kleinfelter's syndrome
"Rudimentary testes"
Bjoreson's syndrome
"Idiopathic unresponders to HCG"
Anorchia

Other
Various chromosomal abnormalities
Isolated or idiopathic
Defective genital tubercle

low LH, even in adolescent subjects beyond the expected age of puberty, implying continued hypogonadotropic hypogonadism as the underlying cause. Only one of five tested responded to a short course of HCG, though three of three subjects given a longer course did respond with an appropriate increase in testosterone. All six of his 15 patients over 13 years of age who underwent 24-hour monitoring of their gonadotropin and testosterone secretion showed a flat-line response without the expected nocturnal elevation of serum LH and testosterone (Boyar et al., 1974). All six of the 15 tested showed a normal response to LHRF, indicating normal pituitary responsiveness (Allen, 1978).

Walsh et al. (1978) have defined two groups of patients with micropenis based on measurement of plasma gonadotropins and results of HCG stimulation. In the first group, LH is undetectable, testosterone response to HCG is normal, and a familial history of hypogonadotropic hypogonadism is present. These findings suggest an abnormality in hypothalamic-pituitary function. In the second group, LH was present in detectable amounts, and no increase in testosterone was noted after a short course of HCG. These findings implied a primary testicular abnormality with diminished testosterone production as the cause (Walsh et al., 1978). Burstein et al. (1979) found that nine of 14 boys with micropenis had hypopituitarism with growth hormone deficiency, gonadotropin deficiency or both. In five of the 14, all prepubertal, no endocrinologic abnormality including gonadotropin deficiency could be identified. In all eight patients tested with HCG, a positive testosterone response could be obtained (Burstein et al., 1979).

In a recent series of patients reported with micropenis, 14 of 45 had central nervous system related abnormalities, 11 had primary gonadal pathology, one had partial androgen insensitivity, three had "idiopathic" micropenis, and in 16 the diagnosis could not be established (Lee et al., 1980). Six of these boys were evaluated for androgen production and androgen binding. Five of the six showed inadequate testosterone production at puberty; two with an inadequate HCG response, two with elevated gonadotropins, and one with Kallmann's syndrome. All showed normal androgen binding in fibroblasts of genital skin (Amrhein et al., 1977). Vanelli's patients could be similarly grouped: 12 of

25 had an underlying hypothalamic or pituitary disorder; five had a suspected testicular cause of their micropenis; and in eight, "isolated" micropenis was diagnosed (Vanelli et al., 1979). In these latter patients, testosterone response to HCG, and LH response to LHRF were significantly reduced however; therefore an underlying gonadotropin deficiency which would become more clinically evident later in life could not be ruled out (Vanelli et al., 1979).

Table 3 summarizes the clinical and endocrine findings in seven of our 15 fully characterized patients with micropenis.* Each had undergone formal evaluation of his hypothalamic-pituitary-gonadal axis following luteinizing hormone releasing factor and HCG administration, 24-hour sleep monitoring of their gonadotropin and testosterone secretion (Boyar et al., 1973, 1974), and evaluation of other pituitary functions. Indications for testing in these adolescent patients were a markedly diminuitive penis conforming to the previous definition of a micropenis, resulting in enough psychologic unrest to prompt physician consultation.

These data serve to reiterate the heterogenous nature of the patient population seen in this syndrome. Though initially it would appear that different populations have been characterized, careful analysis suggests that such may not be the case. It is conceptually useful to categorize these patients as having central nervous system related disease, primary testicular disease or "other" causes of their micropenis, though hypogonadotropic hypogonadism will be seen in a majority of patients. Even this diagnosis may not be entirely reliable based on one evaluation however, as shown by one of our patients who at age nine initially had undetectable LH and FSH levels and low plasma testosterone and was suspected of having hypogonadotropic hypogonadism, only to subsequently have spontaneous LH elevations, puberty onset and penile growth at age 12. Similarly, one of Allen's patients initially described as being hypogonadotropic subsequently developed spontaneous LH elevations (Allen, personal communication).

Endocrine evaluation would best serve to identify patients with a normal hypothalamic-pituitary-

* Kleinfelter's syndrome and anorchic patients not included in this tabulation.

Table 3. Clinical and endocrine findings in seven patients with micropenis

Patient	Chronologic age	Bone age	Pubertal stage	Height/weight percentiles	Testes	ENDOCRINE DATA LH (mIu/ml) baseline	peak++	FSH baseline	peak++	Testosterone (ng/dl) baseline	peak§	Comment
1	9^{10}	9^6	1	25%/60%	Bilateral orchidopexy, both 1 ml	n-d+ *	14.5	n-d+ *	11.5	18	1476	– initially thought to have hypo-gonadotropic hypogonadism – spontaneous LH elevation and penile growth and puberty occurred
2	11^{10}	11^6	1	10%/10%	Left orchidopexy, both 1 ml	2.9+	8.2	2.3+	9.5	10	16	– marked growth retardation – associated midline craniofacial defects – borderline abnormal growth hormone testing
3	12^{10}	12^0	2	80%/95%	Descended both 1 ml	5.7+	10.3	12.3+	17.9	2	68	– marked obesity – brother of patient no. 6 – blunted but reactive LHRF response – other pituitary function tests normal
4	13^{10}	13^0	1	60%/95%	Descended both 1 ml	9.0+	44.4	11.7+	26.7	12	228	– obese – normal endocrine testing
5	15^0	13^0	1	5%/95%	Right minute, left descended, 2 ml	4.2+ (1975) 8.8 (1979)	10.4	1.1+ 14.3	18.6	– 12	– 15	– growth hormone deficiency – blunted LHRF and HCG response, even after chronic HCG administration
6	15^6	15^6	2	10%/95%	Descended, 1 ml	9.4+	65	13.2+	20.2	169	205	– brother of patient no. 3 – normal evaluation – normal penile growth expectation when puberty onset occurs
7	18^0	18^6	3	10%/80%	Bilateral orchidopexy, 2 ml	6.4+ 3.6	– 6.0	5.8+ 2.6	– 7.5	6 35*	26 –	– impaired smell, probable Kallman syndrome

* Random sampling; + 24-hour pooled serum sampling; ++ Following LHRF (100 $\mu g/m^2$); § Following HCG (1500 U × 3 doses); n.d. = non-detectable.

gonadal axis and those with defective testosterone synthesis secondary to a primary testicular problem. Androgen insensitivity (defective end-organ utilization of androgen) seems extraordinarily uncommon as a cause of a diminutive normally formed penis. The remaining group will more than likely have hypogonadotropic hypogonadism. These characterizations may have implications affecting therapy of the micropenis, especially in the newborn where removal of the penis and gender reversal may sometimes be considered. Additionally, identification of associated covert pituitary dysfunction is obviously important.

8. GROWTH POTENTIAL AND THERAPEUTIC MODALITIES

Since the causes of micropenis in these patients are diverse, one might expect that growth potential of these penes may be different. Indeed, in the past a diversity of growth responses has been obtained from various instituted therapeutic methods. More recently, improved overall growth responses have been reported resulting from better understanding of the endocrine pathogenesis of micropenis and standardization of therapy. The basis for these improvements may be found in some recent investigations. The first relates to the understanding that for the most part the micropenis remains androgen-sensitive, at least early in life. In a series of experiments investigating the normal penile growth process in the rat, it was found that neonatal castration would produce a micropenis in the adult, and this could be prevented by simultaneous testosterone or dihydrotestosterone administration (Rajfer et al., 1977). Topical testosterone cream applied to the penis, as well as systemic testosterone, would maintain normal penile size in castrated weanling rats but would not result in a greater than normal penile size in the adult, nor could this therapy increase the adult rat penis beyond the normal (Jacobs et al., 1975, 1977). These findings were also observed in the human. The majority of Allen's treated cases of micropenis were testosterone-responsive (Allen, 1978). All patients in another recent series responded to intramuscular testosterone with eventual normalization of penile size for that age, though in some cases two courses of treatment were required.

Skeletal maturation remained normal in this group (Burstein et al., 1979). These observations contrast with the findings in male pseudohermaphrodites with incomplete male virilization, where androgen insensitivity appears to be not uncommon (Amrhein et al., 1977; Savage et al., 1978; Griffin and Wilson, 1980).

The second important therapeutic consideration relates to the reality that penile growth capacity is age-related, and that there is a progressive loss of growth capacity with increasing age. This intuition for early treatment has pervaded the micropenis literature, but with scant documentation on any factual basis. It has been shown that the ability of fibroblasts from human genital skin (including penile body and prepuce) to convert testosterone to dihydrotestosterone, the biologically active metabolite in the penis, occurs maximally at age three months and falls progressively thereafter (Wilson and Walker, 1969). In this issue, new data are presented showing the progressive linear diminution in 5α reductase capacity and cytoplasmic androgen receptor activity in the rat penis with aging, suggesting that this may be the limiting factor in penile growth (Rajfer et al., chapter 6 of this book). Treatment of the adult rat with testosterone or dihydrotestosterone does not result in a larger than normal penis (Jacobs et al., 1975, 1977; Rajfer et al., 1977). Testosterone administered to normal adult human males fails to increase penile size; if administered to castrated young adults, penile growth will occur normally and then cease (Turner, 1950). Adults with micropenis given systemic testosterone will fail to enlarge their penis (Kogan, personal observation). These observations would seem to confirm the age-limited growth capacity of the penis and would suggest that when testosterone therapy is to be utilized in the treatment of micropenis, it should be utilized early in life.

A third consideration relating to therapy is the recognition that systemic testosterone appears to be the most effective method of treatment. In the past, both topical and systemic testosterone have been used (Guthrie et al., 1973; Jacobs et al., 1975; Klugo and Cerny, 1978). Response to topical therapy is variable. Systemic elevations of plasma testosterone have been documented during topical therapy so the therapeutic response may at least in part be secondary to absorption, and topical testosterone offers no advantage over systemic administration (Jacobs et al., 1975, 1977; Smith, 1977). Certainly, the excellent growth that has been achieved under controlled systemic administration without adversely affecting skeletal maturation attests to the efficacy of this approach. Repeated short courses may be required through early life to maintain normal size until the maximal (pre-determined) growth potential is reached (Burstein et al., 1979). Testosterone may be given in 25–50 mg doses (as the intramuscular preparation) in children every three to four weeks over a 3-month period. Careful monitoring of skeletal maturation during therapy is essential.

HCG has also been used for therapy of micropenis but offers no special advantage. Testosterone responses may be variable; additionally, hypogonadotropic patients may take prolonged periods of time before responding to exogenous HCG (Boyar et al., 1973). Intranasal LHRF, utilized for therapy of undescended testes, may represent a more physiologic means of treating micropenis on a chronic basis, especially in view of the frequent finding of hypogonadotropic hypogonadism. To date this has not been tried, however.

Other considerations beside age and method of treatment which enter into decision-making with each patient are the actual size of the penis and the status of the patient's testes, especially for the neonate. The extreme micropenis without corporal substance will never grow to a useful organ. When associated with rudimentary nubbins of testes, a similar poor prospect for growth can be expected. Conversely, patients with reasonably normal testicular volumes can be expected to have a good response, and some spontaneously virilize at puberty with normalization of penile size (Kogan and Williams, 1977).

If the details of *how* patients should be treated appear well worked out, the details of *which* patients should be so treated remain more evasive.

Disappointing results of past treatment have led some to recommend castration and gender reversal surgery in all but the least extreme cases. In a recent reference to 40 patients with micropenis who had long-term follow up, review of the 30 patients reared as males lead the authors to conclude that these patients would have fared better if they had been reared as females (Jones et al., 1978). This impression is further reemphasized by the findings in long-term psychologic follow up of these patients who have an inadequate organ in adulthood where significant psychopathology has been manifest (Money, personal communication). In the other children where the sex of rearing is well established and where gender identity has been fixed, therapy should be instituted as early in life as possible. The newborn with micropenis represents the problem: to decide what the growth potential of the newborn penis may be, and for its capacity to sustain growth in the future. Extremes of size at either end of the spectrum should constitute no problem in clinical decision making. Intermediate sizes constitute the great problem as to whether maintainence in the male gender with repeated courses of testosterone will result in an "adequate" adult male, or whether early gender reversal offers a more acceptable long range solution. Penile size, associated testicular pathology (structural and/or endocrine) and responsiveness to a diagnostic/therapeutic trial of neonatal intramuscular testosterone constitute the determining factors. The efficacy of this approach, as contrasted with that recommended by those who favor gender reversal, can only be determined after current testosterone treated micropenis patients reach adulthood.

ACKNOWLEDGEMENT

The technical skills of Mr. G. Tannis, Mrs. C. DeVitto and Mr. B. Mordin for their medical photography and medical illustration are acknowledged.

REFERENCES

Allen TA (1978) Microphallus: clinical and endocrinological characteristics. J Urol 119: 750.

Amrhein JA, Myer WJ, Danish RK, Migeon CJ (1977) Studies of androgen production and binding in 13 male pseudohermaphrodites and 13 males with micropenis. J Clin Endocrinol Metab 45: 732.

Bergada C, Cleveland WW, Jones HW Jr, Wilkins L (1962) Variants of embryonic testicular dysgenesis: bilateral anorchia and the syndrome of rudimentary testes. Acta Endocrinol (Copenhagen) 40: 521.

Boyar RM, Finkelstein JW, Witkin M, Kapen S, Weitzman E, Hellman L (1973) Studies of endocrine function in "isolated" gonadotropin deficiency. J Clin Endocrinol Metab 36: 64.

Boyar RM, Rosenbeld RS, Kapen S, Finkelstein JW, Roffwarg

HP, Weitzman ED, Hellman L (1974) Human puberty, simultaneous augmented secretion of luteinizing hormone and testosterone during sleep. J Clin Invest 54: 609.

Burstein S, Grumbach MM, Kaplan SL (1979) Early determination of androgen-responsiveness is important in the management of microphallus. Lancet 2: 983.

Clements JA, Reyes FI, Winter JSD, Faiman C (1976) Studies on human sexual development. III. Fetal pituitary and serum, and amniotic fluid concentration of LH, CG, and FSH. J Clin Endocrinol Metab 42: 9.

Feldman KW, Smith DW (1975) Fetal phallic growth and penile standards for newborn male infants. J Pediat 86: 395.

Flatau E, Josefsberg Z, Reisner SH, Bialik O, Laron Z (1975) Penile size in the newborn infant. J Pediat 87: 663.

Goldman BD, Quadagno DM, Shryne J, Gorski RA (1972) Modification of phallus development and sexual behavior in rats treated with gonadotropin antiserum neonatally. Endocrinology 90: 1025.

Grant DB, Laurance BM, Atherden SM, Ryness J (1976) HCG stimulation test in children with abnormal sexual development. Arch Dis Child 51: 596.

Griffin JE, Wilson JW (1980) The syndromes of androgen resistance. New Engl J Med 302: 198.

Guthrie RD, Smith DW, Graham CB (1973) Testosterone treatment for micropenis during early childhood. J Pediat 83: 247.

Hinman F Jr (1972) Microphallus: characteristics and choice of treatment from a study of 20 cases. J Urol 107: 499.

Jacobs SC, Kaplan JW, Gittes RF (1975) Topical testosterone therapy for penile growth. Urology VI: 708.

Jacobs SC, Judd HM, Gittes RF (1977) Penile growth: topical vs. systemic testosterone therapy in rats. J Endocrinol 73: 189.

Jirasek JE, Raboch J, Uher J (1968) The relationship between the development of gonads and external genitalia in the human fetus. Am J Obstet Gynecol 101: 830.

Jones HW Jr, Park IJ, Rock JA (1978) Technique of surgical sex reassignment for micropenis and allied conditions. Am J Obstet Gynecol 132: 870.

Kaplan JW, Lamm DL (1975) Embryogenesis of chordee. J Urol 114: 769.

Kleintich B, Hadziselimovic F, Hesse V, Schrieber G (1979) Kongenitale Hodendystopien, p 125 Leipzig: VEB Georg Thieme.

Klugo RC, Cerny JC (1978) Response of micropenis to topical testosterone and gonadotropin. J Urol 119: 667.

Kogan SJ, Williams DI (1977) The micropenis syndrome: clinical observations and expectations for growth. J Urol 118: 311.

Laron Z, Sarel R (1970) Penis and testicular size in patients with growth hormone insufficiency. Acta Endocrinol 63: 625.

Laron Z, Kaushanski A, Josefsberg Z (1977) Penile size and growth in children and adolescents with isolated gonadotrophin deficiency. Clin Endocrinol 6: 265.

Lee PA, Mazur T, Danish R, Amrhein J, Blizzard RM, Money J, Migeon CJ (1980) Micropenis. I. criteria, etiologies and classification. Johns Hopkins Med J 146: 156.

Marshall JR, Hammond CB, Ross JT, Jacobson A, Rayford P, Odell WD (1968) Plasma and urinary CG during early human pregnancy. Obstet Gynecol 32: 760.

Najjar SS, Takla RJ, Nassar VH (1974) The syndrome of rudimentary testes: occurrence in 5 siblings. J Pediat 84: 119.

Rajfer J, Coffey DS, Walsh PC (1977) Effects of hormones in newborn period on the development of the penis. Surg Forum 28: 570.

Savage MO, Chaussain JL, Evain D, Roger M, Canlorbe P, Job JC (1978) Endocrine studies in male pseudohermaphroditism in childhood and adolescence. Clin Endocrinol 8: 219.

Schonfeld WA, Beebe GW (1942) Normal growth and variation in the male genitalia from birth to maturity. J Urol 48: 759.

Smith DW (1977) Micropenis and its management. In Blandau RJ, Bergsma D, eds. Morphogenesis and malformation of the genital system, National Foundation-March of Dimes, Birth Defects: Orig Art Ser, Vol XIII, No. 2, p 147 New York: Alan R. Liss.

Troshev K (1969) Contribution to the anthropometric study of the penis in a group of Bulgarian boys from birth to the age of 7 years. Acta Chir Plast (Praha) 11: 140.

Turner HH (1950) The clinical use of testosterone, Thompson WO, ed. Springfield: Charles C. Thomas.

Vanelli M, Chaussain JL, Vassal J, Job JC (1979) L'insuffisance du developpement de la verge (micropenis) Arch Franc Pediat 36: 471.

Walsh PC, Wilson JD, Allen TD, Madden JD, Porter JC, Neaves WB, Griffin JE, Goodwin WE (1978) Clinical and endocrinological evaluation of patients with congenital microphallus. J Urol 120: 90.

Wilson JD, Walker JD (1969) The conversation of testosterone to 5α-androstan-17β-ol-3-one (dihydrotestosterone) by skin slices of man. J Clin Invest 48: 371.

Winter JSD, Faiman C, Reyes FI (1977) Sex steroid production by the human fetus: its role in morphogenesis and control by gonadotropins. In Blandau RJ, Bergsma D, eds. The National Foundation-March of of Dimes, Birth Defects: Orig Art Ser, Vol XIII, No. 2, p 41 New York: Alan R. Liss.

CONCLUDING REMARKS

E. S. E. HAFEZ

1. PHYSIOLOGY OF MORPHOGENESIS AND SEXUAL DIFFERENTIATION

The sex of the fetus is an inherited characteristic carried by the genetic material of the X and Y chromosomes. The combination of the sex chromosomes is fixed at the time of fertilization and is normally transmitted unchanged to all subsequent somatic cells of a given individual. Although a specific sex is thus built into the cells, the transfer of the sex determining genes seems to have been discharged by the formation of the ovary or testis. Whereas the term fetus may indicate immature function of many organ systems, it has a relatively mature hypothalamic-pituitary-gonadal axis. Active testicular function, with the secretion of Müllerian Inhibitory Factor and testosterone, is necessary in early fetal life for male differentiation. At first fetal testosterone secretion is mediated by placental hCG, but in later fetal life pituitary LH also plays a role. Pituitary FSH and LH also appear to be involved in germ cell and Sertoli cell development and testicular descent. Several anomalies of fetal testicular function may lead to ambiguous sexual differentiation, while deficiencies of hypothalamic or pituitary function present in the male with normally formed but hypotrophic genitalia. More subtle disorders of fetal endocrine function may be associated with some unexplained problems of postnatal reproductive function.

Further research is needed to evaluate the extent during fetal life or infancy exposure to exogenous sex steroids and other environmental agents can interfere with the normal pattern of reproductive endocrinology.

The embryonic genital tubercle is situated anterior to the urorectal septum in 10–15 mm embryos (5–6 weeks) and becomes surrounded by the labio-scrotal swellings. The glans becomes evident, and the genital membrane disintegrates revealing the terminal opening of the urogenital sinus at the phallic base (20 mm, 7-week stage). This indifferent appearance of the phallus remains through the 9th week.

Complete differentiation of male external and internal genitalia requires the secretion of three hormones: anti-Müllerian hormone, testosterone, and dihydrotestosterone. Anti-Müllerian factor (MIF) (MIS), and testosterone are secretory products of the fetal testis. Anti-Müllerian hormone causes regression of the Müllerian ducts, the anlage of the uterus, oviducts and upper vagina. Testosterone stabilizes the Wolffian ducts and permits the development of the Wolffian ducts into vasa deferentia, epididymides, and seminal vesicles. For the development of the prostate from the urogenital sinus and the development of the male external genitalia from the genital tubercle, genital folds and genital swelling, dihydrotestosterone is required. Therefore, testosterone acts only as a prohormone and it has to be metabolized peripherally by steroid 5α-reductase to dihydrotestosterone for the development of these structures.

The steroid environment plays a major role in the development of morphology and function of the brain. The various hormone sensitive aspects of human brain development which may be demonstrated in the future will differ in their sensitivity to hormones, the time course of their development, as well as the specific neural loci involved. It is likely that morphological sex differences do exist in the human brain, although even more so than in the laboratory animal, the role of the hormone environment vis-a-vis genomic factors or other environmental influence will be difficult to establish. If brain sexual differentiation occurs prenatally in

S.J. Kogan and E.S.E. Hafez (eds.), Pediatric andrology, 209–213. All rights reserved.
Copyright © 1981, Martinus Nijhoff Publishers bv, The Hague/Boston/London.

man, the existence of protective mechanisms would seem most probable. However, current evidence suggests that α-fetoprotein is not the mechanism since in man this protein does not bind estrogen. The finding that hormonal titers at puberty may influence psychosexual differentiation is consistent with the present view that even in the rat, at least under certain circumstances, the hormone environment well beyond the perinatal period can have permanent, perhaps "morphotropic" effects.

LH-RH, which inhibits gonadotropin secretion, increases MIF production. Replacement with FSH returns MIF values to normal, suggesting indirectly that FSH inhibits the production of MIF, and that, MIF appears to be under the control of the hypothalamic-pituitary axis. MIF secretion is not affected by irradiation during late gestation when germ cells are destroyed but Sertoli cells are spared. There is indirect evidence to support that Sertoli cells produce MIF.

The presence of the Müllerian Inhibiting Factor as a unique fetal regressor has been demonstrated by in vivo and in vitro organ culture techniques. The finding that a human ovarian cancer can respond to fractions that cause Müllerian duct regression in the embryo implies the presence of Müllerian Inhibiting Substance receptors on the tumor. Future research is needed for the isolation, purification, and synthesis of the fetal regressor; not only for better understanding of the congenital anomalies associated with ambiguous genitalia, but also because the purified substance may have potential value as a chemotherapeutic agent for tumors of Müllerian duct origin.

2. CHROMOSOMAL ANOMALIES AND INTERSEXUALITY

Recent advances in chromosome analysis and increased understanding of the principles of sexual development have stimulated interest in problems of intersexuality and encouraged identification and treatment of the intersexual patient at an early age so as to permit a more normal life. Abnormal sexual development has been classified, with emphasis on pathology and neoplastic conditions, into disorders with apparently normal sex chromosomes, and disorders associated with abnormal sex chromo-

somes. For example, female pseudohermaphroditism includes adrenogenital syndrome, administration of progestins or androgens to the mother, and maternal virilizing tumors, whereas male pseudohermaphroditism includes primary CNS defect, testicular regression syndrome, Leydig cell agenesis, defects in testosterone synthesis, defect in Müllerian Inhibiting Substance, androgen insensitivity syndrome (testicular feminization), and 5α-reductase deficiency. Disorders associated with abnormal sex chromosomes include Klinefelter's syndrome, Turner's syndrome, mixed gonadal dysgenesis (MGD) and true hermaphroditism. This classification, based upon gonadal and genital anatomy, chromosomal composition and specific identifiable genetic or metabolic defects, represents the spectrum of intersexual conditions in a comprehensive manner, while grouping those classes of patients who are at high risk for development of neoplasia if their gonads are not removed prophylactically.

The syndromes of male hermaphroditism have been classified according to etiology: (a) chromosomal defects affecting masculinization, (b) defects in the central nervous system affecting the production of gonadotropins; (c) defects of the synthesis of testosterone in the fetal gonads; and (d) defects of the end organ utilization of substrate.

With the discovery of hermaphroditic disorders based on chromosomal constitution or on endocrine production, metabolism, and utilization, it is possible to determine whether or not there is a relationship between any of these etiologic factors and the differentiation and development of gender identity role (G-I/R) in cases of male hermaphroditism. Some infants born as male hermaphrodies have been assigned and reared as males, others as females. Thus, the syndromes of hermaphroditism provide an opportunity to assess the relative contribution of chromosomal, prenatal hormonal, pubertal hormonal and sociocultural events on G-I/R differentiation and erotosexual status.

The syndromes of male hermaphroditism are characterized by ambiguity of the genital organs and the presence of testicular tissue, typically in a 46, XY chromosomal individual. The role of the H-Y antigen explains, in part, testicular development in a 45, X or 46, XX male. Normally the Y chromosome directs testicular organization in the fetal gonad through the action of H-Y antigen, a cell surface, or plasma membrane protein. In some instances, Y chromosomal material is detached from its normal position on cells; the H-Y antigen is expressed nonetheless, organizing testicular tissue in an individual without the expected 46, XY karyotype. There is considerable controversy regarding the presence of H-Y antigen and testicular development in male hermaphroditism.

Male pseudohermaphrodites with steroid 5α-reductase deficiency are remarkable experiments of nature for evaluating the relative influence of androgens (in particular testosterone) as compared to the sex of rearing in determining male gender identity. Testosterone levels in utero, the neonatal period and at puberty are normal; and theoretically testosterone exposure of the brain proceeds as in normal males. However, because of decreased 5α-dihydrotestosterone production in utero, there is such marked ambiguity of the external genitalia at birth that many affected patients are thought to be females and raised as girls. These patients are therefore testosterone exposed and responsive males born with female appearing external genitalia and raised as girls. Normal testosterone exposure of the brain, in utero, the early neonatal period, and at puberty, are important contributing factors in the formation of a male gender identity. Thus, in addition to socio-cultural factors androgens contribute to male gender identity development in man. These patients demonstrate that without physician, family or other socio-cultural factors acting to interrupt the natural sequence of events, the testosterone mediated sex predominates; over-riding the female sex of rearing. Thus male gender identity is not fixed during early childhood but is continually expanding, becoming confirmed during or following the testosterone activation of puberty.

Several in vitro and clinical investigations have been conducted on the H-Y antigen, to evaluate the genetic basis of abnormal gonadal differentiation. In vitro studies included H-Y as the mammalian testis inducer, indications for the H-Y gonadal receptor, and indications for a stable anchorage site for H-Y antigen. The clinical studies H-Y antigen in male pseudohermaphroditism, testicular feminization syndrome (TFS), 17α-hydroxylase deficiency, 5α-reductase deficiency, unclassified male pseudohermaphroditism in 45, X/46, XYq-phenotypic female with ambiguous genitalia, H-Y phenotype:

androgen mediated effects, XX true hermaphrodites, XX males, a note on gonadal growth rates, suppressed production of HY antigen deletion of H-Y genes, mosaicism, loss of receptor binding activity, and mutational deficiency of the H-Y receptor.

3. ANOMALIES OF THE TESTIS

Cryptorchidism, disturbance of testicular descent, is frequently associated with infertility. The main etiologic factor in the development of cryptorchidism is impaired gonadotropin secretion during intrauterine and postnatal life. The transformation of the Wolffian duct into epididymis and its differentiation is responsible for testicular descent, whereas the gubernaculum has no active role in this process. The Leydig cells play a major role in testicular descent. Impaired stimulation of the Leydig cells leads to impared testosterone secretion and cryptorchidism. Endocrine treatment of cryptorchidism is initiated with LH-RH (1.2 mg LH-RH nasal spray daily for 4 weeks).

Maldescended testis comprises two different syndromes: dystopia and ectopia. In dystopia the testis is obstructed at some physiological site during its descent whereas in ectopia the testes are located in a pathological site. The most frequent syndrome is the ectopia epifascialis in which the testicle after passing the outer inguinal ring slips upwards and is palpable as it is lying on the aponeurosis of the musculus abdominis externus directly underneath the skin. The other locations, "ectopia perinealis", "penilis" and "femoralis", are quite rare. Dystopia syndromes are treated hormonally whereas ectopia syndromes are treated surgically.

Spermatogenesis in the undescended testis is already damaged during the second year of life and not between the 5th and 10th year of life as previously stated. Thus hormonal or surgical treatment should be commenced prior to the third year of life if spermatogenesis and future fertility are to be protected. It is possible to manipulate the descent in more than half of the patients by giving gonadotropins alone. Even in patients with unilateral maldescent there are considerable chances of successful treatment with HCG.

Leydig cell tumor of the testis is a non-germinal

neoplasm accounting for 1-2% of all testicular tumors. These endocrine active testicular tumors pose interesting management problems in boys. The distinction between an isolated Leydig cell tumor of the testis and endocrine active testicular tumors associated with congenital adrenal hyperplasia may sometimes be difficult. In addition, the cellular origin of both of these clinical entities has been debated. In order for clinicians to accurately treat both of these disorders, a clear understanding of the distinguishing features is necessary.

4. ANOMALIES OF THE REPRODUCTIVE TRACT

Extensive endocrine and genetic investigations have been conducted on the developmental patterns of urogenital tract with emphasis on the interaction between epithelium and mesenchyme during development and function of urogenital organs. Full comprehension of the mechanisms of urogenital morphogenesis will require the application of a variety of approaches focused upon the role of the extracellular matrix, the cytoskeleton, the nuclear matrix, and the metabolic processes involved in the interacellular processing of sex steroids. Recent progress of cell and organismal biology will have clinical application to several diseases, e.g., benign prostatic hyperplasia, diethylstilbestrol-induced lesions of the male and female genital tracts, carcinogenesis of the prostate, cervix, endometrium and mammary gland, and development of congenital birth defects of the genital system.

Hypospadias, a relatively common anomaly of the lower urinary tract, is characterized by developmental arrest during fetal organogenesis which produces a fusion defect in the urethral tube. The fusion of the urethral folds is induced by fetal testicular androgen; therefore the occurrence of hypospadias is caused by incomplete masculinization of this target structure. This may be a result of either a decline in stimulation caused by decrease in circulating hormones, partial tissue insensitivity or improper chronologic correlation between the hormones, partial tissue insensitivity or improper chronologic correlation between the hormonal level and the critical time for this tissue to respond to androgens. In most patients, hypospadias occurs as a single defect with no apparent or demonstrable

genetic or endocrine disturbance at birth or later in life. However, it may also be a manifestation of more permanent genetic and endocrine derangements, especially if there is ambiguity of external genitalia or the presence of another disorder of male sexual differentiation such as cryptorchidism or well-developed Müllerian duct structures.

Hypospadias in the male seems to be related to epithelial-mesenchymal interactions. Normal morphogenesis of the penile urethra results from fusion of the epithelium of the urogenital folds which bound the urethral groove on the ventral aspect of the penis. Following fusion of the epithelium, the epithelial seam breaks down resulting in the establishment of mesenchymal confluence ventral to the urethra. This process of epithelial fusion followed by breakdown of the epithelial seam is very similar to the process of secondary palate formation. In the palate, the fusion potential of the epithelium is related to the type of subadjacent supporting mesenchyme, since epidermis from tail (a non-fusing epithelium) can be induced to fuse with another epithelial layer when both epithelia are experimentally associated with palatal mesenchyme. The similarities between hypospadias and cleft palate suggest the possibility that certain concepts developed for the morphogenesis of the palate may aid our understanding of development and malformation of the penile urethra.

The incidence of enlarged prostatic utricle is higher in patients with penoscrotal or perineal hypospadias than in the general population (22%), especially if there are associated anomalies in testicular descent. Minor degrees of hypospadias are less frequently associated with this anomaly. Although enlarged prostatic utricles occur frequently in patients with male pseudohermaphroditism, the presence of utricular enlargement in itself does not indicate intersexuality. In patients with hypospadias of any degree, especially if associated with cryptorchidism, the presence of an abnormal cavitation in the prostatic urethra may be due to an enlarged prostatic utricle or a vagina masculinus in continuation with other Müllerian duct derivatives. The presence of a utricle without a cervix would preclude exploratory laparotomy as it would be unlikely that any other Müllerian duct derivatives would be present. Enlarged prostatic utricles, in patients with simple hypospadias and male pseudohermaphroditism as well as vagina masculinus in mixed gonadal dysgenesis, join the prostatic urethra through the verumontanum proximal to the external urinary sphincter in the great majority of cases. Conversely, the vagina in cases of female pseudohermaphroditism, secondary to congenital adrenal hyperplasia, is usually found distal to the external sphincter unless there is complete masculinization (fusion) of the urethra or severe clitoromegaly where it may be proximal.

Congenital anomalies of the mesonephric duct derivatives in the male are more common than previously appreciated, especially in association with cryptorchidism. While the true incidence of these anomalies and their influence on male fertility are unknown, there is a comprehensive classification which permits a prospective study of these anomalies and determination of their importance.

The levels of 5α-reductase and the cAR have been measured in the penis and ventral prostate gland of sexually maturing male rats. In the penis, the level of both 5α-reductase and the cAR decreased with aging, whereas in the prostate, the level of 5α-reductase activity also decreased with aging but the prostatic cAR gradually increased with aging until puberty at which time the receptor concentration began to drop precipitously to about 25% of the pubertal values. It has been concluded that the relative lack of androgenic responsiveness of the adult penis is probably due to the almost complete absence of the receptor at adulthood.

The finding of a minute, but otherwise normally formed penis at birth is noted in a variety of clinical conditions. Common to all these disorders are abnormalities in the fetal production handling of testosterone. Intermediate penile sizes constitute clinical concern as to whether maintenance in the male gender with repeated courses of testosterone will result in an "adequate" adult male, or whether early gender reversal offers a more acceptable long range solution. Penile size, associated testicular pathology (structural and/or endocrine) and responsiveness to a diagnostic/therapeutic trial of neonatal intramuscular testosterone constitute the determining factors. The efficacy of this approach, as contrasted with that recommended by those who favor gender reversal, can only be determined after current testosterone treated micropenis patients reach adulthood. Further research is needed to study normal fetal penile development.

SUBJECT INDEX